THIRD EDITION

HEALTH PROMOTION IN MIDWIFERY

THIRD EDITION

HEALTH PROMOTION IN MIDWIFERY
PRINCIPLES AND PRACTICE

Edited by

Jan Bowden
King's College London, UK

Vicky Manning
King's College London, UK

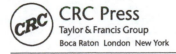

CRC Press
Taylor & Francis Group
Boca Raton London New York

CRC Press is an imprint of the
Taylor & Francis Group, an **informa** business

CRC Press
Taylor & Francis Group
6000 Broken Sound Parkway NW, Suite 300
Boca Raton, FL 33487-2742

© 2017 by Taylor & Francis Group, LLC
CRC Press is an imprint of Taylor & Francis Group, an Informa business

No claim to original U.S. Government works

Printed on acid-free paper
Version Date: 20160217

International Standard Book Number-13: 978-1-4987-2556-9 (Paperback)

Library of Congress Cataloging-in-Publication Data

Names: Bowden, Jan, editor. | Manning, Vicky, RGN, editor.
Title: Health promotion in midwifery : principles and practice / editors, Jan
Bowden, Vicky Manning.
Description: Third edition. | Boca Raton : Taylor & Francis, 2017. | Includes
bibliographical references and index.
Identifiers: LCCN 2016006340 | ISBN 9781498725569 (hardcover : alk. paper)
Subjects: | MESH: Health Promotion--methods | Midwifery--methods | Health
Behavior | Patient Education as Topic--methods | Pregnancy
Classification: LCC RG950 | NLM WQ 160 | DDC 618.2--dc23
LC record available at http://lccn.loc.gov/2016006340

Visit the Taylor & Francis Web site at
http://www.taylorandfrancis.com

and the CRC Press Web site at
http://www.crcpress.com

Contents

Preface

Public health and health promotion aimed at reducing health inequalities and ensuring development and implementation of generational health improvements continues to be a crucial part of health care policy worldwide. Within the United Kingdom, the current government policy and strategy clearly identify midwives as an integral part of its plans. Recent Department of Health data regarding the impact of midwives in public health show that our role is making a vital difference to the women and families in our care.

The role of the midwife in public health and health promotion is not new. It could be argued that almost everything a midwife does has an impact on, or link to, promoting the health of a woman, her baby and her family. This is undertaken against a backdrop of challenges such as changes to welfare services and meeting the health needs of a diverse and, at times, transitory population, coupled with the ultimate aim of providing individualised midwifery care based on the needs of the woman.

The principles of general health promotion, such as good, positive communication and information exchange, with the fundamental understanding of psychology, sociocultural issues, ethics and education are important to the underpinning of good midwifery practice. This book attempts to bring together these concepts in a way that is user friendly and accessible and encourages all midwives to look at their wider public health role as well as working in partnership alongside professionals from many other allied disciplines. Practice issues and frameworks related to providing health promotion within the multidisciplinary team are discussed, and there are links and suggestions for further reading that touch upon wider issues we were unable to cover in this book.

This third edition, and our second as editors, has allowed us to welcome new chapter writers as well as work again with some of our original team. For this edition, each chapter has been revised and new chapters have been developed to meet emerging challenges in clinical practice such as obesity and caring for sexually abused women. This book is intended to be realistic and practical in its suggestions for the promotion of health and for the provision of holistic care that is woman-focused.

Jan Bowden and Vicky Manning
King's College London

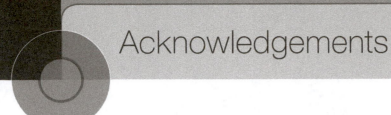

Acknowledgements

We thank our families: Jan sends special thanks to her sister Rae and nieces Ellis and Margaretti (VBF) for their total love and support, and Vicky sends special thanks to her husband for his unwavering support. We also thank our friends who have, in their own distinctive styles, found ways both big and small to encourage; support; and provide advice, much-needed light-heartedness and occasional solace via email, text, telephone and in person; all the chapter writers for their professional expertise and knowledge – working with them has been a unique and valuable experience; and Naomi Wilkinson and Jennifer Blaise from the Taylor & Francis Group for their much-needed help and advice and for giving us the chance to do this all over again.

Chapter 8

I would like to thank my girls, Elizabeth and Imogen.

Eddie West-Burnham

Contributors

Teresa Arias RM, BSc, MSc, PGCEA
Florence Nightingale Faculty of Nursing & Midwifery
King's College London, UK

Louise Armstrong (nee Long) RGN, RM, BSc (Hons), PGCEA, MSc
Midwifery Lecturer
Department of Health Sciences, Faculty of Science
University of York, UK

Jan Bowden RGN, RM, FP Cert BSc (Hons), PGCEA, MSc
Midwifery Lecturer
Florence Nightingale Faculty of Nursing & Midwifery
King's College London, UK

Penny Charles RGN, RM, BA (Hons), PGCEA MSc, PGCEA
Midwifery Lecturer
Florence Nightingale Faculty of Nursing & Midwifery
King's College London, UK

Heather Finlay BA (Hons), MSc, PG Dip PG Cert
Associate Lecturer
Birkbeck, University of London, UK

James M Harris RM, BSc, FHEA, PhD
Midwifery Lecturer
Florence Nightingale Faculty of Nursing & Midwifery
and
King's Improvement Science
King's College London, UK

Sarah Kipps RGN, BA, MSc NFSRH, PG Dip (Med ed), FRT
Clinical Team Leader, Integrated Sexual Health
St. George's NHS Foundation Trust
London, UK

Fabiana Lorencatto BSc, MSc, PhD
Research Fellow
Centre for Health Services Research and Management
School of Health Sciences
City University
London, UK

Mary Malone RN, RM, RHV, PhD
Nurse Lecturer
Head of Department, Adult Nursing
Florence Nightingale Faculty of Nursing & Midwifery
King's College London, UK

Vicky Manning RGN, RM, MSc, PGCEA
Midwifery Lecturer
Florence Nightingale Faculty of Nursing & Midwifery
King's College London, UK

Elsa Montgomery RM, MSc, PGCE, PhD, FHEA
Midwifery Lecturer
Head of Department, Midwifery
Florence Nightingale Faculty of Nursing & Midwifery
King's College London, UK

Emily Nellist
Physiotherapist
King's College Hospital NHS Foundation Trust
London, UK

Ian P S Noonan RMN, AKC, FHEA
Mental Health Lecturer
Florence Nightingale Faculty of Nursing & Midwifery
King's College London, UK

Sheila O'Connor RN, RM, BA, BSc, MA, MPhil
Research Midwife
King's College Hospital NHS Foundation Trust
London, UK

Janette O'Toole BA PG Cert
Clinical Lead Physiotherapist in Women's Health
King's College Hospital NHS Foundation Trust
London, UK

Hannah Rayment-Jones RM, MSc, PGCE, FHEA
Midwifery Tutor
Florence Nightingale Faculty of Nursing & Midwifery
King's College London, UK

Eddie West-Burnham BA, MSc
West Norfolk MIND King's Lynn, UK

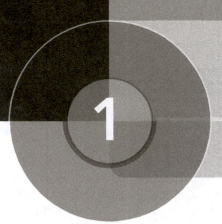

Public health, midwifery and government policy

HEATHER FINLAY

INTRODUCTION

> Public health [is] ... the science and art of preventing disease, prolonging life and promoting health through the organised efforts and informed choices of society, organisations, public and private, communities and individuals....
>
> Wanless (2004, 3)

Midwifery care has always included a public health component, although the emphasis has shifted over the years from an emphasis on reducing maternal and child mortality and the control of contagious diseases at the turn of the twentieth century to a greater emphasis on increasing breastfeeding rates, tackling 'lifestyle' issues such as smoking and obesity and the need for good mental health by the beginning of the twenty-first century (Leap & Hunter 1993; Crabbe & Hemingway 2014). As a profession, midwifery acknowledges childbirth as a psychological and social event rather than a purely clinical event and that optimum outcomes are the result of individual, community and organisational effort. In essence midwives have understood that childbirth and raising a family are more than just a medical event and that the outcomes depend as much on the mother and the family's social, psychological and environmental circumstances as on the input of health professionals.

This chapter will explore how the midwifery model interacts with government policy on public health. To do that, the chapter will start with a brief history of government policy around public health and midwifery. It will then go on to consider the social and economic background to government policy. Current government policy will then be explored in more detail and linked to the factors influencing the ability of midwifery to fulfil its public health role.

BACKGROUND

Through the early years of the twentieth century, midwifery became increasingly focused around institutions and the medicalised model of care, but this focus was starting to be questioned during the 1970s and 1980s with more proponents advocating the benefits of natural birth. The 'natural birth movement' resonated with a move towards a more holistic understanding of the causes of health and illness. The *Health of the Nation* policy document (Department of Health [DoH] 1992) acknowledged the need to promote health as well as to treat illness. This document has been criticised for its emphasis on the role of the individual in maintaining health while minimising the role of external influences; however, despite this, it signalled a belief in the importance of public health. In 1993, the 'Changing Childbirth' report emphasised the need to challenge the medicalisation of childbirth and design services around women and their families rather than institutions (DoH 1993). When the Labour government came to power in 1997, there was an increased recognition of the broader meaning of public health and an acceptance of the influence of disadvantage and inequality on health outcomes. The *Independent Inquiry into Inequalities in Health* (Acheson 1998) established a broad public health agenda that was followed through with *Saving Lives: Our Healthier Nation* (DoH 1999) and *Tackling Health Inequalities: A Cross Cutting Review* (DoH 2002). The public health role of the midwife was specifically mentioned in *Making a Difference: Midwifery Action Plan* (DoH 2001). Both *Choosing Health: Making Healthy Choices Easier* (DoH 2004a) and the *National Service Framework for Children, Young People and Maternity Services* (DoH 2004b; referred to in the text as the NSF) placed midwifery care at the centre of the public health agenda. Both documents acknowledged that placing maternity care in a community context and actively engaging with disadvantaged communities can have positive consequences for the short- and long-term health of women and their children. This approach signalled the beginning of an organised effort to promote health and prevent disease both within communities and among individuals, with a focus (certainly within the NSF) on preventing inequalities even before birth. Thus, midwifery was placed as central to the execution of a broad concept of public health. The Sure Start programme (Department of Education and Employment [DfEE] 1998) and the subsequent Sure Start Children's Centres (Department of Education and Skills [DfES] 2003) were created at a similar time, as part of the drive to improve outcomes for children and families and encourage multi-agency working (House of Commons: Children, Schools & Family Committee 2010). However, in 2010, the Labour government was replaced by a coalition government of Liberal Democrats and Conservatives. This change of government and the subsequent remodelling of the health services in England, alongside the social consequences of the economic crash of 2008, led to a public health environment that has some continuity with what has gone before but at the same time deep differences.

THE PUBLIC HEALTH PICTURE

Government policy from 2010 has been formulated against a background of a society in which obesity has become an increasing public health issue and there are continuing concerns around health inequalities. As a society, the United Kingdom in the early to mid-twenty-first century faces major health challenges, many of which have an impact on the public health role of the midwife. Obesity in both adults and children remains a challenge, and in the 20 years between 1993 and 2013, the number of obese men increased from 13% to 26% and the number of obese women increased from 16% to 24%, provoking fears that being overweight and obese is now becoming normal in the United Kingdom (DoH 2010; Health and Social Care information Centre (HSCIE 2015a). As would be expected, the trend for increased obesity in the general population is also found in women who are becoming pregnant, with an estimated one in five women going into pregnancy with a BMI of >30 kg/m^2 (Soltani 2009 cited in Foster & Hirst 2014). The increase in obesity is taking place alongside large numbers of adults taking less than the recommended amount of exercise and not following dietary guidelines, especially around the '5 a day' fruit and vegetable guidance (HSCIE 2015a). Although the number of smokers in the United Kingdom continues to decrease with only 24% of men and 17% of women smoking in 2013 (HSCIE 2014), there are still women who continue to smoke during pregnancy, with the latest figures showing 11% of women smoking at the time of their delivery (HSCIE 2015b). The common strand between obesity and smoking is that they are more common in some areas of the country and, more specifically, among some communities. For example, the percentage of women smoking in parts of the north-east of England is 19%, whereas in certain parts of London it is 5%. Similarly, the number of people who are obese is higher in the north of England and Scotland than the south (HSCIE 2015a). However regardless of where people live, we know that those who are in the lowest income quantiles are more likely to be obese and to smoke (HSCIE 2014). These statistics demonstrate that when it comes to healthy behaviours and health, there is inequality in those making healthy choices and in health outcomes, with those who are poorest and most vulnerable in our society at most risk of poor outcomes. The poor outcomes mean that those in the poorest areas can expect to die years earlier than those in the wealthiest areas and can further expect to have more years of life with ill health in their old age; this reflects a social gradient in health observed by Marmot (2010) whereby those who are poorest are at risk of worse outcomes. Recent figures suggest that women in the richest part of the country have 13 more disability-free years than women in the poorest parts of the country, and those in the wealthiest areas will live longer overall (NHS England 2013).

MATERNITY INEQUALITIES

The inequalities in health are also apparent during pregnancy, birth and the postnatal period. Although the rates of stillbirths and neonatal deaths continue to improve, there is a wide variation in risk across the United Kingdom. Alongside this regional variation in risk, those who lose their babies are more likely to be living in poverty, to be Black (or Black British) or Asian (or Asian British) (Knight et al. 2014). They are also more likely to be teenagers or aged over 40 (Manktelow et al. 2015). The recent confidential enquiry into maternal deaths also showed that the women who died were more likely to have come from deprived areas, to be older and to have been born outside the United Kingdom (Knight et al. 2014). The reasons why health inequalities persist, and the relative influence of the broader determinants of health is complex and outside the scope of this chapter (Benzeval et al. 2014). But it is becoming increasingly obvious that, at least in countries where there is easy access to health care, the health services around us are not a major influence on our chances of a long and healthy life. Other influences including environment, life chances, genetics and lifestyle are equally important (Public Health England [PHE], 2014a).

This section has highlighted two of the factors that have provided the background to the government policy around public health, namely the increase in obesity in the United Kingdom

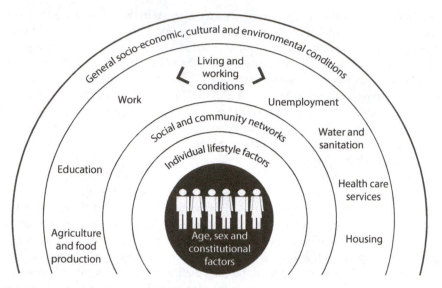

Figure 1.1 The main determinants of health. (From Dahlgren, Goran & Margaret Whitehead. 1993. *European strategies for tackling social inequities in health: Levelling up Part 2.* http://www.euro.who. int/__data/assets/pdf_file/0018/103824/E89384.pdf)

and the realisation that the persistence of health inequalities can only be tackled by an emphasis on the broader determinants of health. The next section will explore the organisational structures and approaches that are meant to make the difference.

ACTIVITY

Before moving onto the next section, see Figure 1.1.

- How could the factors identified in the different sections of the diagram influence your health?
- How could they influence the health of the community in which you live?

ORGANISATION OF PUBLIC HEALTH

The organisation and delivery of health services in United Kingdom have been devolved since 1999, but the differences have become more marked since the changes to the organisation and delivery of health (including public health) in England since the 2012 Health and Social Care Act. This section will look at Scotland, Wales and Northern Ireland first and then outline the major changes that have taken place in England since 2012.

SCOTLAND, WALES AND NORTHERN IRELAND

The factor that unites Scotland, Wales and Northern Ireland is that they have chosen not to have competition, or a market, within their health systems. In Northern Ireland this is due to structural reasons, but for Scotland and Wales it has been an ideological choice.

Scotland and Wales have also abolished the purchaser/provider split in health care, Scotland in 2004 and Wales in 2009, and the previous structure was replaced with health boards. The purchaser/provider split remains in Northern Ireland but only between limited providers (Bevan et al. 2014). In terms of the organisation of public health in these countries, the organisation has not been subject to the radical changes seen in England. In Scotland, public health remains within the purview of the national health system, and it is developed and delivered by a national health board, NHS Health Scotland. In Wales, Public Health Wales was established as an NHS Trust in 2009 and provides strategic and specialist support for local health boards. The Public Health Agency, also established in 2009, fulfils a similar function in Northern Ireland.

ENGLAND

In England, the organisation and delivery of public health was included in the changes to the English health services brought in as part of the 2012 Health and Social Care Act. The act affirmed and consolidated the role of the purchaser/provider split in the delivery of health service, with clinical commissioning groups being at the centre of commissioning health services for the local population.

ACTIVITY

Look at The Kings Fund on-line guide to the changes to the organisation and delivery of health care in England: http://www.kingsfund.org.uk/topics/nhs-reform

- Find out what maternity services are commissioned by your local clinical commissioning group

---

The consolidation of the role of the purchaser/provider split and the central role of the commissioning of services in public health was also introduced in the Health and Social Care Act 2012 (DoH 2012). This Act has seen for the first time Public Health responsibilities in the UK split between the NHS and local authorities. This is to be accomplished under the direction of a new body called Public Health England (PHE). PHE has responsibility for national strategic leadership, while local authorities now commission some public health services such as contraception and sexual health, cervical and breast screening, under the governance of the local Director of Public Health (DoH 2012). These local authority changes have led to the development of local Health and wellbeing boards whose purpose is to plan how to meet the health and social needs of the community. These boards include representatives from the NHS, the local authorities, PHE and user groups (Humphries & Galea 2013). Since the 2012 Act has come into force, there has been a transfer of staff and funds between the NHS and local authorities. Public health provision has the potential to be commissioned from a broader range of organisations, including third sector organisations. An example of this trend is the setting up of 'Health Hubs' in one London borough where a variety of public health services are available, such as stopping smoking services, sexual health services and healthy start information. Although the services are commissioned by the local authority, they are delivered by a third sector organisation. Other services, such as the 'Bump Buddies' service in the same London borough, receive funding from a variety of sources. This service provides support for women during pregnancy and in the postnatal period through mentoring.

Under the new organisation of public health, the commissioning of services that are relevant to maternity services are split between local authorities and the NHS; for example, the Healthy Child Programme up to age five stays under the purview of NHS commissioners, but sexual health and preventing birth defects moves to the ambit of the local authorities. As the examples above illustrate, the services can be delivered by different organisations (Aylett & Donovan 2013), which will require midwives to engage with the changes in their local area to ensure that they understand where the services they use and refer women and families to are now commissioned.

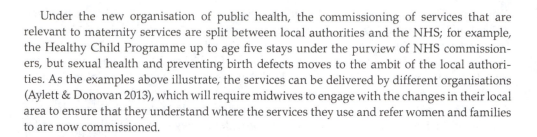

ACTIVITY

Can you identify the public health services available for women and their families in your area?

PRACTICE POINT

Knowing what public health services are available in your area will help you to refer women and their families to the right services

PREVENTION AND INTEGRATION: OVERARCHING AIMS OF THE CHANGES TO THE ORGANISATION AND DELIVERY OF PUBLIC HEALTH

The changes to the organisation of the delivery of public health as highlighted in the Five Year Forward View have a number of stated aims, but they cluster around two major themes (NHS 2014). The first is the need for more preventative services that engage the public in a collective push towards healthier lifestyles, such as weight management services. This is in response to the increase in ill health, for example, type 2 diabetes. In the new organisation and strategy there is an acknowledgement that preventative services can only go so far, and making changes to people's health includes addressing health inequalities and the broader determinants of health. To do this, the changes to the organisation and delivery of public health reflect the belief that this is more likely to be achieved when public health is primarily based within the local community, as represented by the local authority (DoH 2012).

The second theme highlighted emphasises increased integration between the NHS, local authorities, communities and employers to deliver a 'radical upgrade in prevention and public health' (NHS 2014, 8). Within this plan, there are a number of new models of delivering care with a greater emphasis on integrated services. For example, the future of primary care is envisaged as evolving to a point wherein partnerships of GPs and others provide a greater range of services outside of hospitals in 'Multispeciality Community Providers' (MSPs) (NHS 2014, 18). These MSPs could provide a range of community and social care services as well as primary care, and they could also provide a base for those services traditionally provided in secondary care, such as outpatients and diagnostic services. For maternity services, the Five Year Forward View proposes a review of midwifery models of care and configuring the funding of maternity care to make it possible for midwives to set up their own NHS-funded midwifery services. The review of the commissioning of maternity services was announced in March 2015, and this is due to report in early 2016 (NHS England 2015a) with the potential that maternity service provision will change dramatically.

CURRENT POLICY AND THE ROLE OF MIDWIFERY IN PUBLIC HEALTH

The transition to the new public health organisational structure has taken time, and it has only recently become clear how the public health role of the midwife is envisaged in the new organisational structure. The situation is not fixed, and discussions are continuing, including a mapping of the public health role of the midwife based on a review of public health section of Midwifery 2020, including the potential for a future midwifery public health career pathway (DoH 2012; NHS 2014).

The current policy on the public health role of the midwife at the government level has two core components. The first is that midwifery is situated within the idea of a life course framework, as envisaged in the Marmot review (2010). Within a life course framework, disadvantages and related health inequalities start before birth and continue to accumulate throughout life. Hence, action to reduce health inequalities need to start before birth and continue through childhood to tackle the links with disadvantages and health inequalities later in life.

A life course approach to public health is used by PHE in the current framework for 'Personalised Care and Public Health' (PHE 2014b). The midwifery contribution to public health is situated in the 'beginning of life'. The first 1001 days of life from conception are highlighted as a period of life that will make a difference to the rest of an individual's life course and therefore crucial for his or her future. As expected, a healthy pregnancy is emphasised, including interventions such as smoking cessation. But alongside, there is also an acknowledgement that stress in pregnancy can potentially affect neurological development and that secure bonding and attachment are important for future resilience. Figure 1.2 is a suggested service model that shows the integration of maternity services with other services depending on the family need, with the emphasis firmly on the parent–child relationship.

The framework also links to the NICE guidelines on areas such as the 'Transition to Parenthood', 'Maternal Mental Health' and 'Breastfeeding' (PHE 2014b). These links provide more details of what the actual recommendations are for midwifery practice.

The second core component to the public health role of the midwife is that the public health role should take place at three levels, that of the individual, the community and the population. What this means in practice is shown in more detail in the guidance on the *Midwifery Public Health Contribution* produced in 2013 as part of the 'Public health contribution of nurses and midwives: guidance' (PHE 2013a, 2013b).

This guidance, which is shown in Figure 1.3 and as a summary in Figure 1.4, includes the three levels with suggested tasks (Box 1.1). For example, at an individual level, a midwife might prompt women to think about their health needs, such as healthy eating and exercise. At a community level, midwives with a more specialist role might be involved in developing specific public health interventions in partnership with the local community. Then at a population level, midwifery leaders, consultants and specialists (including researchers) could, for example, take on a strategic responsibility and contribute to the implementation and review of health improvement programmes.

This document also includes reference to the wider determinants of health and specifically midwives working in partnership to address health inequalities, which includes working with multi-agency partners, service users, volunteers and user groups. It is worth noting that the time around birth, which has traditionally been part of the clinical role of the midwife, is included in the public health role as well. This acknowledges the effect a traumatic birth can have on mother and child and the need for 'safe, sensitive care' in

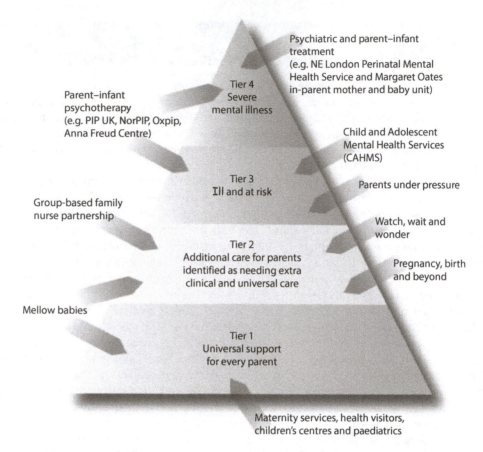

Psychiatric and parent–infant treatment (e.g. NE London Perinatal Mental Health Service and Margaret Oates in-parent mother and baby unit)

Tier 4
Severe mental illness

Parent–infant psychotherapy (e.g. PIP UK, NorPIP, Oxpip, Anna Freud Centre)

Child and Adolescent Mental Health Services (CAHMS)

Tier 3
Ill and at risk

Parents under pressure

Group-based family nurse partnership

Watch, wait and wonder

Tier 2
Additional care for parents identified as needing extra clinical and universal care

Pregnancy, birth and beyond

Mellow babies

Tier 1
Universal support for every parent

Maternity services, health visitors, children's centres and paediatrics

Figure 1.2 Beginning of life: service model. (From PHE. 2014b. *A framework for personalised care and population health for nurses, midwives, health visitors and allied health professionals: Caring for populations across the lifecourse.* https://www.gov.uk/government/uploads/system/uploads/attachment_data/file/377450/Framework_for_personalised_care_and_population_health_for_nurses.pdf)

the intrapartum period. The importance of skin-to-skin contact is also mentioned as is the opportunity for de-briefing after the birth (PHE 2013a, 2013b). This is an ambitious programme which includes many of the expected areas in public health that midwives have been associated with, including mental health issues, domestic violence and safeguarding issues, but it also includes an expectation of midwives working at a community and strategic level to achieve better public health outcomes.

PRACTICE POINT

Understanding the public health frameworks will help to integrate public health into your role

As previously mentioned, public health is devolved in Scotland, Wales and Northern Ireland which means that they have their own strategies for public health. Despite this, the strategies in all four countries are similar with an emphasis on the influence of the early years in life on future health inequalities and deprivation. With the role of the midwife to support healthy choices in all women (e.g. in diet and activity) while also identifying and supporting those more

Midwifery public health contribution to compassion in practice through maximising well-being and improving health in women, babies and families

'Midwives will embrace a greater public health role. Individual midwives and the midwifery workforce will expect support from those who plan and commission maternity services to enable them to meet the challenges of reducing inequalities and improving maternal and family health'. (Midwifery 2020, DH 2010)

Midwives' contribution to outcomes and indicators as specified in the Public Health Outcomes Framework under the four public health domains (DH 2012)

Improving wider determinants of health
Domestic abuse
Social connectedness
Health improvement
Low birth weight of term infants
Breastfeeding
Smoking status at the time of delivery
Under 18 conceptions
Diet
Excess weight in adults
Proportion of physically active and inactive adults
Smoking prevalence
Access to non-cancer screening programmes
Self-reported well-being
Health protection
Chlamydia diagnoses (15–24 years)
Population vaccination coverage
Health care public health preventing premature mortality
Infant mortality
Mortality from causes considered preventable
Suicide

Midwives' contribution to maternity-specific outcomes and indicators

Measurement of women's experiences using patient reported outcomes measures (PROMs)

Midwife as first point of contact and booking by 12 completed weeks of pregnancy

Choice of place of birth

1:1 midwifery care in established labour
Normal birth rate/caesarean section rate

Midwifery public health actions throughout the maternity pathway

Pre-pregnancy: Contraception cessation, nutrition and exercise advice, optimum body mass index, smoking cessation, folic acid supplementation, pre-existing disease management, advice and guidance.

Pregnancy: Direct access to a midwife, which promotes early booking with: Comprehensive information giving and assessment of medical, obstetric and social risk, taking into account the wider determinants of health.

Identification, signposting and appropriate specialist referral of those with
• long-term health conditions including diabetes, epilepsy, asthma, cardiovascular disease, essential hypertension, obesity
• mental health issues
• safeguarding issues
• domestic abuse disclosure and safeguarding issues
• smoking in pregnancy
• drug and alcohol misuse
• learning difficulties
• physical disability
• teenage pregnancy
• sexual health issues

Translation services for non-English speaking women and families

Advice and guidance on healthy nutrition, activity and exercise for all women regardless of body mass index

Promotion of active birth techniques

Supportive and evidence-based guidance on antenatal screening programmes, ensuring informed consent and responsive, efficient care

Education programmes that prepare women and their families for pregnancy, birth and parenthood, and convey clear and informative public health messages

---

Birth
Promoting normality throughout labour and birth within a sensitive and safe birth environment
Psychological and physical care and support throughout labour
Skin-to-skin contact to promote early feeding and bonding
Provision of de-briefing opportunities

Postnatal period
Proactive breastfeeding support and infant nutrition guidance
Safe formula feeding advice and guidance
Maternal nutrition and postnatal pelvic floor and general exercise advice and guidance
Sexual health and contraceptive advice
Provision of newborn screening and supporting vaccination programmes
Unbiased, evidence-based, safe-sleeping and bed-sharing information

---

Midwives' contribution to maximising well-being and improving health outcomes

Every contact will count to influence and maximise the health and well-being of all women, babies, families and communities throughout pregnancy, birth and the postnatal period and beyond.

Midwives will contribute fully to the public health agenda in conjunction with multi-agency partners, service users, volunteers and user groups.

Through partnership working midwives will seek to meet the challenges of reducing health inequalities through improving maternal and population health, ensuring the best start in life, thus contributing to a healthy life expectancy.

Midwives will deliver innovative, evidence-based, cost effective, high-quality care within multi-agency teams across hospital and community-based health and social care settings.

Midwives will facilitate a positive and life-enhancing transition to parenthood for women and their families in collaboration with women and partners, which will be achieved through the provision of trusted support and personalised care, taking into account individual needs, risk and circumstances.

Sensitive, responsive bereavement services will be provided for those who experience poor outcomes to meet the needs of the grieving process and promote long-term health and well-being.

Figure 1.3 Midwifery public health contribution to compassion in practice.

Public health skills and career framework levels of knowledge and competence

Public health research, education and career pathways supporting the midwifery contribution to compassion in practice: maximising well-being and improving health at the three levels of public health practice – individual, community and population

Core Public Health Competencies
Public health skills and career framework (Public Health Resource Unit/Skills for Health 2009)

Surveillance and assessment	Assessing the evidence	Policy and strategy	Leadership and collaborative working

Midwives with strategic responsibility in the field of public health working with local authority public health departments and nationally with Public Health England

Population / Community / Individual

Midwifery leaders: Heads of Midwifery and Local Supervisory Authority
Midwifery Officers
Lead midwives for education
Public health consultant midwives
Research midwives
Named safeguarding midwives
Lactation consultant midwives
Regional screening coordinators

- Contribute to the development and lead on the implementation and review of health improvement programmes across agencies, partnerships and communities
- Needs assessment and population profiling
- Understanding of the commissioning process and its role in improving population health and well-being and reducing inequalities in Public Health service and policy development
- Research into support for the most vulnerable groups
- Research into well-being as a specific outcome of maternity care

Midwives with added responsibility in the field of public health

Community / Individual

Midwifery clinical leaders
Supervisors of midwives
Specialist midwives with primary and secondary health promotion and ill health prevention roles in safeguarding, substance misuse, domestic abuse, teenage pregnancy, ethnic minority issues, smoking cessation, obesity, diabetes
Frenulotomy practitioners
Ante- and postnatal screening co-ordinators

- Plan, implement and evaluate health improvement projects and approaches in partnership with women and their families
- Support women and groups to make and maintain informed choices about improving their health and well-being
- Communicate to relevant people the health concerns and interests of women and communities
- Identify and build on community capacity – tailored interventions specific to public health needs of local maternity populations – impacting on health outcomes

All midwives and maternity support workers

Individual

All midwives and maternity support workers:
Maximising their role and contributing to improving health and well-being through "every contact counts"

- Actively encourage women to think about their own health needs, the health of their babies and families and how this could be improved
- Signpost women and their families to people and agencies that can help them improve their health and well-being

Public health education embedded within and throughout pre- and post-registration midwifery training
NICE public heath guidance and public health research embedded within public health midwifery practice

Defined public health competencies –
public health skills and careers framework (Public Health Resource Unit/Skills for Health 2009)

Health improvement	Health protection	Public health intelligence	Academic health intelligence	Health and social care quality

3 levels of public health practice

Figure 1.4 Public health research, education and career pathways supporting the midwifery contribution to compassion in practice.

BOX 1.1: PHE's outline of midwifery actions at the three levels of public health practice

Individual level

- Individual obstetric, medical and social risk assessment by 12 completed weeks' gestation
- Signposting and referral of individual women with medical risk factors and complex social needs to relevant professionals/agencies, for example, obstetric care, smoking cessation services, dietetic services, safeguarding teams, CAMHs and drug and alcohol services
- One-to-one care in labour to support the promotion of normality and reduction in intervention such as caesarean section rates
- Individualised support and encouragement of breastfeeding with referral to breastfeeding support services for those experiencing problems
- Individualised care pathways to ensure improved maternal physical and mental health and well-being, enabling strong early attachment and maternal and infant well-being

Community level

- Provision of local antenatal and newborn screening programmes meeting key performance indicators
- Smoking cessation carbon monoxide monitoring
- Healthy start vitamin uptakes
- Provision of specialist care pathways for vulnerable women – in conjunction with family–nurse partnerships
- Provision of parent education programmes in preparation for parenthood conveying clear and informative public health messages
- Promotion of breastfeeding in hospitals and at community level – universal baby friendly standard reached by all care staff and 'breastfeeding welcome' promoted in public places

Population level

- Provision of high-quality, responsive maternity services in which women, their partners and families are supported to maintain and improve health and well-being throughout pregnancy, birth, the postnatal period and beyond through the transition to parenthood
- Reduction in maternal and child mortality and morbidity rates resulting from medical, obstetric, social and psychological risk factors
- Provision of regional antenatal and newborn screening programmes, leading to early detection and where possible treatment of congenital abnormalities and disease
- Increase in breastfeeding rates at population level and improved short- and long-term outcomes through improved nutrition, leading to improved obesity rates and related illness in later life

Outcomes of these actions can be measured via the following currently available metrics within the Public Health Outcomes Framework relevant to midwifery

- Low birth weight of term babies
- Breastfeeding, nursing and midwifery actions at the three levels of public health practice
- Under 18 conceptions
- Proportion of physically active and inactive adults
- Smoking prevalence – adults (over 18 years)
- Recorded diabetes
- Infant mortality

Source: PHE (Public Health England). 2013b. https://www.gov.uk/government/uploads/system/uploads/attachment_data/file/208814/3_Levels.pdf

vulnerable families (NHS Scotland n.d.; Public Health Wales 2014). However, there appears to be less emphasis in the policy documents in Scotland and Wales on midwives working at a community and strategic level to achieve change around health behaviours and addressing health inequalities than in England.

> **ACTIVITY**
>
> - Do you believe that your role, or that of your mentor if you are a student, includes a public health component at an individual level?
> - Identify what the clinical area you work for does to address public health at a community and population level, as suggested in Figures 1.3 and 1.4?

BARRIERS TO THE IMPLEMENTATION OF PUBLIC HEALTH POLICIES

Within England, the reforms to the organisation of public health ensure placing parts of the public health system within the communities where inequalities in health are experienced. The aim is to empower local communities and public health professionals to come up with innovative, locally relevant interventions to help tackle the local inequalities in health based on the broader determinants of health. This sounds logical, and it could be argued that the previous system lacked input from communities and users. However, there are a number of issues becoming apparent as the new organisation beds itself in.

First, there is discussion about the role of the Director of Public Health and where they should sit within the local authority and how their power will be mediated and negotiated. This will become apparent over time, but it could lead to variation between local authorities that could impact on the services delivered (Aylett & Donovan 2013). Similarly, there is still uncertainty about how the role of Health and Wellbeing boards will stabilise. There is variation across local authorities, despite most Health and Wellbeing boards being set up and making progress. But their ability to have more influence, especially on commissioning, beyond being a forum for the health services, local authorities and representative of the local community is not clear (Humphries & Galea 2013). This could limit their ability to influence the broader determinants of health, especially in times of financial constraint.

Secondly, there is the issue of funding and the challenge of local authorities to fulfil their public health obligations, especially around the broader determinants of health. Initially, the allocation of funds for public health was ring-fenced, and hence there was a level of protection, preventing its use elsewhere. However, there is now some uncertainty about whether it will remain ring-fenced and thus vulnerable to use in other areas. The allocation of funding for public health to the local authorities is also based on historic precedent rather than need, and hence it varies between local authorities, and there is some concern about how far local authorities are aligning their spending with the issues of public health (NAO 2014). There is also potential for funding to local authorities to be constrained in times when the public budget is cut, as happened in June 2015 when the public health budget was cut by £200 million (LGA 2015).

Uncertainty around funding could impact on how ready local authorities are to commission initiatives that require long-term funding and could add to concerns already expressed about the ability of local authorities to respond to the broader determinants of health that require long-term co-ordinated action, such as warmer and safer homes, transport and secure employment (Buck & Gregory 2013).

These broader determinants of health are also impacted by the central government's policies, for example, on welfare, and it is uncertain how much the public health agenda (or even PHE) will influence central government policy (Buck & Gregory 2013). Since 2010, there has been widening inequalities, which have been shown to have a negative impact on health and well-being (Wilkinson & Pickett 2010; Dorling 2014). Also, the austerity measures that have been applied to public services and welfare have led to some of the poorest and the most vulnerable in society, and those most at risk of poor health outcomes, finding their lives more insecure as the welfare safety net many depended on is reduced. Employment is now more often insecure and low-paid while people are being increasingly called on to do unpaid work to give care that is no longer supplied by the State (Slay & Penny 2013).

Overall, there has been little progress in reducing the numbers of those living in poverty (both adults and children) since 2010 (MacInnes et al. 2014; DWP 2015). The broader policy environment that has been described in this section will make it challenging to pursue a public health agenda designed to reduce the inequalities in health.

BARRIERS SPECIFICALLY AROUND MATERNITY SERVICES

There is no doubt that public health is part of the role of the midwife. The relationship that midwives build with women and their families makes them uniquely placed to work with women and their families around these issues. Also, pregnancy can be a time for people to consider making changes in their lives. Midwives constitute one of the groups that PHE wants to view as public health practitioners (PHE 2013a).

However, for maternity services and the midwives who work within those services, their ability to deliver the public health actions expected of them will be mitigated by a number of factors. The first of these is the number of midwives practising. The Royal College of Midwives estimates that there is a shortage of 3000 midwives, and this will impact on the ability of maternity services to provide more than their core services (Griffiths 2015). This midwifery shortage is also operating within an NHS financial environment where there is both financial insecurity with some Trusts in England operating with large debts and where the promise of increased funding is contingent on efficiency savings (NHS 2014). Funding pressures are also affecting Sure Start Children's Centres which have had a history of being at places where midwives could work with the local community. The spending on children's centres and early year services between 2012–2013 and 2013–2015 was 30% less than the spend in 2011–2012, with 200 centre sites potentially at risk of closure. This is despite centres seeing more families and increasing their involvement in programmes for more vulnerable families, such as the Troubled Families programme (4children 2014).

All the public health organisations in the United Kingdom have 'reduction in health inequalities' as one of their core aims, but there is tension, certainly in England, about the expectations from midwives to be part of this. PHE has an explicit role for midwives in addressing health inequalities (PHE 2013a) which includes, for example, reference to midwives identifying and building on community capacity to develop targeted interventions. But with regard to the more detailed guidance on the actions to be taken by midwives at the three levels (individual, community and population), there is little that midwives do not already do (PHE 2013b). This raises questions about where the public health role of midwives will be placed in the new system in England, especially with the family nurse programme having a prominent role as the support for vulnerable families in the PHE Framework documents (PHE 2014b).

PRACTICE POINT

Understanding the barriers to improvements in public health and the public health role of the midwife will help midwives to influence policy at a strategic level

SUMMARY

- The current emphasis on the public health role of all midwives recognises a strand that has always been present in the role of the midwife
- The unique relationship midwives often have with women and their families makes midwives well placed to include public health in their roles
- Midwives sometimes work with the most vulnerable in society and understand that inequalities in health have consequences for both mothers and babies
- The emphasis throughout the United Kingdom on tackling health inequalities gives midwives opportunities to influence policy at a strategic level
- The changes to the organisation of Public Health can mean new opportunities for midwives around public health
- There are challenges for midwives in fulfilling their public health role:
  - In England, the moving of Public Health out of the NHS means that midwives will have to negotiate the two systems
  - The broader policy environment might challenge the ability of midwives and providers of public health services to affect the broader determinants of health
- Despite the constraints, public health remains an area where midwives can make a difference

REFERENCES

4children. 2014. *Sure Start Children's Centres Census 2014: A national overview of Sure Start Children's Centres in 2014.* http://www.4children.org.uk/Files/6f907ff7-35fe-4c6f-a3a4-a3cb00e1a11c/Children_Centre_Census_2014.pdf

Acheson, Donald. 1998. *Independent inquiry into inequalities in health.* London: HMSO.

Aylett, Laura & Helen Donovan. 2013. Consequences of radical public health reform in England. *Primary Health Care* 23(3): 6–7.

Benzeval, Michaela, Lyndal Bond, Mhairl Campbell, Matt Egan, Theo Lorenc, Mark Petticrew & Frank Popham. 2014. *How does money influence health?* https://www.jrf.org.uk/report/how-does-money-influence-health

Bevan, Gwyn, Marina Karanikolos, Joe Exley, Ellen Nolte, Sheelah Connolly & Nicholas Mays. 2014. *The four health systems of the United Kingdom: How do they compare?* http://www.nuffieldtrust.org.uk/sites/files/nuffield/revised_4_countries_report.pdf

Buck, David & Sarah Gregory. 2013. *Improving the public's health: A resource for local authorities.* http://www.kingsfund.org.uk/publications/improving-publics-health

Crabbe, Katie & Anne Hemmingway. 2014. Public health and wellbeing: A matter for the midwife? *British Journal of Midwifery* 22(9): 634–644.

Dahlgren, Goran & Margaret Whitehead. 1993. *European strategies for tackling social inequities in health: Levelling up Part 2.* http://www.euro.who.int/__data/assets/pdf_file/0018/103824/E89384.pdf

DfEE (Department for Education and Employment). 1999. *Sure Start; making a difference for children and families*. London, The Stationary Office.

DfES (Department of Education and Skills). 2003, *Children's Centres – Developing Integrated Service for Young Children and Their Families*, Nottingham: DfES.

DoH (Department of Health). 1992. *Health of the nation: A strategy for health in England*. London: HMSO.

DoH (Department of Health). 1993. *Changing childbirth: Report of the expert maternity group*. London: HMSO.

DoH (Department of Health). 1999. *Saving lives: Our healthier nation*. London: Stationary Office.

DoH (Department of Health). 2001. *Making a difference: Midwifery action plan*. London: DoH.

DoH (Department of Health). 2002. *Tackling health inequalities: Summary of a cross cutting review*. London: DoH.

DoH (Department of Health). 2004a. *Choosing health: Making healthy choices easier*. London: DoH.

DoH (Department of Health). 2004b. *National service framework for children, young people and maternity services*. London: DoH.

DoH (Department of Health). 2010. *Midwifery 2020 delivering expectations*. https://www.gov.uk/government/uploads/system/uploads/attachment_data/file/216029/dh_119470.pdf

DoH (Department of Health). 2012. *Health and Social Care Act 2012 chapter 7, London, The Stationary Office*. http://www.legislation.gov.uk/ukpga/2012/7/pdfs/ukpga_20120007_en.pdf

DoH (Department of Health). 2012a. *Compassion in practice: Nursing, midwifery and care staff. Our vision and strategy*. http://www.england.nhs.uk/wp-content/uploads/2012/12/compassion-in-practice.pdf

DoH (Department of Health). 2012b. *The new public health role of local authorities*. https://www.gov.uk/government/uploads/system/uploads/attachment_data/file/213009/Public-health-role-of-local-authorities-factsheet.pdf

Dorling, Danny. 2014. Growing wealth inequality in the UK is a ticking time bomb. *The Guardian*. Wednesday 25 October 2014.

DWP (Department for Work & Pensions). 2015. *Households below average income*. https://www.gov.uk/government/uploads/system/uploads/attachment_data/file/437246/households-below-average-income-1994-95-to-2013-14.pdf

Foster, Christine E. & Janet Hirst. 2014. Midwives' attitudes towards giving weight-related advice to obese pregnant women. *British Journal of Midwifery* 22(4): 254–262.

Griffiths, Julie. 2015. The big story: A worry for midwives? *Midwives Magazine*. Sumer 2015.

House of Commons Children, Schools and Families select Committee. *Sure Start Children's Centres. Fifth Report of Session 2009–10*. http://www.publications.parliament.uk/pa/cm200910/cmselect/cmchilsch/130/130i.pdf

HSCIE (Health and Social Care Information Centre). 2014. *Health Survey for England – 2013, Trend tables [NS]*. http://www.hscic.gov.uk/catalogue/PUB16077

HSCIE (Health and Social Care Information Centre). 2015a. *Statistics on obesity, physical activity and diet*. http://www.hscic.gov.uk/catalogue/PUB16988/obes-phys-acti-diet-eng-2015.pdf

HSCIE (Health and Social Care Information Centre). 2015b. *Statistics on women's smoking status at time of delivery, England – Quarter 3, 2014–15*. http://www.hscic.gov.uk/catalogue/PUB16957

Humphries, Richard & Amy Galea. 2013. *Health and wellbeing boards: One year on.* http://www.kingsfund.org.uk/sites/files/kf/field/field_publication_file/health-wellbeing-boards-one-year-on-oct13.pdf

Knight, Marian, Sara Kenyon, Peter Brocklehurst, Jim Neilson, Judy Shakespeare & Jennifer J. Kurinczuk (Eds.). 2014. *Saving lives, improving mothers' care.* https://www.npeu.ox.ac.uk/downloads/files/mbrrace-uk/reports/Saving%20Lives%20Improving%20Mothers%20Care%20report%202014%20Full.pdf

Leap, Nicky & Billie Hunter. 1993. *The midwife's tale: An oral history from handywoman to professional midwife.* London: Scarlet Press.

LGA (Local Government Association). 2015. *Councils respond to £200 million public health funding reduction: Media release.* http://www.local.gov.uk/web/guest/media-releases/-/journal_content/56/10180/7319767/NEWS

MacInnes, Tom, Hannah Aldridge, Sabrina Bushe, Adam Tinson & Theo Barry Born. 2014. *Monitoring poverty and social exclusion 2014.* https://www.jrf.org.uk/report/monitoring-poverty-and-social-exclusion-2014

Manktelow, Bradley N., Lucy K. Smith, T. Alun Evans, Pauline Hyman-Taylor, Jennifer J. Kurinczuk, David J. Field, Peter W. Smith & Elizabeth S. Draper. 2015. *Perinatal mortality surveillance report 2013.* https://www.npeu.ox.ac.uk/mbrrace-uk/reports

Marmot, Michael. 2010. *Fair society, healthy lives: The Marmot review.* http://www.instituteofhealthequity.org/projects/fair-society-healthy-lives-the-marmot-review

NAO (National Audit Office). 2014. *Public Health England's grant to local authorities.* http://www.nao.org.uk/wp-content/uploads/2014/12/Public-health-england%E2%80%99s-grant-to-local-authorities-summary.pdf

NHS. 2014. *Five year forward view.* http://www.england.nhs.uk/wp-content/uploads/2014/10/5yfv-web.pdf

NHS England. 2013. *Promoting equality and tackling health inequalities.* NHS England: Board paper. http://www.england.nhs.uk/wp-content/uploads/2013/12/brd-dec-1.pdf

NHS England. 2014. *Compassion in practice – Two years on. NHS England Report.* http://www.england.nhs.uk/wp-content/uploads/2014/12/nhs-cip-2yo.pdf

NHS England. 2015a. *News: NHS England announces national review of maternity care.* http://www.england.nhs.uk/2015/03/03/maternity-care/

NHS England. 2015b. *The NHS five year forward view: New care models vanguard sites.* http://www.england.nhs.uk/ourwork/futurenhs/5yfv-ch3/new-care-models/

NHS Scotland. n.d. *Maternal and early years for early years workers: Home.* http://www.maternal-and-early-years.org.uk/topic/background

PHE (Public Health England). 2013a. *The midwifery public health contribution: Midwifery visual strategy.* https://www.gov.uk/government/publications/the-midwifery-public-health-contribution

PHE (Public Health England). 2013b. *Nursing and midwifery actions at the three levels of public health practice improving health and wellbeing at individual, community and population levels.* https://www.gov.uk/government/uploads/system/uploads/attachment_data/file/208814/3_Levels.pdf

PHE (Public Health England). 2014a. *From evidence into action: Opportunities to protect and improve the nation's health.* https://www.gov.uk/government/publications/from-evidence-into-action-opportunities-to-protect-and-improve-the-nations-health

PHE (Public Health England). 2014b. *A framework for personalised care and population health for nurses, midwives, health visitors and allied health professionals: Caring for populations across the lifecourse.* https://www.gov.uk/government/uploads/system/uploads/attachment_data/file/377450/Framework_for_personalised_care_and_population_health_for_nurses.pdf

Public Health Wales. 2014. *Raising the profile. The Public Health Wales Nursing and Midwifery Strategy 2014–2017.* http://www2.nphs.wales.nhs.uk:8080/CorporateServicesDocuments.nsf/Public/9B0BA5F9BC43CDFE80257CD80033D032/$file/RaisingTheProfile.pdf?OpenElement

Slay, Julia & Joe Penny. 2013. *Surviving austerity Local voices and local action in England's poorest neighbourhoods.* http://www.neweconomics.org/publications/entry/surviving-austerity

Wanless, Derek. 2004. *Securing good health for the whole population: Final report.* London: HMSO.

Wilkinson, Richard & Kate Pickett. 2010. *The spirit level: Why equality is better for everyone.* Harmondsworth: Penguin.

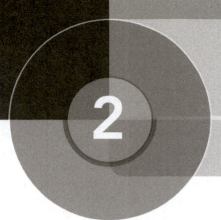

Health promotion: A core role of the midwife

2

VICKY MANNING

INTRODUCTION

Midwives are, by the very nature of the profession, promoters of health. It is written into our code (Nursing and Midwifery (NMC 2015, 5); 2.2 'recognise and respect the contribution that people can make to their own health and wellbeing' and 3.1 'pay special attention to promoting wellbeing, preventing ill health and meeting the changing health and care needs of people during all life stages'. It is also in the definition of the midwife 'the midwife has an important task in health counselling and education, not only for the woman, but also with the family and community' (International Confederation of Midwives (ICM 2011, 1).

In Midwifery 2020, public health is identified as a key area, 'Midwives' unique contribution to public health is that they work with women throughout pregnancy, birth and the postnatal period to provide safe, holistic care' (Midwifery 2020 Programme 2010, 26). So you can see health promotion is not an extended role of the midwife but a core skill. As the lead professional for most of the care provided by the maternity services in the United Kingdom, the midwife is expected to provide a service that helps parents to access health promotion messages and use them effectively to nurture their health as well as that of their family. This chapter, using relevant evidence, looks at the concepts and influences of health, health needs assessment (HNA) of health promotion and the role the midwife plays in the delivery of health promotion.

BACKGROUND

Throughout history, the value of health has been recognised. Virgil, who lived from 70 to 19 BC, was reported to have said 'The greatest wealth is health'. In the past, the determinants of health have been poorly understood and the only main public health tool available was the use of quarantine. The nineteenth century saw great leaps in public health with Edwin Chadwick and Thomas Southwood Smith, pioneers of modern public health, realising that public health was more than preventing the spread of disease, but rather a way to make life better for all. They advocated, along with many others, that for the poor to be able to thrive they needed better living conditions (Moorhead 2002). As public health became more recognised as a force to improve health, many parliamentary acts were passed, a process we still see today with acts such as the Clean Air Act 1993 (United Kingdom Government 1993) or the Health Act 2006 which had smoking in public spaces as one of its elements (United Kingdom Government 2006). Today, in developed countries, the major health problems come less from infectious diseases and more from the degenerative diseases associated with later life and/or poor lifestyle choices, conditions such as heart disease, diabetes and cancer, and disabling illnesses such as arthritis and stroke.

WHAT IS HEALTH?

The word *health* is derived from an old English word *hoelth* meaning a state of being sound. Generally, this was used to infer soundness of body (Dolfman 1973). Our personal understandings of health are influenced by our social and cultural situations (Scriven 2010). The concepts of disease and medical care, health and health promotion do not exist in a sociocultural, institutional or political vacuum (WHO 1986). The way health is thought of in a society reflects the values, beliefs, knowledge and practices that are shared by lay people, health professionals and other influential groups in that society.

There are many ways to think about health. In the Western world, we are most familiar with the 'medical model'. This is when health is defined as the absence of pathology. This is similar to looking at the body as a machine. If health is the absence of pathology, there is an assumption that ill health has a pathology, which needs to be 'healed' or fixed. This is a simplistic way of viewing health as it is identifying ill health, not good health. A further limitation is the lack of acknowledgement of other aspects of a person's life which may have contributed to being unwell or which might reduce or negate the success of a treatment (Green et al. 2015).

On the opposite side of the coin is the' lay concept' of health, which may vary considerably depending on gender, age and culture. This does not tend to focus just on ill health, but good health and well-being. As an example older people may see health and social networks as more important than economic resources (Hill et al. 2007), but young people may see health as being fit, strong and energetic (Blaxter 1990) and may show reluctance in accessing health care (Hagell 2015).

Health professionals now seek to approach health from a more holistic view point. This is looking at the person as a whole, recognising that health is often more than the sum of its parts. Health is seen as a resource for everyday life, not the objective of living (Kumar & Preetha 2012).

The WHO definition of health, 'health is a complete state of physical, mental and social well-being and not merely the absence of disease or infirmity' (WHO 1946, 2), may be seen to incorporate all the concepts above, but there are many arguments against this definition, mainly around the ambiguity of the terms used, for example, what is meant by 'well-being' or how do you measure 'complete' physical, mental and social well-being?

REFLECTION

Consider your own concept(s) of health by thinking about someone you consider 'healthy' and someone else you consider not healthy. Why do you put them in the category you have put them in? How do your thoughts fit into the concepts above?

PREGNANCY AND HEALTH

The definition of health given to us by the WHO can be quite a challenge for midwives as well as for the women themselves. As mentioned above what does 'complete state of well-being actually mean'? Being in a complete state of well-being might be difficult enough when you are fit, well and not pregnant but during pregnancy and the postnatal period, women may not view themselves as in a complete state of well-being. Their idea of 'normal' health may be challenged as concepts of health go beyond the condition that your body is in (Murphy 2015). Women during this time go through a period of physical, sexual, emotional, mental, spiritual and social change. This takes us back to what is mentioned above about profession versus lay person's views of health. The pregnant woman enduring nausea and vomiting, for example, or a newly delivered woman experiencing perineal stitches might view their health as anything but 'healthy'. Midwives, on the other hand, may view all the above as a normal as they see it all the time and see it as normal for pregnancy and childbirth. Alternatively it can be the other way, with women embracing pregnancy and motherhood as healthy and midwives believing in the process as normal only in retrospect. This view from the midwives may originate from the mediatisation of childbirth, which often views pregnancy as a 'non-healthy' condition (Crafter 1997). Considering that one of the midwife's primary roles is 'the detection of complications in mother and child' (ICM 2011) means that deviations from normality are continually looked for and some will almost certainly be found (Crafter 1997). These viewpoints suggest midwives might come from a purely negative or positive standpoint. However in 2010, Midwifery 2020 was published which views childbearing more holistically. It recommends that midwives be the lead professional for all healthy women with straightforward pregnancies (for women with more complex needs the midwife will be the key coordinator of care within the multidisciplinary team) (Midwifery 2020 Programme 2010). With midwives being recognised as lead professionals they are more likely to be encouraged to have a broader interpretation of health, not purely a negative or positive view. There are challenges to giving holistic care as the birth rate increases, there are more older women giving birth and the number of women with complex health or social needs is rising. Midwives can be caring for a wide spectrum of women, some with no specific health issues at all to caring for others entering pregnancy with life-threatening health or obstetric problems or complex social problems and everything in between. However this is what midwives do, they work within the continuum of normality and high risk pregnancies, providing supportive, facultative care, including health promotion, seeking medical support as and when needed (Bowden 2006).

WHAT IS HEALTH PROMOTION?

ACTIVITY

What does the term health promotion mean to you? Write your own definition before you look at the WHO and other definitions given below.

Health promotion, as a branch of medicine, has emerged with the increasing realisation that health can and should be improved for everyone. 'Health promotion action aims at reducing differences in current health status and ensuring equal opportunities and resources to enable all people to achieve their fullest health potential' (WHO 1986, 1). Biomedical interventions alone will not guarantee better health (Kumar & Preetha 2012). The WHO (1986) defines health promotion as:

the process of enabling people to increase control over, and to improve, their health. It moves beyond a focus on individual behaviour towards a wide range of social and environmental interventions. (1)

Other definitions of health promotion include:

The science and art of promoting and protecting health and well-being, preventing ill-health and prolonging life through the organised efforts of society (Faculty of Public Health 2010, 1).

Public health is about helping people to stay healthy, and protecting them from threats to their health (Public Health England 2015).

The WHO definition is the most widely used, but all definitions have a common theme, recognising that health is specific for the individual, but also involves the whole of society and where they live. To be able to encompass these definitions, the term health promotion is used as an umbrella term, which then has under it specific aspects for the promotion of health (see Figure 2.1).

The Millennium Development Goals attempt to fight poverty on many levels and have identified key health promotion issues, including maternal and child health, communicable diseases

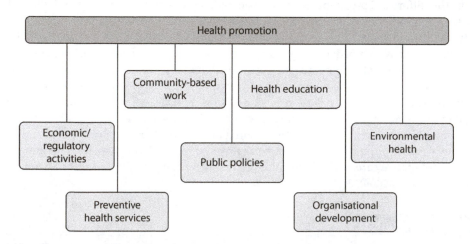

Figure 2.1 Activities encompassed within health promotion. (Adapted from Bowden, Jan. 2006. Health promotion and the midwife. In *Health promotion in midwifery: Principles and practice*, edited by Jan Bowden and Vicky Manning. London: Hodder Arnold. p. 17.)

and social, economic and other determinate factors as well as non-communicable diseases (NCDs) such as smoking, obesity/diet and lack of exercise (United Nations 2015). Within developed countries, the area of NCD tends to be primarily a health promotion focus, which narrows the view of health promotion considerably. Health promotion may seem to focus on healthy lifestyles and/or health education, but if you look at the WHO definition, it suggests not only helping people to be empowered to take more control of their health but also recognises that there are wider social and environmental issues to be considered, which will be discussed later.

ACTIVITY

List some of the health promotion activities you do in your practice.

INFLUENCES OF HEALTH

When considering health, it is imperative to explore and understand what influences health. There are factors that affect health both positively and negatively. As you can see from Figure 2.2, good or poor health is a result of many interwoven factors.

The WHO identified that the two main determinants of health are social and economic factors. The 2008 WHO report 'Closing the gap in a generation; health equality through action on the social determinates of health' looks at the causes and consequences of social and economic disadvantages on health (WHO 2008). The report clearly identifies that the social condition

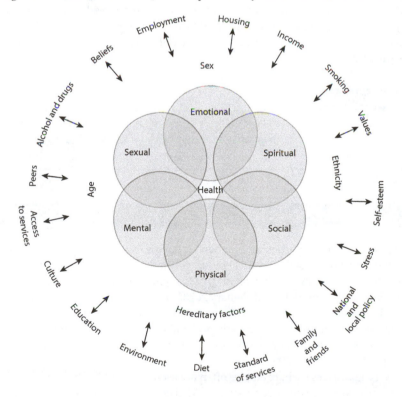

Figure 2.2 Dimensions of health and influencing factors.

into which people are born, live and work is the single most important determinants of good or ill health. A baby girl born in some countries, for example Malta, can expect to live to the age of 80 but less than 45 years if born in other countries such as Sierra Leone (WHO 2015). The 2008 WHO report identified the lack of female voices and recognised the role women play in the early years of their child's life. The early years are key to a healthy adulthood, a theme also recognised in a UK report 'Fair Society Healthy Lives' (Marmot 2010). Public Health England (PHE) (2014, 8) has used the WHO 2008 report and the Marmot 2010 report to identify the following determinates of health to focus on in the United Kingdom:

- Good employment
- Higher educational attainment
- Safe, supported and connected communities
- Poor housing and homelessness
- Living on a low income
- Social isolation, exclusion and loneliness
- Stigma and discrimination

However, social and environmental elements are not the only determinants of health; age, sex, new and re-emerging diseases, mental health issues and NCDs all require urgent responses (Kumar & Preetha 2012). 'The truth is that healthcare has a relatively limited impact on our health. The environment around us, our genetic inheritance, how we live our lives and the opportunities we have together largely determine our health' (PHE 2014, 6). You may feel that midwives can make little impact on the determinants of health, but the fact remains that they can, and they do. Midwives have a role in providing optimal care and optimising health during pregnancy and the postnatal period. Maternal health in pregnancy, postnatally and the early neonatal period will influence the health of a baby, and this influence will continue throughout the baby's life (DoH 2010).

PRACTICE POINT

Although midwives cannot influence a person's genes or his or her age, they can influence the beginning of a person's life by supporting the mother to be as healthy as she can be during pregnancy and beyond.

MIDWIVES AND HEALTH PROMOTION

'Maternity care providers, particularly midwives, have a window of opportunity to influence pregnant women about positive health choices' (Marmot 2010, 1). The importance of the relationship between public health and midwifery is highlighted in Midwifery 2020 with public health as a key area for midwives (Midwifery 2020 Programme 2010). The standards for maternity care (RCOG 2008) have public health as standard 1.1, 'All commissioners and providers of maternity services, in collaboration with local authorities, should ensure local multi-agency health promotion for pregnancy so all women of reproductive age are empowered to be as healthy as possible' (RCOG 2008, 11). Midwives constantly undertake health promotion but do not always recognise it as such. Examples often not seen as health promotion are breastfeeding drop-in centres, whereas smoking cessation initiatives, antenatal screening and good contraceptive advice that support birth spacing are all examples of health promotion (Biro 2010).

The theory of salutogenesis offers midwives a way of thinking about how they can support women to move towards health and well-being rather than avoiding disease. Salutogenesis is a model created by Antonovsky (1996) who identified that individuals are in a state of balance, which when upset because of physical or psychosocial stressors activate the regulatory mechanisms. A person's salutogenic response is termed as a sense of coherence (SOC) that empowers him or her to continue moving towards optimal health (Sinclair & Stockdale 2011).

When people experience an SOC, Antonovsky (1996) proposed that they would:

- Wish to and be motivated towards coping (meaningfulness) – life's trials and tribulations are worthy of commitment and life has some emotional sense to it. The individual must see coping as a desirable skill.
- Believe that the challenge is understood (comprehensibility) – the level to which an individual organises his or her world to bring understanding, meaning, order and consistency to it.
- Believe that the resources to cope are available to them (manageability) – the individual believes that support and resources are effortlessly found and straightforwardly accessible when needed.

The idea is for the midwife to ask, 'How can I facilitate this person in moving towards better health?' This is a more positive way of looking at health than looking to avoid ill health, supporting a vulnerable woman to identify the positive factors that help maintain her balance between health and poor health continuum, as suggested by Antonovsky (1996). The identification of these positive factors then supports women to build on these and regain balance. Salutogenesis also helps midwives to understand better how some women may struggle to make health choices or be aware that a poor choice may have more of an impact than it might have for another woman. The salutogenic model has been adopted by the Royal College of Midwives (RCM) for enhancing normality in pregnancy and child birth (Sinclair & Stockdale 2011).

The Marmot report (2010) recognised that midwives have a big part to play in closing the inequality gap. An example of how midwives can play their part is the 1000 Days Movement which is an international initiative that is working to raise awareness of the necessity of good nutrition in a child's life from conception to the child's second birthday to break the cycle of poverty. Midwives play a part in this, maybe unknowingly, by encouraging women to eat well in pregnancy and then encouraging breastfeeding where the woman chooses to breastfeed or to help women understand how to use formula feeds safely (1000 Days 2015). This then goes on to midwives discussing returning to a healthy postnatal weight ready for a further pregnancy, or a continued healthy life (see Chapter 13).

Figure 2.3 is from the Midwifery 2020 Programme (2010) health promotion review and shows the role midwives play in health promotion. Look back at your list of health promotion activities and see how they will fit into Figure 2.3.

The challenge is not to see public health as an extra task but as an integrated core role of the midwife (Kaufmann 2000). The need of the hour is to ensure midwives are provided with the requisite training, skills and time to undertake health promotion.

PRACTICE POINT

Midwives have a window of opportunity to influence pregnant women about positive health choices. Make every contact count by giving bite sized pieces of information and keep thinking about how to move women towards optimal health.

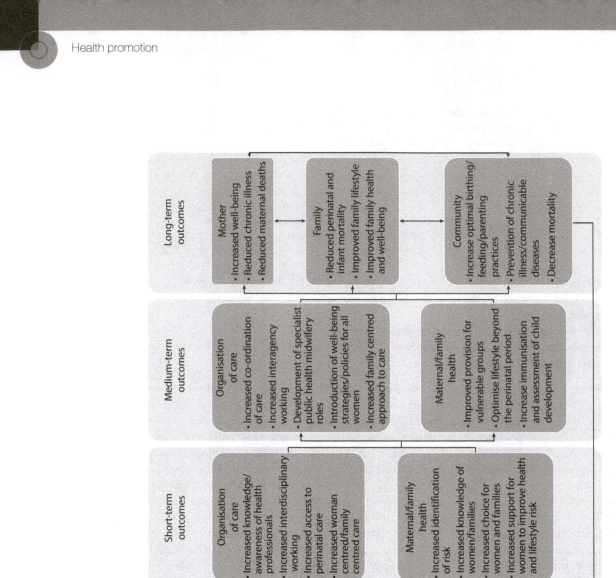

Figure 2.3 The logic model. (From McNeill, J. et al. *BMC Public Health* 12, 955, 2012.)

NEEDS IN HEALTH PROMOTION

The first element of any health promotion intervention is to establish what the needs are. Bradshaw taxonomy of need (1972) defines four types of needs:

1. *Normative need:* a desirable/expected standard specified by the professional, often in the form of a policy or recommendation.
2. *Felt need:* what people actually want. This may eventually become an expressed need.
3. *Expressed need:* that is, the service requested/demanded by an individual, group or community.
4. *Comparative need:* occurs where the recipients of a service are compared with assess gaps and inequality in service provision. The need is to bring about equality and fairness.

Often needs are identified by the health professionals or the government who undertakes a health needs assessment (HNA). An HNA is a systematic method for reviewing health issues facing a community. It is a recommended public health tool that provides evidence to address health issues and social inequalities. It relies on the analysis of a given population or group using epidemiology and demographic data. Social and environmental needs of the population or group also need to be addressed when undertaking an HNA (Green et al. 2015; Mooney et al. 2011). These data then influence local commissioning decisions. This is considered a top-down approach – meaning it is in the control of the health professional(s) or the local or national governments, and it may be a disadvantageous approach because what a health care professional or government department identifies with their data as a glaring health need may not be considered so by the local population of that area. This is because definitions of need vary depending on whose perception, interpretation and values are in play. Having needs identified by the service user – a bottom-up approach – may raise a different set of needs to those identified by the local authorities. A basic way of looking at needs comes from Liss (1990). 'A need for health care exists when an assessor believes that health care ought to be provided' (cited by Mooney et al. 2011). Who that assessor is may make a difference to what is identified.

PRACTICE POINT

There are tensions to HNA. Who is doing the assessment? Their view of health such as biomedical or social models all play a part in the assessment. Being aware of these issues can support better evaluation of the health needs of an individual or group or area.

ACTIVITY

Think of a health need you have seen implemented in your practice area.

- Who identified the need for this intervention?
- How was the HNA undertaken?
- Do you think different needs might have been identified if another agency had been involved in the HNA?

PHE (2014) has set out seven health need priorities (normative need). The following four are specific to the midwife.

1. Tackling obesity particularly among children, for example, baby friendly initiative, encouraging women to breastfeed.

2. Reducing smoking and stopping children from starting, for example, smoking cessation programmes in the antenatal period with ongoing support postnatally.
3. Reducing harmful drinking and alcohol-related hospital admissions, for example, discussing alcohol intake during pregnancy.
4. Ensuring every child has the best start in life, for example, optimising maternal health during pregnancy, encouraging breastfeeding.

The last three are relevant to all health care professionals, including midwives.

- Reducing the risk of dementia, its incidence and prevalence in 65- to 75-year-olds
- Tackling the growth in antimicrobial resistance
- Achieving a year-on-year decline in tuberculosis incidence

However, lists such as these do not fully explain what policies are involved in making these priorities work. The policies required could include:

- Tackling obesity in children by providing finances to support breastfeeding initiatives and even financial incentives to women, thereby leading to an increase in the breastfeeding rate and a reduction in the number of obese women entering the maternity services several years down the line (Harder et al. 2005).
- Trying to ensure every child has the best start in life. This could result in monies being provided for preconception care and encouraging midwives to undertake contraception training (Atrash et al. 2006).
- Trying to lower the teenage birth rate and improving educational attainment; this may eventually lead to improved health in the women accessing the maternity services (LGA 2013).

Needs are like health, the whole is more than the sum of their parts. There is an element of subjectivity with what the needs might be and what the goals are. A formula to present needs might be:

'A' needs 'X' in order to 'G', for example, 'A' = a woman who wants to breastfeed, needs 'X' = breastfeeding support, in order to 'G' = breastfeed successfully (Green et al. 2015).

This formula maybe too simplistic (Green et al. 2015), but whenever a health promotion activity is developed, it starts with identification of the need, which starts with an HNA. For midwives, identification of a need can be challenging, where is the need coming from, a pressure group or your manager? If several needs are identified, whose need should be met first? There are many pitfalls with needs identification and seeking support, and clarification is an essential part of beginning the road to creating an intervention. The success and longevity of health promotion interventions depend on the identification of a genuine health need. On the contrary, it may fail if the identified health need is not deemed important by those it is intended for.

PRACTICE POINT

The identification of health needs is an essential part of setting up a health promotion intervention. Seek support and clarification at every step to ensure that the need identified is one that is considered equally important by the service users as well as the service providers.

SUMMARY OF KEY POINTS

- Health promotion is part of their role with midwives undertaking a lot of activities they do not always recognise as health promotion; vaccinations, screening programmes, breastfeeding support, discussing diet or alcohol use during pregnancy are just a few examples.
- Health has many different meanings and how someone defines health can change over their lifetime.
- Health is affected by different aspects such as where you live, what you eat, your genetic code, your gender, etc. Midwives can use this information to target health messages.
- The identification of needs is an essential part of a successful health promotion intervention. It can be affected by who is identifying the need and by the HNA which may not always acknowledge the social and environmental issues pertinent to that specific area.
- Midwives undertake a large amount of health promotion. Salutogenesis may provide a model to support midwives in this task.

REFERENCES

Antonovsky, Aaron. 1996. The salutogenic model as a theory to guide health promotion. *Health Promotion International* 11(1): 11–18.

Atrash, Hani, Kay Johnson, Myron (Mike) Adams, José F. Cordero & Jennifer Howse. 2006. Preconception care for improving perinatal outcomes: The time to act. *Maternal and Child Health Journal* 10(Suppl 1): 3–11.

Biro, Mary. 2010. What has public health got to do with midwifery? Midwives' role in securing better health outcomes. *Women and Birth* 24: 17–23.

Blaxter, Mildred. 1990. *Health and lifestyles*. London: Routledge.

Bowden, Jan. 2006. Health promotion and the midwife. In *Health promotion in midwifery: Principles and practice*, edited by Jan Bowden and Vicky Manning. London: Hodder Arnold, pp. 13–24.

Bradshaw, Jonathan. 1972. The concept of social need. *New Society* 19: 640–643.

Crafter, Helen. 1997. *Health promotion in midwifery: Principles and practice* (1st ed.). London: Hodder Arnold.

DoH (Department of Health). 2010. *Healthy lives, healthy people: Our strategy for public health in England*. London: TSO. https://www.gov.uk/government/uploads/system/uploads/attachment_data/file/216096/dh_127424.pdf

Dolfman, Michael. 1973. The concept of health: A historic and analytical examination. *Journal of School Health* 43(8): 491–497.

Faculty of Public Health. 2010. *What is health promotion?* http://www.fph.org.uk/what_is_public_health

Green, Jackie, Keith Tone, Ruth Cross & James Woodall. 2015. *Information needs. In Health promotion, planning and strategies*. London: Sage.

Hagell, Anne. 2015. *Promoting young people's health literacy and understanding their help-seeking behaviour*. AYPH Exploring Evidence series, *March 2015*. Association of Young People's Health, Public Health England. http://www.youngpeopleshealth.org.uk/wp-content/uploads/2015/07/628_Health-literacy-EE-format-Updated-by-AH-march.pdf

Harder, Thomas, Renate Bergmann, Gerd Kallischnigg & Andreas Plagemann. 2005. Duration of breastfeeding and risk of overweigh: A meta-analysis. *American Journal of Epidemiology* 162: 397–403.

Hill, Katherine, Karen Kellard, Sue Middleton, Lynne Cox & Elspeth Pound. 2007. *Understanding resources in later life views and experiences of older people.* York: Joseph Rowntree Foundation.

ICM (International Confederation of Midwives). 2011. *ICN international definition of the midwife.* http://www.internationalmidwives.org/assets/uploads/documents/Definition%20 of%20the%20Midwife%20-%202011.pdf

Kaufmann, Tara. 2000. Public health: The next step in woman-centred care. *RCM Midwives Journal* 3(1): 26–28.

Kumar, Santosh & Gnanadhas Preetha. 2012. Health promotion: An effective tool for global health. *Indian Journal of Community Medicine* 37(1): 2–12.

Liss, Per-Eric. 1990. *Health care need: Meaning and measurement.* Aldershot: Avebury.

LGA (Local Government Association). 2013. *Tackling teenage pregnancy, local government's new public health role.* London: LGA.

Marmot, Michael. 2010. *Fair society, healthy lives. The Marmot review.* London: Marmot Review Team. http://www.instituteofhealthequity.org/projects/ fair-society-healthy-lives-the-marmot-review

McNeill, J., Fiona Lynn & Fiona Alderdice. 2012. Public health interventions in midwifery: A systematic review of systematic reviews. *BMC Public Health* 12: 955.

Midwifery 2020 Programme. 2010. *Midwifery 2020: Delivering expectations.* London: Midwifery 2020.

Mooney, Gavin, Stephen Jan & Virginia Wiseman. 2011. Measuring health needs. In *Oxford textbook of public health.* Free medical textbooks. https://medtextfree.wordpress. com/2011/12/18/12-2-measuring-health-needs/

Moorhead, Robert. 2002. William Budd and typhoid fever. *Journal of the Royal Society of Medicine* 95(11): 561–564.

Murphy, Dominic. 2015. *Concepts of disease and health.* http://plato.stanford.edu/entries/ health-disease/

NMC (Nursing and Midwifery Council). 2015. *The code.* London: NMC.

PHE (Public Health England). 2014. *From evidence into action: Opportunities to protect and improve the nation's health.* London: PHE.

PHE (Public Health England). 2015. *Public health.* https://www.gov.uk/government/topics/ public-health

RCOG (Royal College of Obstetricians and Gynaecologist). 2008. *Standards for maternity care, report of a working party.* London: RCOG, Hobbs. https://www.rcog.org.uk/globalassets/ documents/guidelines/wprmaternitystandards2008.pdf

Scriven, Angela. 2010. *(Ewles and Simnett's) Promoting health: A practical guide* (6th ed.). China: Bailliere Tindall.

Sinclair, Marlene & Janine Stockdale. 2011. *Achieving optimal birth using salutogenesis in routine antenatal education.* Royal College of Midwives. https://www.rcm.org.uk/learning-and-career/ learning-and-research/ebm-articles/achieving-optimal-birth-using-salutogenesis

United Kingdom Government. 1993. *The Clean Air Act 1993.* London: HMSO.

United Kingdom Government. 2006. *The Health Act 2006.* London: HMSO.

United Nations. 2015. *The Millennium Development Goals report 2015.* New York: United Nations Department of Social and Economic Affairs.

WHO (World Health Organization). 1946. Preamble to the Constitution of the World Health Organisation as adopted by the International Health Conference, New York, 19 June–22 July 1946; signed on 22 July 1946 by representatives of 61 States (Official Records of the WHO, no 2, p100) and entered into force on 7 April 1948. http://who.int/about/definition/en/print.html

WHO (World Health Organization). 1986. *The Ottawa charter for health promotion*. Geneva: WHO.

WHO (World Health Organization). 2008. *Closing the gap in a generation; health equality through action on the social determinates of health*. Geneva: WHO.

WHO (World Health Organization). 2015. *World Health Statistics 2015*. http://apps.who.int/iris/bitstream/10665/170250/1/9789240694439_eng.pdf?ua=1&ua=1

1000 Days. 2015. http://www.thousanddays.org/

FURTHER READINGS

Lindstrom Bengt, Monica Eriksson. 2010. The hitchhiker's guide to salutogenesis: Salutogenic pathways to health promotion Helsinki Fokhalsan Health Promotion Research.

Public Health England. 2014. Public health contribution of nurses and midwives: guidance. https://www.gov.uk/government/collections/developing-the-public-health-contribution-of-nurses-and-midwives-tools-and-models

Royal College of Midwives. Public health and health promotion online resources http://rcm.redactive.co.uk/midwives/by-subject/public-health/

Stockdale, Janine. 2011. Achieving optimal birth using salutogenesis in routine antenatal education. https://www.rcm.org.uk/learning-and-career/learning-and-research/ebm-articles/achieving-optimal-birth-using-salutogenesis

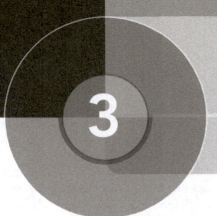

Factors affecting health promotion: What makes women different?

3

HEATHER FINLAY

INTRODUCTION

Making people aware of their ability to make healthy choices and how they can be supported to do this within their lives is problematic. How to achieve this has been a major point of discussion and debate in the field of health promotion and public health. Over the years, the understanding of how we all make choices about actions that can impact on our health has become more sophisticated. Chapter 6 elaborates in more detail about the health behaviour theories and models that seek to address this problem. But one thing that many theories and models have in common, for example, the Theory of Planned Behaviour (Ajzen 2012) and the Stages of Change Model (Prochaska & DiClemente 1984), is acknowledging that there are factors that influence or mediate our ability to make healthy choices. This chapter seeks to explore in more detail the mediating factors that disproportionately influence women's ability to make healthy choices in reaction to health promotion or public health interventions. It then seeks to explore how these mediating factors can be influenced in a positive way through health promotion and public health interventions, which will involve considering two other health promotion approaches: empowerment and social change.

FAMILY AND HOUSEHOLD

The mediating factors that influence women's decision making around making healthy choices are less a product of women's life choices and more a product of their life chances or circumstances. These life chances or circumstances will be a reflection of women's interaction between themselves and among their family, community and environment (Currie & Weisenberg 2003). The first area that can moderate a woman's ability to make healthy choices is the role women play within the household. Although the expectations of the role women play in the household vary from family to family and community to community, gender stereotypes can designate women as the carer within a household. This reflects a cultural acceptance that it is more natural for women to be 'nurturing'. Women's normal responsibilities within the home can be extensive and include preparing nutritious meals, caring for family members (including elderly and disabled individuals) and keeping the home clean (Currie & Weisenberg 2003).

Data from the various European countries show that even when women work more than 30 hours a week, they still do the majority of their housework. In the United Kingdom, women are reported to do between 65% and 70% of the housework (ESS 2013). This is borne out when looking at the literature on women's choices around their health behaviours where the expectations of them as a mother and their family commitments are frequently seen as barriers to having a healthy lifestyle (MacFarlane et al. 2010). One woman, in the study by Withall et al. (2011, 7), commented, 'I would go to a gym or fitness classes, if I knew if I could get someone to have the children. I would do it, I would'; worry about childcare was identified as a particular barrier in this study. Highlighted elsewhere is the role that women finding time for their own needs within a family context can play in them making healthy choices. For example, with regard to exercise, women cite 'being time poor' as an issue but some women also feel guilty about spending time away from the family to focus on their personal needs (Sport England 2015). Indeed, women of childbearing age, especially if they have children, are particularly at risk of weight gain, physical inactivity and poor diet (MacFarlane et al. 2010). Having said this, women's role as the primary purchaser and provider of food for the family helps a woman to make healthy choices to buy and serve healthy food for the good of the family (MacFarlane et al. 2010). Plus, the drive to remain healthy to care for the family can be a factor in supporting healthy activity; another participant, in the study by Withall et al. in 2011, commented, 'I want to make sure I'm healthier for my kids, that I don't get ill from my diabetes or anything, if I don't control my weight properly' (6).

The encouragement from family and partners can also be a motivating factor for women in making healthy choices (Cleland et al. 2013). Although the role of family in encouraging healthy behaviours can be limited by a number of factors including guilt at giving the family food they do not want, low income and cultural norms. Some of these will be discussed in more detail later. Overall, women's situation within households can mediate their ability to make healthy choices in a number of ways. On the negative side, many women report, due to their caring commitments, being time poor. But for many women, the encouragement and motivation that comes from being part of a family group help them to begin or maintain activities or choices that are good for their health.

PRACTICE POINTS

- Awareness of women's responsibilities and the impact on attendance needs to be considered when planning health promotion or public health activities.
- Being thoughtful about times and providing childcare can help all women attend.

BEING A WOMAN IN SOCIETY

A person's gender is based on a social construction of individuals as male and female, and it includes beliefs about behaviour and relationships (Naidoo & Wills 2009). These beliefs can influence the ability of both women and men to make healthy choices. This section will continue the focus on women and discuss in more detail the influence that beliefs about gender have on women's ability to make healthy choices could, although it needs to be noted that beliefs about gender are not static and vary from community to community. Generally, there are societal norms about how women should look and behave, what is meant by being feminine and these can be a barrier to some healthy choices, such as exercise. Young girls and women have a complex relationship with physical activity. Many young girls enjoy physical activity but they feel constrained by wanting to appear feminine, and Spencer et al. (2015) cite a number of studies that show getting sweaty and dirty without the time to shower and get ready after doing physical activity can leave young women feeling self-conscious, vulnerable and uncomfortable. This matters as lacking confidence in physical activity when young can influence the chances of a woman exercising as an adult. Women generally seem to prefer to exercise in groups and can be reluctant to go on their own. This reluctance can be due to a lack of confidence. In one study, women commented, 'If I was to come on my own I don't think I would because I'm not a very confident person' (Withall et al. 2011, 7). Alongside issues around confidence, this preference for group exercise also reflects the value many women put on the social nature of exercise (Withall et al. 2011).

The recent work by Sport England also found that some women do not exercise because they fear being judged. The related insecurity can range from not feeling the right shape, weight or age to not being fit enough 'I'm self-conscious going to a gym. There are fit women on the treadmill and big men' (Sport England 2015, 21). The feeling of being judged and found wanting reflects common norms about what a fit healthy woman looks like. This is being challenged by the Sport England campaign – 'This Girl Can', which uses images of real women to promote women in sport (This Girl Can n.d.).

In this section, exercise has been used as an example to explore how societal norms about how women should look and behave can influence women's ability to make healthy choices. It should be borne in mind that shame or the fear of being judged, due to not fitting in to societal norms in some way or the other, can be particularly be acute for women and can limit their ability to access a wide range of public health initiatives. Including those addressing issues around obesity and addictions (Brown 2006, cited in Hernandez and Mendoza 2011).

ACTIVITY

- Review the current guidelines for exercise by accessing the NHS Choice website: http://www.nhs.uk/livewell/fitness/pages/physical-activity-guidelines-for-adults.aspx
- Do you stick to the guidelines?
- If you do not, what prevents you from exercising?

POWER AND CONTROL

There is an increasing acknowledgement of the role of power and control in mediating women's decisions to adopt healthier behaviours. Despite the change in the relationship between the genders in recent years in the United Kingdom, for some women there are still issues around power and control. There are women who are marginalised from decision making, both within a family setting and at a community level. Also, some women are subject to various forms of physical or sexual violence. Accurate figures for domestic violence are difficult to get as those affected might be reluctant to report their ordeal, and there can be many incidents before the abuse is finally reported (Walby and Allen 2004 cited by Howard et al. 2010). It is likely that 30% of women and 16% of men will experience domestic violence in their lifetime in the United Kingdom, the figures for domestic violence have remained steady since 2008–2009 (Gay & Bardens 2015). Partner abuse/violence is discussed in more detail in Chapter 15. But aside from partner abuse and violence, there are other ways in which power and control can affect women's ability to make healthy choices. For example, whether women feel safe when walking in their area makes a difference to whether they will exercise or not (Timperio et al. 2015).

But a lack of control and the influence of various forms of power over some women's lives can manifest itself in many ways, such as lack of financial control, physical or psychological coercion and expectations of women's behaviour or not being permitted to access knowledge around healthier choices. This could mean, for example, that a lack of control over household finances would make it difficult to buy good-quality food or even fill prescriptions, or a lack of money for fares may prevent a woman from attending appointments or result in sporadic attendance. Similarly, the decision to seek preventive screening, health care or reproductive choices may not be the woman's alone (Collier & Quinlivan 2014).

The powerlessness that can result from a feeling of lack of control could have consequences for women's ability to make choices. The locus of control theory suggests that having an external locus of control, where events in one's life are perceived as being governed by powerful others or 'fate', will reduce a person's ability to see the value of trying to change the situation (or health) (Tones 1991). For example, women report an inability to think clearly or make choices or decisions when subject to domestic violence (Boothroyd 2002). Thus, women disempowered by their situation may feel that it is hopeless to try to adopt healthy choices, even if they are aware of them. This section illustrates how women's responses to health promotion are mediated by their particular experiences and life situations and that there are many psychological and practical issues that prevent women from making healthy choices.

PRACTICE POINT

When a woman is making choices around changing her behaviour, a midwife needs to offer an opportunity for the woman to talk about that decision in the context of her wider situation.

POVERTY

Poverty can affect the ability of women to make healthy choices both as an individual and through the practical consequences of poverty. Like domestic violence, poverty can affect anyone but women are disproportionately affected. The Fawcett Society (2013) found that the austerity agenda in place since the 2010 election has had more of a negative effect on women than men through what they term 'triple jeopardy'.

The triple jeopardy results first from cuts to the public sector, where women make up two-thirds of the workforce and so are more vulnerable to losing secure, well-paid jobs; this is then combined with women appearing not to benefit from job creation in the private sector to the same extent as men.

The second aspect of the triple jeopardy is cuts to benefits where three-quarters of the money being cut come from the money for women. Single parents (who are predominantly women) are particularly hard hit, with an estimated 16% loss in their income (Rabindrakumar 2013).

Third, a contraction in public services that women are more likely to rely on means that women may have to pay for services they would have previously received free or they have to spend time giving care that would previously have been given by the state. Overall, the consequences of the austerity agenda have left women more likely to be poor and in low-paid part-time work than men with fewer financial assets to protect themselves with (Fawcett Society 2014).

In the Gingerbread study 'Paying the price' (Rabindrakumar 2013), women graphically describe their situation:

- I work full time at minimum wage and have to work 60+ [hours] a week to cover rent, bills and food. (25)
- We are not going to be able to heat our house as much as we probably would like because it's just going to cost so much. We can't afford to put ourselves in any more arrears. (17)

It is inevitable that being in poverty challenges a woman's ability to make healthy choices, and poverty is another mediating factor in women's response to health promotion. Women facing such situations are more likely to override their own health needs and can be at more risk of being subjected to factors around power and control (Howard et al. 2010). In addition, being poor brings its own practical constraints on women's ability to make healthy choices. For example, a lack of money may make it difficult to follow health education guidelines on diet (especially in pregnancy). The Gingerbread study 'Paying the price' (Rabindrakumar 2013) has numerous examples of women faced with poverty struggling to afford to eat well:

- I regularly have to choose 'buy gas or buy food'. (13)
- Sometimes the boys will say, 'Why've you got so little food, Mum?' … Sometimes there's not enough to go round, you just have to limit it because they need it much more than I do. (35)
- I let them eat the healthy and nutritious things, and I'll get the big plate of mashed potato. (35)

It seems that women's response to poverty is often to go without food themselves, so that the rest of the family can have more (Rosenblatt & Rake 2003).

A lack of money may also mean that women and their families are unable to take advantage of facilities outside their immediate area (or even inside their immediate area unless they are free). One response from the study by Withall et al. in 2011 when thinking of going to the local leisure was: 'I just couldn't afford it. Every time I thought oh I'll go put some money on my card and then it's like oh no I've got to buy nappies, oh no I've got to do this, oh no the phone bill needs paying' (26).

Facilities outside the immediate area that women might be prevented from accessing could include getting to food shops with more choice or accessing free healthy activities or screening (Rabindrakumar 2013). The cost of transport may be prohibitive and the facilities for claiming fares back retrospectively does not solve the problem when there is no money before the journey is started, or if a woman has no recourse to public funds and her status in the United Kingdom is unclear. These examples show how the practical consequences of poverty can reduce the ability of those affected to make healthy choices. However, alongside this, there is the impact on the individual of being poor.

For many of those living in poverty, there is a feeling that there are negative stereotypes applied to those who are poor, resulting in many of those living in poverty feeling stigmatised in the media, in parts, adding to these negative stereotypes (Skeggs 2004; Larsen & Dejgaard 2013; McKenzie 2013). This can then affect how confident women feel about mixing with those outside their area or social group. One woman in the study by McKenzie commented on how she felt going along to her local Gingerbread group for single parents:

> Well I thought the people were posh people do you know what I mean the way they looked at me I felt really small I had to come out and my kids were playing up basically but I felt they were looking at me cos I was white and they [my kids] were mixed-race … no one talked to me.

> McKenzie (2013, 1348)

The fear of being treated differently or stigmatised for being poor could prevent women from taking part in group activities even when they are free or it could prevent poor women from using services where they feel that they are treated differently.

Poverty brings with it many practical limitations to choices, such as an inability to afford a nutritious diet that may make some health education messages unrealistic for many women. However, it also has a more corrosive effect that can prevent women from accessing services that are available to them. Having said that, it is important to remember that individual experiences can differ and while the practical limitations of poverty are very real, many women refuse to be stigmatised for being poor and are active in defining themselves and their community in a positive way. This will be discussed in more detail later.

ACTIVITY

- Access the Fawcett Society website to find out more about how far we have come towards financial equality between women and men: http://www.fawcettsociety.org.uk/
- There are also resources around pregnancy discrimination and maternal employment

PRACTICE POINT

- Health promotion initiatives that take into account the cost of access, such as travel and childcare, would facilitate a broader mix of women attending.
- Moving initiatives closer to these populations would increase the numbers accessing them.

ETHNICITY

The influence of ethnicity on women's ability to engage with health promotion messages is complex. However, it is worth noting that black and minority ethnic (BME) women and families are subject to the same pressures as other women and families, but these pressures intersect with their experience of being part of a BME community in the United Kingdom. There are many examples where custom-based behaviour within some BME groups promotes healthy behaviours, such as not smoking and not drinking alcohol being the cultural norms for women. Many BME communities also prefer preparing food using fresh ingredients; for example, Chinese and Afro Caribbean communities consume a higher proportion of fruit and vegetables than other groups (Leung & Stanner 2011). There is also some suggestion that living around others from the same community can help improve maternal and infant outcomes for some communities (Pickett Kate et al. 2009). Alongside this, there are various initiatives coming from within communities to help improve their health outcomes; one example is the long running Day-mer Turkish and Kurdish community centre in London that has, among others, a women's service that provides a health promotion information service.

However, the picture is mixed with some BME custom-based behaviour not promoting healthy behaviours (Leung & Stanner 2011). For example, one study of the Somali population living in London found a low level of fruit and vegetable consumption (McEwen et al. 2009). It can also be the case that when individuals behave in a way that is outside the norms of custom-based behaviour in their community, they can feel they have to hide their behaviour from their community, and this limits their ability to access health promotion initiatives and other support (Hurcombe et al. 2010). This can be a particular problem for women because of the fear of the shame their behaviour could bring to their families or community. For example, one study of Bangladeshi women who used illicit drugs found that the women faced more discrimination due to expectations around gendered behaviour in their community, and this was a barrier to the women getting help and support (Cottew & Oyefyesi 2005).

Some BME communities are disproportionately affected by poverty, and households headed up by someone from an ethnic minority are more likely to be classified as having a low income, with households headed by someone of Bangladeshi or Pakistani heritage particularly at risk of having low income (DWP 2015). This will leave these communities at risk of the effects of poverty and negatively impact on their ability to make healthy choices, as described earlier in this chapter.

ACTIVITY

Before looking at Box 3.1, identify your definition of the terms refugee and asylum seeker. Refugees and asylum seekers from various BME communities are an especially at-risk group when it comes to poverty and poor health outcomes. Many refugee and asylum-seeking women and families can have complex health and social care needs, while at the same time they can also be disadvantaged and face barriers in accessing health care and health promotion/public health initiatives. These barriers include an uncertainty about eligibility and how to access services that alleviate poverty. Women asylum seekers and refugees are at risk of poor birth outcomes and have lower than expected take up of breast and cervical cancer screening services (Aspinall & Watters 2010). Although there are interventions in place to include this group, one example is the health and maternity streams of the 'City of Sanctuary' initiative which supports refuges and asylums seekers through building on the expertise and experience within their communities (Haith-Cooper & McCarthy 2015; City of Sanctuary, n.d.).

Overall, when considering the relationship between health promotion, public health and BME groups in the United Kingdom, there are a number of core messages. The first is that BME

BOX 3.1: Definition of a refugee and an asylum seeker

Refugee: A person who 'owing to a well-founded fear of being persecuted for reasons of race, religion, nationality, membership of a particular social group, or political opinion, is outside the country of his nationality, and is unable to or, owing to such fear, is unwilling to avail himself of the protection of that country' as stated in Article 1, 1951 Convention Relating to the Status of Refugees (UNHCR 2010, 14).

Asylum seeker: Persons become asylum seekers when they have applied for asylum and they are waiting to see if they will be granted refugee status (UNHCR n.d.).

groups in the United Kingdom are very diverse, with the health-related behaviours in different groups being similarly diverse. Second, individuals within those BME groups might or might not observe the custom-based behaviour of their communities. It is also the case that many of the custom-based behaviours in BME communities support healthy behaviours and reflect many health promotion and public health messages, while other custom-based behaviours might be at odds with health promotion and public health messages. For some of these communities, there is also a particular problem in accessing services and getting support for individuals who step outside the accepted custom-based behaviours in their communities. Issues around stigma and shame might prevent them from sharing their issues. When considering the needs of women and families from BME communities in relation to health promotion, it is important to acknowledge the lived experience of particular communities and ensure that the community is included and active in the development and delivery of health promotion or public health interventions (Ochieng 2011).

ACTIVITY

- Find out whether your trust/organisation consults with representatives from the local communities when developing health promotion/public health initiatives. Focus particularly on initiatives for women and families.
- Does your trust provide guidance on the rights of refugees and asylum seekers to access maternity care?
- Review them and identify what they mean for your practice?

BEING PREGNANT

So far, this section has largely focused on women in general; however, although many of the barriers are applicable to both pregnant and non-pregnant women, there are aspects that are specific to being pregnant that make engaging with healthy choices difficult. Fatigue appears to be a major issue for many pregnant women, as also feeling unwell, especially when considering participation in exercise (Duncombe et al. 2009; Haakstad et al. 2009). Family beliefs, both positive and negative, around activities such as exercise and diet in pregnancy also influence how comfortable pregnant women feel in making healthy choices (Johnson et al. 2013). One study with South Asian women found that the advice given by health professionals around diet and exercise was at odds with advice from their family (Greenhalgh et al. 2015). Also, many women had unaddressed apprehensions about the appropriate exercise in pregnancy. (Duncombe et al. 2009; Connelly et al. 2015). Women with a high body mass index (BMI), particularly when characterised as obese (BMI >30), faced particular issues. Many midwives were unsure about how to approach the subject in a sensitive and productive way. There was also a worry that it would upset the bond between the woman and the midwife: 'I think if you do it wrong you are up against a brick wall because you've got that woman in a position where she thinks you are being judgmental and not giving advice for the right reason…' (Foster & Hirst 2014, 258). Some obese women reported feeling stigmatised in the maternity system although many wanted help to adopt a healthier lifestyle. Obese women also felt uncomfortable in situations, such as aqua natal classes, where they had to wear swimsuits in front of other women but at the same time felt pressurised by the media to adopt an unrealistic weight both during and after pregnancy (Johnson et al. 2013).

WHAT DO WE KNOW?

So, it seems that when it comes to making healthy choices and being able to put them into practice, women have particular barriers, and some facilitators, that mediate their response to models of health promotion based on education or attempts to change behaviour. Women's choices appear to be constrained by time and their obligations to others. Women are also more likely than men to be constrained by poverty and the power and control others might have over them. However, women's place in the family can give them the support and motivation to make healthy choices for both themselves and their families, with women also preferring to have the company of others, for example, when starting something new. Pregnancy also has extra challenges for women making healthy choices in terms of physical changes and the expectations of others. Women from BME communities also have to manage the intersection of their lived experience with general health promotion messages and provision. So, helping women to make healthy choices is complex and needs to address the particular experience of individual women. The next section will outline some schemes that have tried to do this – some using an educational or behaviour change approach and others using an empowerment or social change approach.

PRACTICAL CHANGE: MAKING HEALTHY CHOICE EASIER AND LISTENING TO WOMEN

Sport England in its document, 'Go Where the Women Are' acknowledges that when planning exercise interventions you have to build it around women's lives; they do not always have the time to do things separately (Sport England 2015). There are increasing examples of schemes where this idea is at the core of the intervention, including postnatal exercise groups, where the baby is included, such as buggy classes, or training where babies are brought along; these can be expensive but are publically funded and free in some areas. Other examples of interventions designed to fit into women's lives include providing text messages to remind or prompt pregnant women to make healthy lifestyle choices with texts such as: 'Eat for you, not for two' and 'If you're feeling tired remember that exercise can give you a real energy boost' (Soltani et al. 2012).

Even health promotion schemes relying on giving women the tools to change their behaviour are being trialled with inputs from women to make sure that the intervention fits into women's lives. One example is a project in a more deprived area of the North of England. Here, pregnant women were given information on pregnancy through a 'lifestyle course' that women would continue to use in pregnancy and even after the baby is born. The initial feasibility phase seemed positive and the women responded well to a 10-week scheme that included sessions on healthy eating, relaxation sessions and inbuilt exercise sessions. However, some parts of the scheme such as daily diaries and the use of pedometers were discontinued as the participants did not find them useful. The scheme included women from a wide range of backgrounds and relies on the impact of the information and techniques given to prompt behaviour change. After a year, the majority of those taking part had an awareness of a healthy lifestyle, although the number making changes for a healthy lifestyle were smaller (Smith et al. 2015). This illustrates how health promotion interventions that are designed in partnership with women and their families can help achieve better results.

For many women, including vulnerable women, caseload midwifery can provide a myriad of benefits, including midwifery support, in making healthy choices through the midwives and women establishing a relationship (Rayment-Jones et al. 2015). Some National Health Service best practice tool kits have recently been produced as part of the London Maternity Strategic Clinical Network for care in London (NHS 2015). One of the tool kits also advocates increasing continuity of care. These tool kits identify areas of good practice in order to facilitate good outcomes for all pregnant women and babies. One study on case-loading in London from the best practice tool kit achieved 30% homebirth rate and 88% exclusive breast feeding at 6 weeks. This demonstrates that the organisation of midwifery care can also influence public health outcomes, such as breast feeding.

EMPOWERMENT AND SOCIAL CHANGE

Some health promotion interventions go beyond attempting behaviour change or education and have a specific empowerment agenda. Empowerment can be self-empowerment, where people are supported in taking control of their lives, and making changes to their behaviour as they choose to (Naidoo & Wills 2009). This approach can include 'critical consciousness raising', wherein participant's awareness of the broader causes of ill health, including inequality, is enhanced (Tones 1986 cited in Naidoo & Wills 2009). There is also community empowerment where community development work is undertaken to help groups of people identify their concerns and put in place a plan to address them. These concerns can encompass a broad definition of 'health' including such areas as housing and might aim for some level of social change. These types of intervention can arise spontaneously in communities and are more likely to be 'bottom up' rather than responding to an agenda decided outside the community or group. Although empowerment, and possible social change, is part of the midwifery role, it has prompted debate within the profession (Hall 2012). However, some of the public health guidance includes a broader, more strategic role for some midwives around social change, mainly to address the social risk factors for maternal and infant mortality and morbidity (PHE 2013). For further information about models and approaches in health promotion, refer to Chapter 4.

An example of self-empowerment is a young parents' group project in Scotland that was set up by a Sure Start midwife. The aim of this project is to facilitate mutual support for vulnerable parents and to increase their confidence in their role as parents. Here, the parents who attend are active participants in the development and review of the group. The issues addressed were the ones relevant to their lives at that time and reflected their experience (McKenzie et al. 2010).

There are other examples of schemes that include elements of community empowerment such as co-operatives providing fresh food and vegetables at affordable rates that mothers can pick up when they pick up their children from school. For example, the East London Food Access (ELFA) scheme that operates at a number of venues in East London (East London Food Access n.d.). This scheme is an example of a health promotion intervention that is based around empowering communities and prompting social change. ELFA is a social enterprise and not for profit organisation with an aim to 'develop a local infrastructure to reduce "Food Poverty," and to encourage local residents within the communities to improve their own and others health and well-being' (ELFA n.d.). This is the sort of project information that the local midwives might share with the women and families they work with to increase the families' access to fresh fruit and vegetables at affordable rates.

Even more radically, some groups call directly for social change to address inequalities and improve health. One example of this is the 'Focus E15' mothers who took possession of empty social housing in Newham where they lived when they were told that they would have to move to the Midlands or North West to be housed. The group's focus is on 'decent housing 4 all' with an emphasis on the provision of social housing. The group and others like them challenge the local authorities and the government to provide homes for all (Focus E15 Mothers n.d.)

All the above examples illustrate how varied health promotion interventions can be; this variability reflects the variety in women's lives (and the lives of their families). If health promotion interventions have to succeed, there has to be an appreciation of the things that mediate women's ability to make healthy choices. Midwives are ideally placed to work alongside women and their communities to design and implement health promotion activities that work alongside women's complex lives.

ACTIVITY

- Find examples of health promotion activities and initiatives for women and families run by midwives or other organisations within your area.
- Identify the approach you think they are aimed at:
  - Changing behaviour
  - Education
  - Empowerment

SUMMARY

Women's ability to make healthy choices is mediated by their lives in a number of ways such as:

- Their situation within a household and expectations of their role within that household. These expectations can support women to make healthy choices or it can be a barrier.
- Women are also subject to beliefs about gender that can influence their ability to make healthy choices, such as exercise, or to access health promotion or public health initiative when their behaviour is interpreted as outside the norm in their community. Beliefs about gender are not static and vary from community to community.
- Women are disproportionately affected by factors around poverty and power and control which can limit their ability to make healthy choices and take advantage of health promotion or public health initiatives.
- Within BME communities, the ability of people to make healthy choices can be supported by custom-based behaviour or some behaviour can be a barrier.
- It cannot be assumed that everybody in a community will adopt the custom-based behaviour prevalent in that community.
- Pregnant women have additional hindering factors, such as tiredness, that can affect their ability to make healthy choices and take advantage of health promotion or public health initiatives.
- Health promotion and public health initiatives need to take into account the lives of the women, families and communities with whom they work. Ideally, these initiatives should be developed in consultation with, or with the involvement of, the women, families and communities to whom the initiatives are addressed.

REFERENCES

Ajzen, Icek. 2012. The theory of planned behaviour. In *Handbook of theories of social psychology: Volume one*, edited by Paul A. M. Van Lange, Arie W. Kruglanski and E. Tory Higgins, 438–460. London: Sage.

Aspinall, Peter & Charles Watters. 2010. *Refugees and asylum seekers; a review from an equality and human rights perspective.* Equality and Human Right Commission. http://www.equalityhumanrights.com/sites/default/files/documents/research/refugees_and_asylum_seekers_research_report.pdf

Boothroyd, L. 2002. Domestic violence: Implications for children. *MIDIRS Midwifery Digest* 12(Suppl 2): S9–S11.

City of Sanctuary. n.d. *Home Page.* http://cityofsanctuary.org/

Cleland, Verity, Alba Granados, David Crawford, Tania Winzenberg & Kylie Ball. 2013. Effectiveness of interventions to promote physical activity among socioeconomically disadvantaged women: A systematic review and meta-analysis. *Obesity Reviews* 14: 197–212.

Collier, Rachael & Julie A. Quinlivan. 2014. Domestic violence is a leading risk factor in default from colposcopy services. *The Journal of Obstetrics and Gynaecology Research* 40(6): 1785–1790.

Connelly, Megan, Helen Brown, Paige van der Pligt & Megan Teychenne. 2015. Modifiable barriers to leisure-time physical activity during pregnancy: A qualitative study investigating first time mother's views and experiences. *BMC Pregnancy and Childbirth* 15: 100.

Cottew, Gillian & Adenekan Oyefyesi. 2005. Illicit drug use among Bangladeshi women living in the United Kingdom: An exploratory qualitative study of a hidden population in East London. *Drugs: Education, Prevention and Policy* 12(3): 171–188.

Currie, Dawn H. & Sara Weisenberg. 2003. Promoting women's health-seeking behaviour: Research and the empowerment of women. *Health Care for Women International* 24: 880–899.

Duncombe, Dianne, Eleanor H. Wertheim, Helen Skouteris, Susan J. Paxton & Leanne Kelly. 2009. Factors related to exercise over the course of pregnancy including women's beliefs about the safety of exercise during pregnancy. *Midwifery* 25: 430–438.

DWP (Department for Work & Pensions). 2015. *Households below average income.* https://www.gov.uk/government/uploads/system/uploads/attachment_data/file/437246/households-below-average-income-1994-95-to-2013-14.pdf

East London Food Access. n.d. *About ELFA.* http://www.elfaweb.org.uk/

ESS (European Social Service). 2013. *Exploring public attitudes, informing public policy selected findings from the first five rounds.* http://www.europeansocialsurvey.org/docs/findings/ESS1_5_select_findings.pdf

Fawcett Society. 2013. *Cutting women out.* http://www.fawcettsociety.org.uk/2013/03/cutting-women-out/

Fawcett Society. 2014. *The changing labour market 2: Women, low pay and gender equality in the emerging recovery.* http://www.fawcettsociety.org.uk/wp-content/uploads/2013/02/The-Changing-Labour-Market-2.pdf

Focus E15 Mothers. n.d. *Facebook page.* https://www.facebook.com/pages/Focus-E15-Mothers/602860129757343

Foster, Christine E. & Janet Hirst. 2014. Midwives' attitudes towards giving weight-related advice to obese pregnant women. *British Journal of Midwifery* 22(4): 254–262.

Gay, Oonagh & John Bardens. 2015. *Domestic violence: Commons Briefing papers SN06337.* http://researchbriefings.parliament.uk/ResearchBriefing/Summary/SN06337

Greenhalgh, Trisha, Megan Clinch, Nur Afsar, Yasmin Choudhury, Rita Sudra, Desirée Campbell-Richards, Anne Claydon, Graham A. Hitman, Philippa Hanson & Sarah Finer. 2015. Socio-cultural influences on the behaviour of South Asian women with diabetes in pregnancy: Qualitative study using a multi-level theoretical approach. *BMC Medicine* 13: 120.

Haakstad, Lene, Nanna Voldener, Tore Henriksen & Kari Bø. 2009. Why do pregnant women stop exercising in the third trimester? *Acta Obstetricia et Gynecologica* 88: 1267–1275.

Haith-Cooper, Melanie & Rose McCarthy. 2015. Striving for excellence in maternity care: The Maternity Stream of the City of Sanctuary. *British Journal of Midwifery* 23(9): 648–652.

Hall, Alice. 2012. Health promotion: To educate or empower? *British Journal of Midwifery* 20(3): 156.

Hernandez, Virginia R. & Carmen T. Mendoza. 2011. Shame resilience: A strategy for empowering women in treatment for substance abuse. *Journal of Social Work Practice in the Addictions* 11: 375–393.

Howard, Louise M., Kylee Trevillion & Roxane Agnew-Davies. 2010. Domestic violence and mental health. *International Review of Psychiatry* 22(5): 525–534.

Hurcombe, Rachel, Mariana Bayley & Anthony Goodman. 2010. *Ethnicity and alcohol: A review of the UK literature.* https://www.jrf.org.uk/report/ethnicity-and-alcohol-review-uk-literature

Johnson, Maxine, Fiona Campbell, Josie Messina, Louise Preston, Helen Buckley Woods & Elizabeth Goyder. 2013. Weight management during pregnancy: A systematic review of qualitative evidence. *Midwifery* 29: 1287–1296.

Larsen, Christian A. & Thomas E. Dejgaard. 2013. The institutional logic of images of the poor and welfare recipients: A comparative study of British, Swedish and Danish newspapers. *Journal of European Social Policy* 23(3): 287–299.

Leung, Georgine & Sara Stanner. 2011. Diets of minority ethnic groups in the UK: Influence on chronic disease risk and implications for prevention. *British Nutrition Foundation Nutrition Bulletin* 36: 161–198.

MacFarlane, Abbie, Gavin Abbott, David Crawford & Kylie Ball. 2010. Personal, social and environmental correlates of healthy weight status amongst mothers from socioeconomically disadvantaged neighbourhoods: Findings from the READI study. *International Journal of Behavioural Nutrition and Physical Activity* 7: 23.

McEwen, Andy, Lianne Straus & Helen Croker. 2009. Dietary beliefs and behaviour of a UK Somali population. *Journal of Human Nutrition and Dietetics* 22: 16–121.

McKenzie, Karen, Rebecca Wade & Linda Davidson. 2010. The young parents' group: Supporting vulnerable parents. *British Journal of Midwifery* 18(9): 584–597.

Mckenzie, Lisa. 2013. Narratives from a Nottingham council estate: A story of white working-class mothers with mixed-race children. *Ethnic and Racial Studies* 36(8): 1342–1358.

Naidoo, Jennie & Jane Wills. 2009. *Foundations for health promotion* (3rd ed.). London: Baillière Tindall.

NHS. 2015. *Maternity best practice toolkits. Ensuring equally good outcomes for all pregnant women and families.* http://www.londonscn.nhs.uk/wp-content/uploads/2015/06/mat-suite-of-toolkits-062015.pdf

Ochieng, Bertha, M. N. 2011. Black families' perceptions of barriers to the practice of a healthy lifestyle: A qualitative study in the UK. *Critical Public Health* 23(1): 6–16.

Pickett, Kate, Richard Shawa, Karl Atkin, Kathleen E. Kiernan & Richard G. Wilkinson. 2009. Ethnic density effects on maternal and infant health in the Millennium Cohort Study. *Social Science & Medicine* 69: 1476–1483.

PHE (Public Health England). 2013. *Nursing and midwifery actions at the three levels of public health practice improving health and wellbeing at individual, community and population levels.* https://www.gov.uk/government/uploads/system/uploads/attachment_data/file/208814/3_Levels.pdf

Prochaska, James O., Carl C. DiClemente. 1984. *The transtheoretical approach: crossing traditional boundaries of therapy*. Homewood IL: Dow Jones/Irwin.

Rabindrakumar, Sumi. 2013. *Paying the price: Single parents in the age of austerity*. http://www.gingerbread.org.uk/uploads/media/17/8737.pdf

Rayment-Jones, Hannah, Trevor Murrells & Jane Sandall. 2015. An investigation of the relationship between the caseload model of midwifery for socially disadvantaged women and childbirth outcomes using routine data – A retrospective observational study. *Midwifery* 31(4): 409–417.

Rosenblatt Gemma, Katherine Rake. 2003. *Gender and poverty*. London, the Fawcett Society.

Skeggs, Beverley. 2004. *Class, self and culture*. London: Routledge.

Smith, Debbie M., Wendy Taylor, Melissa K. Whitworth, Stephen Roberts, Colin Sibley & Tina Lavender. 2015. The feasibility phase of a community antenatal lifestyle programme [The Lifestyle Course (TLC)] for women with a body mass index(BMI) >30 kg/m². *Midwifery* 31: 280–287.

Soltani, Hora, Penny Furness, Madelynne A. Arden, Kerry McSeveny, Carolyn Garland, Helena Sustar & Andy Darden. 2012. Women and midwives perspectives on the design of a text messaging support for maternal obesity services: An exploratory study. *Journal of Obesity* 2012: 1.

Spencer, Rebecca A., Laurene Rehman & Sara F. L. Kirk. 2015. Understanding gender norms, nutrition, and physical activity in adolescent girls: A scoping review. *International Journal of Behavioural Nutrition and Physical Activity* 12: 6.

Sport England. 2015. *Go where women are insight on engaging women and girls in sport and exercise*. https://www.sportengland.org/media/806351/gowherewomenare_final_01062015final.pdf

This Girl Can. n.d. *Home page*. http://www.thisgirlcan.co.uk/

Timperio, Anna, Jenny Veitch & Alison Carver. 2015. Safety in numbers: Does perceived safety mediate associations between the neighborhood social environment and physical activity among women living in disadvantaged neighborhoods? *Preventive Medicine* 74: 49–54.

Tones, Keith. 1991. Health promotion, empowerment and the psychology of control. *Journal of International Health Education* 29: 17–26.

UNHCR (Office of the United Nations High Commissioner for Refugees). 2010. *Convention and protocol relating to the status of refugees*. http://www.unhcr.org/3b66c2aa10.html

UNHCR. n.d. *Asylum in the UK*. http://www.unhcr.org.uk/about-us/the-uk-and-asylum.html

Withall, Janet, Russell Jago & Kenneth T. Fox. 2011. Why some do but most don't. Barriers and enablers to engaging low-income groups in physical activity programmes: A mixed methods study. *BMC Public Health* 11: 507.

Health promotion models and approaches

4

JAN BOWDEN

INTRODUCTION

Health promotion has been a contested field of study, mainly because of its broad field of action, incorporating many professions, such as medicine, public health, education, the third sector and midwifery, and because its focus changes. The focus of health promotion can change and shift due to international sways, for example, the World Health Organization (WHO), national authority such as the Department of Health (DoH) and local power such as the public health unit which now is a subsidiary of the local government. With its wide scope of practice and multitudes of influences, the approaches that underpin health promotion have also come from various disciplines, namely psychology, sociology, management, consumer behaviour and marketing to name a few (Nutbeam & Harris 2010). Although approaches and models have been used in disciplines such as medicine and nursing for some time, within midwifery their development and use have not been as swift. This may be due to the unique and individual situations of pregnancy and childbirth, which do not always lend themselves to categorisation of women, their families or their needs. Midwifery's resistance may also be the result of our belief in our own autonomy as practitioners and in a more holistic approach to care. Most models used within midwifery have been adapted from nursing and medicine, which historically have illness as a starting point. However, for public health to be recognised as a core skill of the midwife as indicated in midwifery's public health contribution (DoH 2013), the midwife must have a full understanding of the approaches and models used in health promotion to enhance the way that they deliver care.

Within this chapter, the approaches developed by Ewles and Simnett (2003) will be high-lighted, and the models developed by Downie et al. (1996) and Taylor (1990) identified alongside the model designed by Piper (2005) specifically for midwives and their application to practice explored.

BACKGROUND

The turning point for what is now termed health promotion was the Lalonde Report published in 1974. This report was released by the then Canadian Minister for Health, Marc Lalonde. This report identified for the first time the term health promotion and identified activities that worked towards improving health. It recognised the complicated connections between biology, lifestyles, environment and health care provision. It also provided the foundation that facilitated the exploration of the roles that government, societies and the individual have in maintaining good health for all (Lalonde 1974). On the back of the Lalonde Report, academics and researchers have studied and examined health promotion to identify its key concepts and common themes. This has led to the development and design of theoretical frameworks and models, providing those engaged in health promotion with effective knowledge and guidance on which to practice. However, as Nutbeam and Harris (2010) highlight, not all of these have been rigorously tested.

WHY USE MODELS AND APPROACHES IN HEALTH PROMOTION?

Health promotion as identified in Chapter 2 can be defined in many varied ways. There is no straightforward unity about the ideas that underpin health promotion or a single attempt to define what the principal goals of health promotion should be. Health promotion is neither neutral nor value free, and it cannot be. The main protagonists, including midwives, have differing views about the priorities and strategies that are influenced by their personal views of the concept (Cribb & Duncan 2002). These views are based on values, beliefs and experiences about health and health promotion developed with time and experience. The importance of these differing views becomes apparent when working in a team where values are shared and made explicit. It is essential that health promoters listen to each other so that they can work towards the same goals.

The development of unified models and approaches in health promotion and midwifery practice can therefore help us to communicate with each other more effectively and strengthen initiatives, which benefits everybody. The more sophisticated models and approaches will also allow for individual, holistic expression for both the midwife and the woman being cared for.

PRACTICE POINTS

- The use of health promotion models has not been swift in midwifery as in other health care professions.
- Midwives should be aware of the impact of their personal views and experiences.
- Differing views between midwives or health care teams can affect the ability to work towards a shared health goal with a woman.

Before reading the next part of the chapter on approaches in health promotion, think about the last client with whom you undertook health promotion, for example, one-to-one breastfeeding support in the postnatal period or discussion around the newborn heel prick test.

What approaches do you think you used in that health promotion conversation?

APPROACHES IN HEALTH PROMOTION

There is a plethora of approaches currently being used within health promotion. This is perhaps testimony to the speed with which the philosophy of health promotion is advancing, and the need for theorists to develop their own framework to understand and explain, in as simple terms as possible, the relationship between the theory and the practice of health promotion. Some have argued that this identifies the status of health promotion as a profession and as a field of study that is a relatively 'new kid on the block' (Cribb & Duncan 1999; Nutbeam & Harris 2010), while others have highlighted this rapid development of numerous approaches as a natural part of the topography of health promotion, which is large, loosely defined and under continuous development (Katz & Perberdy 2001; Scriven 2010). Some approaches are better known than others, often because they are more frequently quoted and used in health promotion practice. The health promotion approaches developed by Ewles and Simnett in 1985 fall into this criteria, along with the ease in which they can be applied to midwifery health promotion.

EWLES AND SIMNETT'S APPROACHES IN HEALTH PROMOTION

Ewles and Simnett, in 1985, developed a framework of five approaches to health promotion, which were further elaborated on in 1992 (Ewles & Simnett 2003; Scriven 2010) (Table 4.1). They are considered seminal pieces of work within nursing and midwifery health promotion literature and provide significant examples of mapping health promotion practice.

Alongside the approaches, Ewles and Simnett recognised that an intervention could be developed to improve health at the population level, the community level and the individual level. They were clear that there was no one single approach that was correct but the ideal would be a combination of them all:

In our view there is no 'right' aim for health promotion, and no one right approach or set of activities. We need to work out for ourselves, which aim and which activities we use, in accordance with our own professional code of conduct (if there is one), our own carefully considered needs and our own assessment of our clients' needs.

Ewles and Simnett (1992, 37)

These approaches identified by Ewles and Simnett are not without quandaries. They can be seen as rather idealistic and simple in their layout. They do not necessarily address the issue of values, attitudes and beliefs held by both the health promoter, in this case the midwife, and the woman and/or her family, which will have a significant impact on their use.

The authors themselves have identified that these approaches are not perfect and need to be questioned and challenged 'as part of a healthy debate on the theory and practice of

Table 4.1 Different approaches to health promotion

The medical approach

The concept here is based within the WHO definition of health. The clearly identified aim is that of being free from medically defined diseases, illnesses and disabilities. This approach involves active medical participation to prevent or improve ill health and reduce morbidity and premature mortality. The medical approach takes physical well-being as a marker on which to show success, with little or no reference to the psychological, social or economic aspects of the cause and effect of disease. It values preventative medical procedures, and evidence shows that this has been successful, lending itself to the measurement of success better than the other approaches in the form of such things as clinical trials and randomised control trials (Donaldson and Scally 2009). An element of paternalism (one person deciding what is best for another) is involved because compliance is necessary on the part of the client/patient.

There has been much debate in recent years on the suitability of the medical approach in normal pregnancy and childbirth (DoH 2001; RCM 2000; Sinclair & Stockdale 2011). However, this approach is still used within midwifery, for example, the screening for syphilis at booking and routine urinalysis and blood pressure checks for eclampsia and the heel prick test for newborns.

The behaviour change approach

This approach is probably the most familiar to a midwife. Here, the approach takes as its premise that an individual will, when faced with a behaviour that is impacting on her health, for example, poor diet or smoking, alter her poor behaviour for a healthier one. Most of the health service provisions worldwide are investing time and effort on this approach (Nutbeam & Harris 2010; Thompson 2014). It is cost-effective in terms of the outlay by governments and in terms of the savings made to the health service.

An element of paternalism can be argued as being visible in this approach, but compliance is necessary for behaviour change.

The educational approach

In its most traditional sense, the aim of this approach is that the educationalist, that is, the midwife, will give the facts and information, with as few personal values as possible. The recipient, that is, the woman, of this information is free to use it in whatever way she chooses – to continue with or abandon attitudes and behaviours as she wishes. The educationalist's responsibility is to raise issues. However, today this approach is seen very much as a two-directional approach, in that the midwife will provide information about a health issue and a woman will ask for information.

This approach is considered the first approach when engaging in health promotion (Thompson 2014; Upton & Thirlaway 2014). It has the capacity to reach a large number of people, and evidence shows that never before have so many people been so well informed about health and the development of illness and disease (Donaldson & Scally 2009; Thompson 2014). However, the midwife needs to be aware that health knowledge on its own will not change an unhealthy behaviour that would be far too simple. This approach should not be undertaken in isolation but in an environment where the woman's values and attitudes can be explored to help in her decision-making process.

The client-centred approach

This approach is also known as the empowerment approach and lies as a key ethos for health promotion in the Lalonde Report (Lalonde 1974). The aim of this approach is for the individual or community to take charge of their health and set their own goals to achieve that change. Here, the individual or community works in collaboration with the health promoter, who assumes in this instance the role of a facilitator (Piper 2005; Thompson 2014).

(Continued)

Table 4.1 *(Continued)* Different approaches to health promotion

The client-centred approach

Here, the woman decides her health issues and sets the agenda. This is considered to be a 'bottom-up' rather than a 'top-down' approach in which those in power and authority set the agenda. The woman is seen as an equal and the knowledge and skills that she brings to the interaction are valued. The theme of self-empowerment is pivotal. Available data show this approach to be a successful one (McLoughlin 2000; Donaldson & Scally 2009; Upton & Thirlaway 2014).

However, this approach does not provide 'quick wins'; it requires a steady long-term approach to ensure success. This can be troublesome when looking at the finances and services required to support the individual or community to achieve change. The midwife may also find herself at the mercy of health targets, causing her to revert to approaches that are more easily achieved and measured.

The societal change approach

This is the only approach by Ewles and Simnett that does not directly concern the individual. Society is seen as central to health in that changes need to be made on social and environmental fronts, making the 'healthier option' easier to achieve for most of the population. An example of this societal change within the United Kingdom can be seen in the current discussions about banning smoking in private cars which have children as passengers (UK Government 2014). This approach has had increasing credence within the United Kingdom which made local governments review the impact of the health of the communities they served when deciding their economic and social policies. This has been further strengthened with the move of some of the commissioning of health promotion services from the NHS to local authority control in England (see Chapter 1).

It is not without its problems, with some seeing it as an invasion of privacy and the development of a 'nanny' state (Donaldson & Scally 2009), with the potential to change depending on the party in power at the time.

health promotion' (Ewles & Simnett 2003, 46). However, the delineation of the approaches is clearly very useful in developing health promotion theory and helping midwives to understand these approaches as well as clarifying their aims and values when using them.

PRACTICE POINTS

- The five approaches by Ewles and Simnett provide examples of mapping in health promotion.
- It is usual to use several approaches in order to gain success.
- They might be identified as too simplistic and do not address issues such as values, attitude and beliefs, and their impact on health promotion.
- They have made inroads into the development of health promotion theory and facilitate challenge and debate in this area.

ACTIVITY

Reflect on the activity you were asked to do prior to reading the section on approaches in health promotion.

Look at the list of approaches you were asked to identify, and using the approaches of Ewles and Simnett identified above pinpoint what approach/approaches you used.

MODELS IN HEALTH PROMOTION

On scrutinising the available literature from various disciplines that use models, it soon becomes very apparent that many terms of reference are used loosely and interchangeably. Examples of such terms are models, theories, conceptual frameworks, approaches, paradigms, taxonomies and ideologies. Within this section, the term 'model' will be used unless an original author refers to his or her ideas by a different term.

A model is a single physical representation of a set of ideas, often diagrammatic, that provides assistance for our thinking and understanding of the underlying philosophical issues of both theory and practice. A model aims to be objective and gives shape to a theory and will either conform to a pattern or reveal a pattern. Within disciplines, such as health promotion and medicine, models are used equally in reference to theory and/or philosophy. However, in midwifery, the term model has, to a certain degree, been adopted to define the mode of care given to women, for example, one-to-one care or case loading.

The models by Downie et al. (1996) and Taylor (1990), and the midwifery-specific model by Piper (2005) will be explored.

DOWNIE ET AL. MODEL OF HEALTH PROMOTION

Developing earlier work by Tannahill (1985), Downie et al. (1996) designed a model that explored the issues surrounding positive health, life skills, self-esteem, participation and dimensions of health, choice and behaviour. The authors identified that:

> The modern approach uses a broad information base and sound educational principles, and recognises the importance of the sociopolitical factors in health and health related behaviours. It is a participatory model.
>
> **Downie et al. (1990, 48)**

Downie et al. (1996) developed this further and endorsed a model of health promotion, which maps out the various possible domains of health promotion.

Three areas were identified:

1. Health education
2. Health prevention
3. Health protection

These three areas frequently overlap (as shown in Figure 4.1), and within these overlapping circles lie the seven possible domains into which health promotion activities may fall.

HEALTH EDUCATION

This is defined as 'all influences that collectively determine knowledge, belief and behaviour related to the promotion, maintenance and restoration of health in individuals and communities' (Smith 1979; cited in Downie et al. 1996, 27). This includes incidental as well as intentional education, and Downie and his co-authors also acknowledge the two-way communication process of education, where teaching and learning can come from and to both the midwife and the woman.

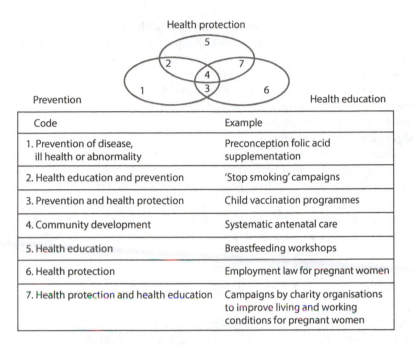

Code	Example
1. Prevention of disease, ill health or abnormality	Preconception folic acid supplementation
2. Health education and prevention	'Stop smoking' campaigns
3. Prevention and health protection	Child vaccination programmes
4. Community development	Systematic antenatal care
5. Health education	Breastfeeding workshops
6. Health protection	Employment law for pregnant women
7. Health protection and health education	Campaigns by charity organisations to improve living and working conditions for pregnant women

Figure 4.1 A model of health promotion. (Reproduced from Downie, R. S., et al. *Health promotion: Models and values* (2nd ed.). Oxford: Oxford University Press.)

HEALTH PREVENTION

This encompasses avoiding, or reducing, the risk of different forms of diseases, accidents and other forms of ill health. Within this sphere would fall the role of the midwife in contraception, sexual health and breast and cervical cancer screening. Downie et al. (1996, 51) went on to define the four aspects of prevention as:

1. Prevention of the onset or first manifestation of a disease process or some other first occurrence through risk reduction, for example, promotion of healthy eating and reducing the risk of Type 2 diabetes.
2. Prevention of the progression of a disease process or other unwanted state through early detection, for example, assessing mental health and the early detection of postnatal depression.
3. Prevention of avoidable complications of an irreversible, manifest disease, or some other unwanted state, for example, health promotion for Type 1 diabetes.
4. Prevention of the recurrence of an illness or other unwanted phenomenon, for example, an eating disorder such as anorexia nervosa.

HEALTH PROTECTION

This incorporates the environmental aspects safeguarding health by political, legislative and social control, which uses a number of mechanisms to achieve positive health by attempting to make the environment hazard free, such as regulation, policy and voluntary codes of practice.

In their model, Downie and his co-authors include both individual and community action in health promotion but exclude curative medicine. They acknowledge overlap in all of the three areas of health promotion that they describe and see community action as the ultimate in health promotion because it broadly incorporates health education, prevention of disease and health protection. This model offers the health promoter many permutations; however, it does not make explicit the principal political or social values in each approach. Nor does it reveal the authors' preferences as to the methods. Perhaps in not doing so, the model offers the health promoter a greater autonomy than other models and approaches do, and this makes it more appealing to midwives who value their professional autonomy.

The model by Downie et al. (1996) takes the perspective of health outcomes rather than the perspective of the health promoter which the Ewles and Simnett approaches tend to focus on. It encourages community-based health care and includes an educational approach which acknowledges all influences that lead to learning in clients and communities. Downie et al. do not include a medical approach in the curative sense (although they do acknowledge preventive medicine) and their model is distinct from the approaches developed by Ewles and Simnett in this respect. Nor does the model include the client-centred and behaviour change approaches of Ewles and Simnett. A possible weakness is that in attending to outcomes, or products of health promotion, the process by which success is measured is missing, and the model is being seen as a 'top-down' approach to health promotion, whereby the promotion is led by those in 'power', the government or the health care professional (Bowden 2006).

TAYLOR'S MODEL OF HEALTH PROMOTION

Taylor (1990) provides a more sociological model to what she refers to as health education, although on examining the breadth of her perspectives in today's terms, she could be said to be referring to health promotion. Her ideas take the form of a paradigm map as shown in Figure 4.2.

RADICAL HUMANISM

The perspective of radical humanism is that of self-development, particularly through personal growth, but with outreaching effects for community development. Removal from social regulation as far as possible is necessary and in some cases health professionals may be seen as social regulators, in that they are required to work strictly by rules and laws. A group of breastfeeding mothers running their own support group could be considered an example of the radical humanist approach.

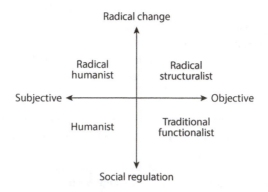

Figure 4.2 Perspectives of health education. (Reproduced from Taylor, V. 1990. *Health Education Journal* 49: 13–14.)

RADICAL STRUCTURALISM

Similar to radical humanism, radical structuralism is about moving towards change in the organisation of society, and indeed is more concerned with changing society to remove barriers to health than changing the individual. Radical structuralism may be exemplified by a nationwide campaign to encourage breastfeeding, including legislation to improve maternity leave, an advertising campaign among the public to improve attitudes towards breastfeeding and the provision of widespread facilities for breastfeeding mothers.

TRADITIONAL FUNCTIONALISM

The traditional functionalist may be seen as the professional who possesses the expertise that is passed on to the layperson, who can then progress to healthier behaviours. An example of traditional functionalism is the existence of antenatal classes aimed at promoting breastfeeding.

HUMANISM

The humanist is concerned with personal autonomy and empowering individuals through development of life skills. A network of NHS breastfeeding counsellors illustrates the humanist quarter of the map. Within Taylor's model, there are elements of medical and behaviour change approaches proposed by Ewles and Simnett, and radical structuralism has some common ground with the health protection approach of Downie et al., in that it is concerned with political and societal changes to improve the health of the public. However, overall, the sociological background to Taylor's paradigm is so different from the more clinical frameworks set by Ewles and Simnett and Downie et al. as to make these three systems impossible to compare (Bowden 2006).

This model acknowledges that the approaches within the model are top-down in nature, that is, they are in the control of those in power, for example, the DoH or the health care professional. Ideally, a bottom-up approach is preferred in health promotion. The bottom-up approach puts the health promotion within the control of the client/s and tends to have at its heart the client-centred, empowerment perspective. It is often seen as having more success and longevity as the approach is client driven and more likely to meet the needs of the client (Donaldson & Scally 2009).

PIPER'S MODEL OF HEALTH PROMOTION

The model of health promotion designed by Stuart Piper is unique in that it is one specifically made for the midwife. Based on the work by Beattie (1991), this is similar to that of Taylor as it encompasses both a top-down and a bottom-up approach. This model identifies the midwife as a behaviour change agent, an empowerment facilitator, a strategic health promotion practitioner and a collective empowerment facilitator (see Figure 4.3). The model is then split by an intersection, basically a power continuum between subjective knowledge and objective knowledge, with an axis dividing the individual and the population. This then creates four distinct models of health promotion.

> **ACTIVITY**
>
> Review the Piper's model (Figure 4.3). Think of which of the roles identified you fall into; i.e., are you a strategic practitioner or an empowerment facilitator. What skills did you use to achieve this role?

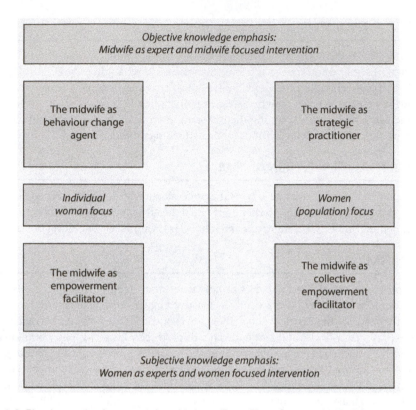

Figure 4.3 Piper's practice framework for midwives. (From Piper, Stewart. 2005. *British Journal of Midwifery* 13(5): 284–288.).

THE MIDWIFE AS A BEHAVIOUR CHANGE AGENT

This reflects a more traditional health promotion role of the midwife. The model places the midwife in a position of power and reflects a more medical and top-down approach to health promotion and can be applied to all three levels of health promotion (Table 4.2):

1. *Primary:* where health promotion is used to recognise or prevent the development of a health issue, for example, the mental health questions asked at the booking visit; they are asked of every woman.
2. *Secondary:* where health promotion is used to prevent/limit complications occurring from the health issue or recognising a vulnerable woman, for example, the mental health questions to identify a woman with previous postnatal depression.
3. *Tertiary:* where health promotion is used to optimise outcomes and limit complications when they occur.

The intended outcomes are healthy women and babies with no complications and are based on the assumption that women will make the right decisions about their health when given health promotion information. However, this is a little simplistic and does not necessarily acknowledge the factors that impact on changing behaviours (see Chapter 6).

Table 4.2 Midwife as a behaviour change agent

Aims	To encourage women to change unhealthy behaviours that may impact on their health either at the present time or sometime in the future
	Encourage compliance with treatments
	Attend the services they are referred to
Methods	Parent education classes, information giving
Impact	Increase the women's awareness, confirm the advice given and correct the unhealthy behaviour, increase uptake in the services offered
	Can been seen as paternalistic in its approach
	Issues around compliance, especially if unsuccessful
Outcome	A medically healthy mother and baby with no/minor complications
	Possible issues with guilt and stereotyping if outcome not achieved

Source: From Piper, Stewart. 2005. *British Journal of Midwifery* 13(5): 284–288.

THE MIDWIFE AS AN EMPOWERMENT FACILITATOR

This area of the model is in complete contrast to that identified above. This sees the midwife in the role of the facilitator, the aim of which is to assist a woman, or groups of women, achieve her identified health promotion needs (Table 4.3). This should be accomplished in a way that is non-hierarchical, non-coercive and empowering for the women. The midwife advocates for the woman, maximising the woman's opportunities for decision making and increasing self-esteem and confidence with regard to her health and health promotion.

This part of the model fits the current consumer culture within the NHS and the shift in the balance of power to the service user (Sturgeon 2014).

THE MIDWIFE AS THE STRATEGIC PRACTITIONER

This can be seen as taking the midwife outside her usual sphere of health promotion, which is usually undertaken with an individual woman or a small group of women (Table 4.4). However, with the development of the role of the consultant midwife with public health as a specialty, this part of Piper's model takes as its premise the wider issues involved in health and health promotion such as socio-economic inequalities, environmental improvements and legislations such as welfare provision and provision of maternity leave.

Table 4.3 The midwife as an empowerment facilitator

Aims	To act as an advocate and support women as they become empowered
Methods	Advocacy, informed choice and informed consent. Client-centred engagement within a non-hierarchical framework
Impact	The woman leads her own health agenda with support from the midwife. A more bottom-up approach with, possibly, better success and longevity
Outcome	Increase in confidence and self-esteem. Women feel in control with improved decision-making skills
	Strengthen coping strategies and make childbirth a more positive experience
	An approach more favoured by the WHO and the RCM

Source: From Piper, Stewart. 2005. *British Journal of Midwifery* 13(5): 284–288.

Table 4.4 The midwife as the strategic practitioner

Aims	Influencing policy development and health care provision within Public Health – within the job description of a consultant midwife with public health as a specialty
Methods	Lobbying, clinical audits and practice development
Impact	Organisational change, setting of professional/clinical standards at the national or local level
Outcome	Reduction in women and children's premature mortality and morbidity at national and local levels
	Reduction in the negative factors that impact on the health of a community or population
	Midwifery input at a strategic level and also at the development and pressure stage when supporting professional body and/or aligning with a pressure group

Source: From Piper, Stewart. 2005. *British Journal of Midwifery* 13(5): 284–288.

It is fair to say that not all midwives will engage with this part of the model on a regular basis unless their role indicates a strategic public health focus. However, every midwife has the ability to be involved in supporting/changing current public health policies and strategies. This can be accomplished either by lobbying the power holders via their professional organisations, for example, the Royal College of Midwives, or by associating themselves with pressures groups, such as the National Childbirth Trust, that aim to address issues such as poverty and women, breastfeeding and employment.

THE MIDWIFE AS COLLECTIVE EMPOWERMENT FACILITATOR

This can be seen as in direct opposition to the previous role as a strategic practitioner (Table 4.5). Here, the midwife will work in a more bottom-up approach, working with a collective group of women in response to their expressed health needs. The midwife in this role is able to encourage and support the development of social networks and improve social capital for all women, particularly those who are most vulnerable, for example, young single mothers or women whose first language is not English (Thompson 2014).

Table 4.5 The midwife as collective empowerment facilitator

Aims	Facilitating the building of social networks and social capital
	Supporting communal action by women with regard to 'their' expressed health needs
Methods	Public health consultation and intervention development led by women. A bottom-up approach with all its usual benefits of greater success and longevity
Impact	Developing and strengthening of social networks, especially for those women from the most vulnerable areas of society. Develop service user involvement and assist in 'opening doors' to power holders. Building self-confidence, self-esteem and empowerment
Outcome	Increased collective empowerment
	Social capital strengthened and developing the model to the linking stage
	A more fruitful project developed with a stronger chance of success and a longer time frame

Source: From Piper, Stewart. 2005. *British Journal of Midwifery* 13(5): 284–288.

This chapter has explored some of the available approaches and models used in the practice of midwifery. The examples given are common to midwives. Midwives can use these approaches to understand individuals' different outlooks and work towards a minimum standard of high-quality health promotion practice.

SUMMARY OF KEY POINTS

- Health promotion models and approaches provide a spur to examine and re-examine practice and its underlying assumptions.
- The plethora of models and approaches currently in use is often criticised for being perplexing and ineffectual.
- Creators of models and approaches must aim, as far as possible, to design very broad frameworks that acknowledge the political dimension of health care administration, as well as recognise the day-to-day practicalities for health promoters working with individuals in the community.
- Effective models and approaches serve to state the relationship between the theory and practice of health promotion. There is a moral requirement for the midwife to be clear about this relationship because, where an attempt is made to change people's behaviour, the ethical dimensions of such professional practice can be immense.
- Models and approaches in health promotion can help us to communicate more effectively by concentrating discussion on shared values and beliefs relevant to professional practice, and putting these into a framework that explicitly states acceptable standards of practice, to both the midwife and the women in her care.
- The application of health promotion models and approaches to some aspects of midwifery practice can offer a means by which agreed evidence-based frameworks standardise good practice.
- The study and application of various health promotion models and approaches to midwifery practice can help us understand different outlooks and develop innovative strategies suited to particular communities.

REFERENCES

Beattie, Alan. 1991. Knowledge and control in health promotion: A test case for social policy and social theory. In *The sociology of health service*, edited by Gabe, Jonathon, Calnan Michael and Bury Michael. New York: Routledge.

Bowden, Jan. 2006. Using health promotion models and approaches in midwifery. In *Health promotion in midwifery principles and practice* (2nd ed.), edited by Bowden, Jan and Vicky Manning. Malta: Hodder Arnold.

Cribb, Alan & Peter Duncan. 2002. *Health promotion and professional ethics*. London: Blackwell Science.

DoH (Department of Health). 2001. *Making a difference: the nursing, midwifery and health visiting contribution, the midwifery action plan*. London: The Stationary Office.

DoH (Department of Health). 2013. *Midwifery public health contribution to compassion in practice through maximising wellbeing and improving health in women, babies and families*. https://www.gov.uk/government/uploads/system/uploads/attachment_data/file/208824/Midwifery_strategy_visual_B.pdf

Donaldson, Liam J. & Gabriel Scally. 2009. *Donaldson's essential public health* (3rd ed.). Cornwall: Routledge.

Downie, R. S., Carol E. Fyfe & Andrew Tannahill. 1990. *Health promotion: Models and values.* Oxford: Oxford Medical Publications.

Downie, R. S., Carol Tannahill & Andrew Tannahill. 1996. *Health promotion: Models and values* (2nd ed.). Oxford: Oxford University Press.

Ewles, Linda & Ina Simnett. 1985. *Promoting health: A practical guide.* London: Baillière Tindall.

Ewles, Linda & Ina Simnett. 1992. *Promoting health: A practical guide* (2nd ed.). London: Baillière Tindall.

Ewles, Linda & Ina Simnett. 2003. *Promoting health: A practical guide* (5th ed.). London: Scutari Press.

Katz, Jeanne & Alyson Perberdy. 2001. *Promoting health knowledge and practice* (2nd ed.). London: Palgrave Macmillan.

Lalonde, Marc. 1974. *A new perspective on the health of Canadians.* Ottawa: Ministry of National Health and Welfare.

McLoughlin, Aileen. 2000. Empowerment and childbirth. In *Community health promotion challenges for practice*, edited by Kerr, J., 65–81. London: Baillière Tindall.

Nutbeam, Don & Elizabeth Harris. 2010. *Theory in a nutshell* (3rd ed.). North Ryde, NSW: McGraw Hill Education.

Piper, Stewart. 2005. Health promotion a practice framework for midwives. *British Journal of Midwifery* 13(5): 284–288.

RCM (Royal College of Midwives). 2000. *The midwife's role in public health.* Position Paper No. 24. London: RCM.

Scriven, Angela. 2010. *Ewles and Simnett's promoting health: A practical guide* (6th ed.). London: Bailliere Tindall.

Sinclair, Marlene & Janine Stockdale. 2011. *Achieving optimal birth using salutogenesis in routine Antenatal Education.* https://www.rcm.org.uk/learning-and-career/learning-and-research/ebm-articles/achieving-optimal-birth-using-salutogenesis

Sturgeon, David. 2014. The business of the NHS: the rise and rise of consumer culture and commodification in the provision of health care services. *Critical Social Policy* 34(3): 405–416.

Tannahill, Andrew. 1985. What is health promotion? *Health Education Journal* 44: 167–168.

Taylor, Vicki. 1990. Health education – A theoretical mapping. *Health Education Journal* 49: 13–14.

Thompson, Susan R. 2014. Approaches and models used in health promotion. In *The essential guide to public health and health promotion*, edited by Thompson, Susan R., Croydon: Routledge.

UK Government. 2014. *Smoking in private vehicles carrying children-consultation on proposed regulations to be made under the Children and Families Act 2014.* London: DoH. https://www.gov.uk/government/uploads/system/uploads/attachment_data/file/329885/Smoking in_cars_carrying_children.pdf

Upton, Dominic & Katie Thirlaway. 2014. *Promoting health behaviour: A practical guide* (2nd ed.). Oxford: Routledge.

FURTHER READING

Fahey, Jenifer O. & Edmond Shenassa. 2013. Understanding and meeting the needs of women in the postpartum period: The perinatal maternal health promotion model. *Journal of midwifery and Women's Health* 56: 613–621.

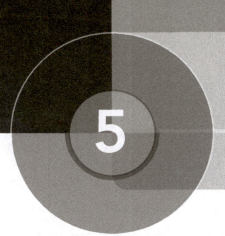

Evaluation in health promotion

5

JAN BOWDEN

INTRODUCTION

The drive to evaluate all aspects of health to ensure a strong evidence base and high-quality care is a key component of modern day health care services. Within the National Health Service (NHS), that drive to evaluate health extends to public health and health promotion, and rightly so. Considering the junior status of health promotion as a profession and field of study, there is added impetus for evaluation to take place to prove its worth. However, evaluation in health promotion is not as straightforward as it seems. The waters are often muddied by a combination of factors, such as the long timescale of projects, the numerous kinds of activities involved in a health-promoting project and the many stakeholders working in partnership, all of whom may have their own different objectives. Within health, the gold standard for evaluating success is the randomised control trial (RCT). However, this adds a further complication to evaluating health promotion as health promotion does not fit neatly into the RCT model. In this chapter, the meaning of evaluation, for whom it is done and why it is undertaken, as well as focusing on the process and challenges of evaluating a health promotion activity will be examined.

BACKGROUND

In the early years of the NHS, there were no formal comprehensive processes by which to evaluate health care. It was naturally and perhaps simplistically thought that every health care practitioner would work to the highest professional standard and provide a uniform level of high-quality care to the benefit of their patients (Donaldson & Scally 2009). This, plus the complex nature of defining and measuring quality in health care, left the NHS without a formal and rigorous evaluation framework for most of its existence.

In the 1980s and 1990s, a series of highly publicised events altered this thinking forever. These included the cases of Beverley Allitt (a children's nurse) and Harold Shipman (a general practitioner) – both convicted of murdering patients in their care and scandals at the Bristol Royal Infirmary's Children's Cardiac Surgery Department and the Alder Hey Children's Hospital in Liverpool (Table 5.1). These scandals led to a radical overhaul of the NHS and the development of formal evaluation frameworks (Donaldson & Scally 2009).

Within England, this led to the formation of the Care Quality Commission (CQC) in 2009, an independent regulator for health and social care. Their main aim is to monitor, inspect and regulate services to ensure that they meet the agreed fundamental standards of quality and safety in health care, and this includes public health.

PRACTICE POINT

Historically, evaluation in all aspects of health care was not considered necessary. Recent NHS scandals have led to the formation of the CQC where there is an agreed level of quality and safety in public health and health promotion as well as other aspects of health care.

Table 5.1 NHS scandals

Beverley Allitt	Employed as a nurse on a children's ward: She killed three children and further grievously harmed six others. The subsequent Clothier Inquiry and Report (1993) laid out a framework for the evaluation of near miss and poor outcome care. It also set in place 12 safeguarding points for children while in hospital. From then on, all wishing to commence health care training needed occupational health and criminal record clearance first.
Harold Shipman	Employed as a general practitioner: he was convicted of murdering 15 patients, although the subsequent Shipman Report (2005) indicated that it may have been as many as 250. The Shipman Inquiry and Report indicated major flaws in the processes of registering deaths and prescription of medications.
	Services Users were now 'employed' by the General Medical Council (GMC) after the report added that the GMC appeared to look after the interests of doctors and not patients.
Children's Cardiac Surgery Unit, Bristol Royal Infirmary	In the late 1990s, 29 babies died undergoing heart surgery. Parents asked questions for which answers were not forthcoming and following intense parent and media pressure the Kennedy Inquiry was set up. The report, published in 2001, identified a lack of performance monitoring, a lax approach to clinical safety and secrecy about surgeons' performances.
	The outcome of the report led to the development of the commission of health improvement and subsequently the setting up of the CQC.
	The inquiry also led to a further scandal with regard to the storage of human tissue, bodies and whole bodies – The Alder Hey Organ Scandal.
Alder Hey Children's Hospital Liverpool	At the Alder Hey Children's Hospital in Liverpool, the tissues and body parts of some 850 infants were uncovered along with 1,500 foetuses/babies that had been miscarried, aborted or stillborn.
	The Redfern Inquiry and Report (2001) uncovered 104,000 samples of tissue, body parts or whole bodies of miscarried and aborted foetuses or stillborn infants in 210 NHS facilities.
	The outcomes were to provide a framework evaluating the coroner's system within the United Kingdom and the development of the Human Tissue Act 2004.

WHAT IS EVALUATION AND WHY DO IT?

The *Oxford Dictionary of English* (Stevenson & Soanes 2010) defines evaluation as 'the process of assessing and appraising'. It is a process in which we are involved daily both as professionals and as individuals. We are involved in that process whenever we reflect upon our actions and either alter or continue them (Bowden 2006).

Within health promotion, the simplest purpose of evaluation is to assess if the activity achieved what it set out to. In today's health care climate of ensuring public funds are used sensibly and to good effect, this simple view may be good enough. However, to show success in health promotion, the World Health Organization (WHO) clearly identifies that evaluation has a crucial role in capacity building and improving the abilities of 'individuals, communities, organisations and governments to address important health issues' (Naidoo & Wills 2009, 9).

Evaluation must be completed during the planning cycle of an intervention as well as after the intervention has been completed. It must look at what worked or not, and if it worked, in what conditions and to what benefit to the population targeted within the intervention (Green et al. 2015). An ethical evaluation must also be undertaken to ensure no harm has been done (McFarlane 2014; Naidoo & Wills 2009).

Evaluation is guided by two essential principles: identifying and ranking the criteria (value and aims), and gathering data and information that will make it possible to measure to what degree these criteria are being, or have been, met. There are different criteria that can be used when a health promotion activity is being judged on its worth.

EFFECTIVENESS

This evaluation explores whether the activity has accomplished what it set out to do and to what extent the aims and objectives were met. It is essential to realise that, although in practice the terms 'aims' and 'objectives' are used interchangeably, it is vital to know that there is an important difference. Aims tend to be general and may be divided into particular objectives. Objectives contribute to the aims and are the 'nuts and bolts' of the planned project. Both are vital to the evaluation process. Poor identification of aims and objectives within a project will make evaluation impossible (Bauman & Nutbeam 2012; Naidoo & Wills 2009).

APPROPRIATENESS

This is assessing the relevance of the intervention to the needs. The perception of needs differs depending on who is defining them: the individual/group requiring the health promotion project or the health care professionals who develop the project (Bradshaw 1972; Scriven 2010).

ACCEPTABILITY

This assesses whether the project is being carried out in a sensitive way. This is sometimes overlooked and a health promotion project may have ethical and moral values that affect its use either in the community for which it was intended or when the project is used in another community. For example, a considerable quantity of the initial health education information on HIV and AIDS in the 1980s in the United Kingdom portrayed the genesis of HIV firmly in Africa and the developing world. This promoted racist typecasting and caused immense distress to many black and ethnic minority communities which impacted on the uptake of testing and compliance with treatment (Katz & Perberdy 2001; Naidoo & Wills 2009).

EFFICIENCY

This considers whether time, finances and resources have been well spent given the benefits of the project. In recent years, the ratio of costs to benefits has increased in importance. Assessment needs to involve *cost-effectiveness analysis* (the comparison of the financial costs of similar projects) and *cost–benefits analysis* (the comparison of the cost of the project with the financial benefits, resulting from achieving the goal) (Bauman & Nutbeam 2012; Katz & Perberdy 2001).

EQUITY

This measures how accessible a project is. It goes beyond the identification of the numbers that a project reaches. Equity evaluates the social composition that the project has reached. Some have stated that health promotion should go all out for equity over equality by not always aiming for equal access but intentionally aiming at those in socially excluded groups (Edelman et al. 2014; Fredriksen-Goldsen et al. 2014; McFarlane 2014; Trinh-Shevrin et al. 2015).

For an evaluation to be successful, it must be built into the health promotion project from the planning stage and be ongoing and explicit at all times during the lifetime of that project. The complexity comes in when this process of evaluation becomes formalised and with it the potential for it to become 'public', in that it is open to inspection and criticism by others (Bauman & Nutbeam 2012). A further difficulty arises in the fact that health promotion can be an ambiguous affair with no assurances that specific effects will follow particular inputs (Bauman & Nutbeam 2012).

> **ACTIVITY**
>
> Identify why evaluation is an essential element of health promotion: Compare your list with Figure 5.1.

So why evaluate? Evaluation provides the best sort of feedback on which to develop health promotion projects. If the responses of users of the service are considered as essential to achieving aims, their opinions and comments can serve only to help the health promoter – in this case the midwife – to develop health promotional work.

In recent years, there has been much debate about the reasons for the development of this evaluation culture within health. Some argue that it has a political and ideological function to legitimise the actions of governments (Bauman & Nutbeam 2012; Scriven 2010). Irrespective of this debate, there are many possible reasons about why evaluation is required within health promotion, and Figure 5.1 identifies possible reasons for evaluation. It is important to stress that Figure 5.1 offers only some suggestions and is not finite, and you may well be able to add more.

Evaluation is undertaken for many reasons, as seen in Figure 5.1, and from this it can be argued that there are several groups and individuals for whom evaluation is beneficial and necessary. Ideally, evaluation is best undertaken in a way that will allow each of the different stakeholders involved in the project to see if their aims and objectives have been met.

FINANCIAL BACKERS

Those providing the financial backing for the project may want the evaluation to show the efficiency of the project and its cost-effectiveness. This would allow them to see if their money

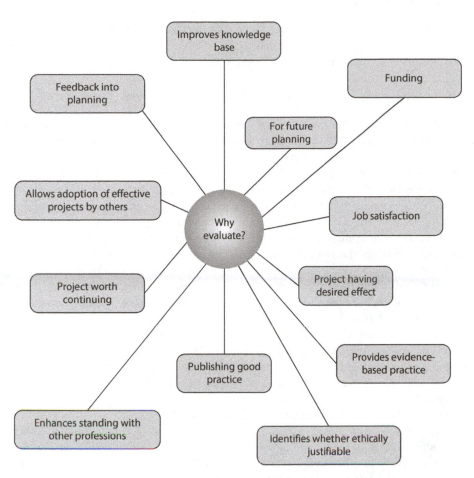

Figure 5.1 Why evaluate? Who is it for and who should do it? (Adapted from Katz, Jeanne and Alyson Perberdy. 2001. *Promoting health knowledge and practice* (2nd ed.). London: Palgrave Macmillan.)

has been well spent during the course of the project and to assess whether it requires continued longer-term funding or a possible reduction in funding.

HEALTH PROMOTERS

The health promoters may want the evaluation to show that their objectives have been met and that the project identified an acceptable way of working with the clients/community groups. They may also use it to 'push' for the project to be rolled out to other communities within their trust areas or further afield. Health promotion managers may look upon evaluation as a way to assess performance and productivity (Bauman & Nutbeam 2012; Green et al. 2015).

SERVICE USERS

The users may use the evaluation as a way of signifying some degree of control over health-related aspects of their lives and of gaining ownership of the project. A lack of service user

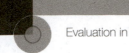

evaluation may show a lack of engagement with the target population on the part of the health care professionals, which could have a potentially negative impact on the project in terms of success, longevity and funding (Bauman & Nutbeam 2012; Thompson et al. 2014).

POLICY MAKERS

Finally, the policy makers, for example, local government, national government or international organisations, such as the WHO, may use the evaluation to justify their policies and strategies for health (Katz & Perberdy 2001; Scriven 2010).

After identifying for whom the evaluation may be required, it is essential to examine who is going to evaluate the project and the impact it can have on the evaluation process. Most evaluation processes are undertaken internally, and this is an accepted practice within health promotion. Internal evaluation allows for a more continuous process of evaluation to take place, because those evaluating are always available. It is seen as non-threatening; so all stakeholders are truthful about the project. However, internal evaluation does have its problems. Evidence suggests that evaluation does not always fully evaluate a project due to issues such as lack of time and inexperience of the person undertaking the evaluation, and the findings are less likely to be made 'public', that is, open for inspection (Bauman & Nutbeam 2012; Thompson et al. 2014).

This means that poor projects are not always properly evaluated, which in turn means that a valuable learning experience is lost. Newburn (2001) identified the concept of pseudo-evaluation and identified five types (Figure 5.2). Equally, good projects are not brought to closer or wider attention and the knowledge and practice base are not enhanced (Bauman & Nutbeam 2012).

External evaluation is seen as more beneficial because it tends to be carried out by individuals who are well-versed in the practice of evaluation, for example, UK Breastfeeding Initiative, CQC. It also tends to be more thorough with all stakeholders being asked their viewpoints. However, it is likely to suffer from issues associated with the evaluators being seen as outsiders and the stakeholders perhaps putting on a 'united front' and may also be more expensive (Bauman & Nutbeam 2012; Valente 2002). Table 5.2 attempts to identify more of the advantages and disadvantages of internal and external evaluation. Irrespective of whether evaluation is internal or external, 'a warts and all' approach to evaluation must be considered within health promotion to gain vital learning experience from both good and not so good health promotion projects (Bauman & Nutbeam 2012; McQueen 2002).

Types	Meaning
Eyewash	The evaluation focus is on the surface/outward appearance of the project only.
Whitewash	The aim of the evaluation here is to completely cover up an intervention's failure.
Submarine	The evaluation is used by the power holders, for example the government, to undermine the intervention.
Posture	This is a tick box exercise; evaluation is undertaken as it is expected but there is little to no intention to use the findings in any way.
Postponement	This is where the evaluation is sidestepped as a means of avoiding the outcomes to be identified and addressed.

Figure 5.2 Pseudo-evaluation. (Adapted from Newburn, T. 2001. *Children and Society* 15(1): 5–13.)

Table 5.2 Advantages and disadvantages of internal and external evaluation

Internal evaluation	External evaluation
Knows background of project	Fresh viewpoint
Known and therefore accepted more readily	More objective
Easier to establish networks of communication	No allegiance to the project
Knowledge about the community for which the project is intended and therefore awareness of any issues	Unbiased attitude
Usually has some idea of weaknesses and strengths of the project	More likely to have research expertise
Financially beneficial as usually cheaper	More likely to have experience in evaluation
Too involved in the project	More likely to be made 'public'
Biased towards proving the success of the project	More likely to be thorough
Less likely to have research expertise	More likely to access the views of all the stakeholders including the users
Less likely to have experience in evaluation	More likely that all the stakeholders will receive the evaluation report
Time constraints prevent a thorough evaluation	Less accepted as seen as outsiders
Users may not be so honest with their evaluation because they know the evaluator	Networks of communication more difficult to establish
	More expensive than internal evaluation
	Lacks knowledge about the project and the community for whom it is intended
	Stakeholders may portray a 'united front' for the external evaluation

Source: Adapted from Naidoo, Jennie and Jane Wills. 2009. *Health promotion foundations for practice* (3rd ed.). London: Baillière Tindall; Katz, Jeanne and Alyson Perberdy. 2001. *Promoting health knowledge and practice* (2nd ed.). London: Palgrave Macmillan.

USER EVALUATION

Health promotion is a complex process of intervention in an individual's or community's life at varying levels. Therefore, it must be justified and evaluated by the individual and community at whom it is aimed, allowing them to have their story heard. In recent years, the Department of Health (DoH), the NHS Executive and various research charities and funding bodies have emphasised the importance of user involvement (DoH 2010, 2014). However, have users been included merely to satisfy regulations from the DoH and other funding bodies or is there a genuine conviction that their views are valuable to the evaluation process? By being used actively within the evaluation process, users will, similar to external evaluation, provide a fresh perspective on the health promotion project. It will provide ownership of the project and allow the user to shape and guide the project and alter its organisational culture and structure (Farr 2012). Active user evaluation will add value and legitimacy to a project and potentially generate knowledge that could increase its significance and acceptance to other user groups (Farr 2012).

If users are given only a token involvement in evaluation, their role will be different, and it is less likely that their story will be fully told, leaving them frustrated at not being heard or being allowed to be heard. Ownership of the project will be with the 'experts', and the organisational culture and structure will remain firmly within a professional remit. This, in turn, may affect the validity of the project and its sustainability within the community at which it is aimed at (Beresford 2002).

To facilitate user involvement within the project and the evaluation process, consideration must be given to include users from the inception of the project and for them to undertake some training about their role within the project. Training for professionals must also be considered to allow them to understand lay perspectives and to work effectively with users in different situations (Smith et al. 2008; Staniszewska et al. 2012).

HOW BEST TO EVALUATE SUCCESS?

As identified earlier, evaluation in health promotion helps build a foundation of research and enquiry that allows health promotion to demonstrate its success in meeting its aims and objectives. It allows effective health promotion practices to be identified and used by others. It also allows these health promotion practices to be further developed and enhanced. This evidence-based practice, which is defined as 'the conscientious, explicit and judicious use of current evidence in making decisions about the care of the individual patient' (Sackett et al. 1996, 42), has already been established in other areas of health, such as midwifery, nursing and medicine, where RCTs have been used to identify the most effective treatment and care for the most number of people. However, the RCT is not a tool that can be neatly fitted into health promotion. It is problematic for the following reasons:

- It is impossible to isolate the effect of a health promotion project owing to the multiplicity of factors involved.
- A project's success is in some part due to its spread to other groups beyond the target group.
- The length of time that many projects take.
- The number of stakeholders, each with their own aims, objectives and viewpoints which they want to achieve.
- The awareness of health promoters of the social and cultural context in which they carry out their work.

PRACTICE POINTS

- The RCT approach is not applicable when evaluating health promotion interventions.
- However, it does share the RCT requirement that the aims and objectives of a project must be SMART:
  - Specific
  - Measurable
  - Achievable
  - Relevant
  - Timed

Therefore, a more social science approach to evaluation suits health promotion. It would allow for a much broader use of different methodologies from both the quantitative and the qualitative approaches. The different stakeholders and their individual viewpoints would also be taken into account, making the evaluation pluralistic (Green et al. 2015). This of course may lead to criticisms that there is a lack of methodological rigour and that the pluralistic approach is complex and lacks clarity (Bauman & Nutbeam 2012).

The difficulties in evaluating health promotion led Nutbeam and his colleagues to develop a six-stage model demonstrating an evaluation hierarchy which identifies how best to evaluate success in health promotion (Bauman & Nutbeam 2012; Nutbeam & Harris 2010). These stages are:

1. *Problem definition:* This draws upon the data used to identify the health issue which the health promotion project has to improve. This information relies on epidemiological data and needs appraisal to define the problem, the factors influential to the problem and the scope for change.

2. *Solution generation:* This explores the behavioural and social research to expand the knowledge of the targeted population and the breadth of personal, social, environmental and organisational features that may need to be adapted to form the basis for the project. It will also help to explain and predict change in those features as well as clarify the potential content and approaches for the intervention. Stages 1 and 2 will help with the success and sustainability of the project developed.

3. *Testing innovation:* This stage incorporates three areas that need to be considered and judged:

   a. *Process evaluation:* This is concerned with the assessment of the implementation and maintenance of the activity. Sometimes called formative or illuminative evaluation, it also focuses on the perception and responses of the participants to the health promotion project (Bauman & Nutbeam 2012). Moreover, it attempts to identify the factors that have hindered the project, as well as ascertain those that have supported it. Process evaluation is a useful mechanism to gauge the acceptability as well as the appropriateness and equity of a health promotion project. Interviews, diaries and observations are some of the 'soft' qualitative methods that process evaluation uses to gain details about a project. However, the use of qualitative evaluation methods is often dismissed because they lack the 'scientific' credibility of the 'hard' quantitative evaluation approaches and are often criticised for being unrepresentative (Naidoo & Wills 2009).

   b. *Impact evaluation:* The evaluation of a health promotion project must include identification of the effects of the project. The easiest and therefore the most popular way to undertake this is by assessing the immediate effect that the activity has on the recipients' knowledge, attitudes, behaviour and short-term health change (Scriven 2010). The midwife often collects these data at the time of finishing the activity or shortly thereafter. Data collected tend to be of a quantitative nature, with all the usual criticisms.

   c. *Outcome evaluation:* This is considered the real test of whether the initial aims and objectives have been achieved. Outcome evaluation is more difficult and complex because it looks at evaluating the longer-term impact of the health promotion project. This may mean the midwife having to contact clients a year after the project has finished. However, despite these issues, outcome evaluation tends to be much preferred. It attempts to evaluate changes that have stood the test of time. This evaluation often uses control groups and data that are expressed numerically, which increases its credibility because it is seen as more accurate and more like the quantitative approach (Bauman & Nutbeam 2012).

4. *Intervention demonstration:* This stage changes emphasis slightly from the assessment of process, impact and outcome, and looks more closely at the conditions for success or lack of thereof. It will assess the achievement of the project under ideal circumstances and then look at whether the desired outcomes of the project can be achieved in a more 'real' environment. This is particularly relevant to the communities that are targeted for the project, as well as the health promoters, because it looks at the achievability of the project in everyday life. It will also take into account the unpredictable facets of health promotion practice and identify what basics need to be in place for it to be a success.

5. *Intervention dissemination:* In this fifth stage, the emphasis is further moved to look at ways in which successfully evaluated projects can be disseminated. This dissemination would advance evidence-based practice by investigating what others have done and, through use of their experiences, aid other health promotion projects. Understanding how individuals and communities adopt and maintain a healthier lifestyle and what support is needed to assist this, determining what basics need to be in place to facilitate the success of a project as well as highlighting what needs to be done, by whom, to what criterion and to what cost would be some of the benefits of intervention dissemination. However, it is rarely undertaken.

6. *Programme management:* In the final stage, evaluation is tasked with assessing the maintenance of the project. Evaluation will incorporate the monitoring of the project's delivery in relation to its optimal conditions for success and, of course, value for money. The project's sustainability and longevity will be continuously evaluated.

LEARNING ACTIVITY

Before reading the next section, consider: What could impact on the results of a health promotion project?

CHALLENGES TO EVALUATION IN HEALTH PROMOTION

A midwife will face many issues when evaluating the midwife's role within health promotion or a health promotion project based or led by midwifery. Naidoo and Wills (2009) identified the following challenges that will be faced by the health professional – in this case the midwife – when involved in health promotion evaluation:

- What needs to be measured?
- Are the effects entirely the result of the health promotion project?
- When to evaluate?
- What signifies success in a project?
- Is the effort worth it?
- What ethical issues are related to evaluation?

WHAT NEEDS TO BE MEASURED?

The essential tenet has to be measurement of the objectives identified in the planning stage of the health promotion project. This appears to be reasonably straightforward; however, on reviewing the literature, the midwife may find numerous published studies that breach this simple golden rule (Naidoo & Wills 2009; Seedhouse 2003). The biggest problem appears to be a lack of consensus between the stakeholders about the suitable measures; for example, trying to measure the involvement of a community in relation to breastfeeding or showing an increase in breastfeeding rates as a result of the development of breastfeeding workshops is not easy because of the other factors that may be involved, for example, influence of peers, family and media.

ARE THE EFFECTS ENTIRELY THE RESULT OF THE HEALTH PROMOTION PROJECT?

Health promotion does not provide a 'quick win' to improving health. The constantly changing situation makes it very difficult to be confident that the results of a health promotion project are solely the result of the input of that project (Seedhouse 2003). Health promotion is a long-term process and, during that period of time, health-related knowledge, attitudes and behaviours can change both for the health promoter and the targeted population. Society also continually reacts to varying factors; so the success of a health promotion project may be caused more by societal change than the actual project (Naidoo & Wills 2009); for example, the success of smoking cessation workshops for pregnant women who smoke may not be the result of the workshops themselves so much as society's changing views on smoking. A project's success is also in some part the result of its spread to other groups beyond the target population. It would be very difficult to prevent the health promotion project 'seeping out' beyond its target population (Naidoo and Wills 2009).

WHEN TO EVALUATE?

As a result of the process of health promotion, a project may have different outcomes at different times in its lifetime. Timing is vital when evaluating the success of a health promotion project, for example, a breastfeeding promotion project may have the following outcomes (Naidoo & Wills 2009):

- Improvement in women's knowledge of breastfeeding.
- Increase in numbers of women attending breastfeeding workshops.
- Increase in local (and perhaps national) media coverage on breastfeeding.
- Persuasion of local restaurants, cafes and shops to advertise that women may breastfeed within their environs.
- Encouragement of various organisations to adopt pro-breastfeeding measures, that is, local employers.
- Reduction in the number of babies admitted to hospital with formula feed–related gastroenteritis.

Each of these outcomes will need to be evaluated at different times to be able to prove the project's success or indeed identify its failure. However, there is no clear guidance to assist with the solution to this timing issue, and health promoters tend to work on their own previous experience or the experience of other projects as to when to evaluate. For example, when working through the evaluation of the above-mentioned breastfeeding promotion project, the midwife may consider the following:

- An immediate evaluation of the project to ascertain the improvement in women's knowledge of breastfeeding.

- An interim evaluation at 3–6 months to identify the outcomes regarding the numbers of women attending the breastfeeding workshops and to assess whether there is an increase in media coverage, local or national.
- A longer-term evaluation (maybe as long as 5 years) may be needed to assess if local businesses are adopting more pro-breastfeeding measures, café and shops are advertising breastfeeding-friendly status and if there is a reduction in the number of babies admitted to hospital with formula feed–related gastroenteritis.

This raises the issue of whether the success of the project is the result of the project alone or of changes within the community or society.

> **PRACTICE POINTS**
>
> - There are many challenges that can affect the outcome of a health promotion project, such as when to plan evaluation to collect appropriate data, the impact of peers and family.
> - Midwives need to be aware of these as many are outside the influence of a midwife, for example, the media.

WHAT SIGNIFIES SUCCESS IN A PROJECT?

Investigation of what others have done and the use of their experiences to aid other health promotion projects is one way of proving effectiveness. Effectiveness reviews assist health promotion in two ways: first by evaluating the quality of the research and second the quality of the health promotion project (Bauman and Nutbeam 2012). They also identify a means by which a foundation of knowledge is cultivated to pinpoint what the reasonable expectations of a successful project are. This in itself is problematical on several counts:

1. Health promotion's aim of changing health knowledge, behaviours and attitudes on many different levels over a sometimes lengthy time period. It therefore requires a multi-pronged evaluation process that is fraught with difficulties.
2. The preferred 'gold standard' of an RCT does not fit well in health promotion where feelings, behaviours, attitudes and changes to these are not easily expressed numerically.
3. Effectiveness reviews are the least common research found in the health promotion literature, partly due to a lack of interest in this area of research and partly due to the limited number of projects that have reached a stage of development that allows an effectiveness review to be undertaken (Bauman & Nutbeam 2012; Glasgow et al. 2003).

IS IT WORTH THE EFFORT?

Appraising the value of one's work is an essential component of being a reflective practitioner. However, in light of all the difficulties that evaluation in health promotion faces, a decision to undertake a more formal evaluation of that work and making it 'public' is not so easy. The dilemma of what to measure, how to measure, when to measure and what constitutes success is faced by all health promoters who undertake evaluation of their projects. For a midwife, measuring her own effectiveness in delivering a small-scale health-promoting project, reliability and validity are of little consequence. However, for larger project evaluation, these concepts must be addressed to make sure that the results obtained are genuine.

It is worth the effort, if the evaluation is built into the health promotion project from the planning stage and is ongoing and explicit at all times during the lifetime of that project. Also, it is worthwhile, if the evaluation is explicated and fed back into the project and to all those involved.

WHAT ETHICAL ISSUES ARE RELATED TO EVALUATION?

There are a number of ethical issues that deserve consideration. The first is whose interests does the evaluation serve? The politics of vested interests in choosing an evaluation technique and the issue of who receives the findings, and what they do with them, are very much pertinent when evaluating a health promotion project. Evaluation can be time-consuming for those involved and frustrating if they do not see any change in spite of the comments that they have given (Brett et al. 2012). Although future recipients may benefit from previous evaluations, if the information gained was made use of, they will not benefit if the evaluator has not done anything with the findings.

This often happens if the evaluation highlights information that is difficult to interpret as a result of poor identification of the aims and objectives. It also occurs when the evaluation gives such a wide range of feedback that it is impossible to decide the effectiveness of the project or identify where improvements should be made.

Given that an evaluation has been reasonably well carried out and conclusions drawn, decisions must be made about who holds responsibility for incorporating the findings in future practice. If the conclusions recommend the investment of further resources, it may be impossible for the non-budget-holding evaluator to act. Aims and objectives almost always include an element of behaviour change, which may cause personal discomfort and have an effect on the recipients' relationships with family and friends. The effect of education cannot be predicted and, as seen in the film *Educating Rita*, where Rita's new knowledge leaves her abandoned by her husband and old friends and feeling misunderstood by her family, it can be a double-edged sword (Bowden 2006).

PRACTICE POINTS

- Like any other aspect of health care, public health and health promotion has ethical considerations.
- Not just with regard to how ethical the health promotion project is but also with regard to the ethical impact on the individual, the family and the community as a whole.

SUMMARY OF KEY POINTS

- Within the health care services, there is a drive to evaluate all aspects of health to ensure that all practices, including health promotion, are providing evidence-based care that does no harm to those being 'cared' for.
- As health promotion is a junior health care profession, there is added impetus for evaluation to take place to prove the worth of health promotion.
- Evaluation is formed of two essential parts: identifying and ranking the criteria (value and aims) and gathering data and information that will make it possible to measure to what degree these criteria are being, or have been, met.
- When judging the worth of a health promotion project, effectiveness, appropriateness, acceptability, efficiency and equity must be considered.

- Health promotion is concerned with changing health knowledge, behaviours and attitudes on many different levels, sometimes over a lengthy time period. It therefore requires a multi-pronged evaluation process that is fraught with difficulties.
- The preferred 'gold standard' of RCT does not fit well with health promotion, where feelings, behaviours, attitudes and changes to these are not easily expressed numerically.
- Evaluation must include assessment of the ethical issues the project highlights.
- Evaluation within health promotion is a complex, difficult endeavour which is often undertaken poorly.

REFERENCES

Bauman, Adrian & Don Nutbeam. 2012. *Evaluation in a nutshell* (2nd ed.). North Ryde, NSW: McGraw Hill Education.

Beresford, Peter. 2002. User involvement in research and evaluation liberation or regulation. *Social Policy and Society* 1(2): 95–105.

Bowden, Jan. 2006. Evaluating health promotion activities. In *Health promotion in midwifery principles and practice*, edited by Jan Bowden & Vicky Manning (2nd ed.). London: Hodder Arnold.

Bradshaw, Jonathan. 1972. The concept of social need. *New Society* 19: 640–643.

Brett, Jo, Sophie Staniszewska, Carol Mockford, Sandra Heron-Marx, John Hughes, Colin Tysall, & Rashida Suleman. 2012. Mapping the impact of patient and public involvement on health and social care research: a systematic review. *Health Expectations and International Journal of of Public Participation and Health Care an Health Policy*, 17(5): 637–650.

DoH (Department of Health). 2010. *Healthy lives, healthy people: Our strategy for public health in England*. https://www.gov.uk/government/publications/healthy-lives-healthy-people-our-strategy-for-public-health-in-england

DoH (Department of Health). 2014. *NHS public health functions agreement 2015–2016 public health functions to be exercised by the NHS England*. London: DoH.

Donaldson, Liam J. & Gabriel Scally. 2009. *Donaldson's essential public health* (3rd ed.). Cornwall: Routledge.

Edelman, Carole, Elizabeth Kudzma & Carol Mandle. 2014. *Health promotion throughout the life span* (8th ed.). St. Louis, MO: Elsevier Mosby.

Farr, Michelle. 2012. Collaboration in Public Services: Can service users and staff participate together. In *Critical perspectives on user involvement*, edited by Marian Barnes & Phil Cotterell. Bristol: The Policy Press.

Fredriksen-Goldsen, Karen, Simoni Jane, Kim Hyun-Jun, Karina Wates, Joyce Yang, Ellis Hoy Charles & Anna Muraco. 2014. The health equity promotion model – Reconceptualisation of lesbian, gay, bisexual and transgender (LGBT) health disparities. *American Journal of Orthopsychiatry* 84(4): 653–663.

Glasgow, Russell, Lichtenstein Edward & Alfred Marcus. 2003. Why don't we see more translation of health promotion research to practice. Rethinking the efficacy to effectiveness transition. *American Journal of Public Health* 93(8): 1261–1267.

Green, Jackie, Keith Tone, Ruth Cross & James Woodall. 2015. *Information needs in: Health promotion, planning and strategies*. London: Sage.

Katz, Jeanne & Alyson Perberdy. 2001. *Promoting health knowledge and practice* (2nd ed.). London: Palgrave Macmillan.

McFarlane, Vanessa. 2014. The same or different? Health promotion in ethically diverse communities. In *The essential guide to public health and health promotion*, edited by Susan R. Thompson. Croydon: Routledge.

McQueen, David V. 2002. The evidence debate: Evaluating evidence for public health interventions. *Journal of Epidemiology and Community Health* 56: 83–84.

Naidoo, Jennie & Jane Wills. 2009. *Health promotion foundations for practice* (3rd ed.). London: Baillière Tindall.

Newburn, Tim. 2001. What do we mean by evaluation. *Children and Society* 15(1): 5–13.

Nutbeam, Don & Elizabeth Harris. 2010. *Theory in a nutshell* (3rd ed.). North Ryde, NSW: McGraw Hill Education.

Sackett, David L., William Rosenberg, J. A. Muir Gray, Brian Haynes & W. Scott Richardson. 1996. Evidence based medicine: What it is and what it isn't. *British Medical Journal* 3: 71–72.

Scriven, Angela. 2010. *Ewles and Simnett's promoting health: A practical guide* (6th ed.). London: Baillière Tindall.

Seedhouse, David. 2003. *Health promotion philosophy, prejudice and practice.* Chichester: Wiley.

Smith, Elizabeth, Fiona Ross, Sheila Donovan, Jill Mounthorpe, Sally Brearley, Peter Sitzia & Peter Beresford. 2008. Service user involvement in nursing, midwifery and health visiting research: The review of the evidence & practice. *International Journal of Nursing Studies* 45(2): 298–315.

Staniszewska, Sophie, Mockford Carole, Gibson Andy, Herron-Marx Sandy & Rebecca Putz. 2012. Moving forward: Understanding the negative experiences and impact of patient and public involvement in health service planning, development and evaluation. In *Critical perspectives on user involvement*, edited by Marian Barnes & Phil Cotterell. Bristol: The Policy Press.

Stevenson, Angus & Catherine Soanes. 2010. *Oxford English Dictionary* (3rd ed.). Oxford: Oxford University Press.

Thompson, Susan R, Claire Novak & Kate Thompson. 2014. Programme planning. In *The essential guide to public health and health promotion*, edited by Susan R. Thompson. Croydon: Routledge.

Trinh-Shevrin, Chau, Nadia Islam Smiti Nadkarni, Rebecca Park & Simona Kwan. 2015. Defining an integrative approach for health promotion and disease prevention: A population health equity framework. *Journal of Health Care for the Poor and Underserved* 26(2): 146–163.

Valente, Thomas W. 2002. *Evaluating health promotion programs.* New York: Oxford University Press.

FURTHER READINGS

Bauman, Adrian & Don Nutbeam. 2012. *Evaluation in a nutshell* (2nd ed.). China: McGraw Hill Education.

Nutbeam, Don & Elizabeth Harris. 2010. *Theory in a nutshell* (3rd ed.). China: McGraw Hill Education.

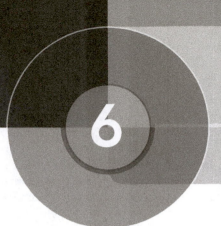

Health, healthy lifestyles and behaviour change

6

JAN BOWDEN

INTRODUCTION

The impact of lifestyle and health behaviours on the individual is a complex one. When a poor lifestyle choice, such as smoking in pregnancy, and a premature birth cause possible negative impacts on a woman's health, one of the most common questions asked by the woman, her family and the health care professionals is 'What could have be done to prevent this?'

Prior to a negative impact happening, the threat of that poor lifestyle choice might be ignored or its relevance considered unimportant by the woman and her family. It may also be considered beyond the remit of the health care professionals. Midwives have public health and health promotion as a central tenet of their scope of practice (ICM 2013; Midwifery 2020 2010; NMC 2015). The issues of lifestyles, health behaviours and the impact on health are a conundrum that causes midwives puzzlement and frustration both professionally and personally.

This chapter will explore the background of health and lifestyle and the theories of health behaviours and examine factors that impact on changing health behaviours. The way midwives may act and react when exploring healthy behaviour and the impact on the women and their families will be explored, along with some application to practice.

BACKGROUND

The link between health and lifestyle has long been recognised. Pythagoras (570–495 BC) noted 'No man, who values his health, ought trespass beyond the boundaries of moderation'

(Haslam 2007, 32). Hippocrates (460–370 BC) went on to identify that 'those very fat are more liable to sudden death than those who are thin' (Donaldson & Scully 2009, 117).

By the late eighteenth century and early nineteenth century, the issue of lifestyle and behaviour was overtaken by the birth of a public health policy in the United Kingdom. This policy had at its centre the new science of the identification of organisms and their control by medicine. This resulted in a decline of infectious diseases and the development of a strong vaccination programme (Donaldson & Scully 2009). However, there are sufficient data to argue that improvements to sanitation, nutrition and housing stock have also played a part (Donaldson & Scully 2009; Upton & Thirlaway 2014).

Public health evidence shows that within the United Kingdom, life requires less effort than ever before (DoH 2011). The living and working environments are safer, with travel, household tasks and even shopping requiring less effort than for our forebears (DoH 2010); this coupled with cheap processed foods and alcohol have made a significant impact on the population's lifestyle (Barbor et al. 2010; Bouine et al. 2009).

In the late twentieth and early twenty-first centuries, the spotlight has returned to the importance of healthy behaviours and in particular the impact of poor lifestyle choices on health and the increased workload of the National Health Service (HM Government 2010).

HEALTH AND HEALTHY BEHAVIOURS: WHAT DO THEY OFFER?

Behaviours that improve the health of an individual, a community or a whole population can affect society in general. Improving health behaviours has the potential to promise health benefits and ultimately reduce health service expenditure. Potentially, it has the possibility to provide benefits that are cost-effective, efficient and low risk (Dunn & Rollnick 2003; Kerr et al. 2005). However, approaches that concentrate on healthy behaviours can be acknowledged as being in direct opposition to the more expensive biomedical approach. The healthy behaviour approaches do not focus on just a cure but have roles in prevention and the reduction of complications where a health issue already exists. They require a more psycho-social understanding of health and the need to work in collaboration with all health-related services and the clients.

Improving health by changing behaviour can be seen as a less costly approach to health by the government and the health services, with the focus moved from a societal responsibility to an individual one. Some argue this is as it should be; the Self Care forum – an organisation that believes that people should be empowered to be more informed and to look after their own health and only access medical intervention when necessary – feels strongly that health is the responsibility of the individual and not a responsibility that should be given away to others such as the government (Webber et al. 2015). However, this can lead to a 'blame culture', when poor lifestyle choices lead to significant health issues, and a more inward focus to health (Cherrier 2012; Upton & Thirlaway 2014).

PRACTICE POINT

Behaviour change can offer a cost-effective, client-led approach to health promotion, which can strongly complement the traditional biomedical approach.

LIFESTYLE BEHAVIOURS

Upton and Thirlaway (2014) acknowledge that behaviours are:

- Multifaceted
- Altered and changed depending on age, environment, social network and personal beliefs
- Usually seen as pleasurable in the beginning, with the future impact on health not considered

Upton and Thirlaway (2014) also elucidate that they play a crucial part in the development and maintenance of:

- Social networks
- The ability to cope with stress
- The building and development of resilience

TYPES OF BEHAVIOURS

ACTIVITY

Identity the different types of behaviour, then look at Table 6.1 and compare what you have listed to those in the table.

A certain behaviour could take more than one form; for example, a routine behaviour such as smoking is also an addictive behaviour, and it may also be traditional or custom based (the norm for a family or a social group). A one-time behaviour such as breastfeeding may also be traditional or custom based (Upton & Thirlaway 2014).

At the onset of the behaviour, it may be considered as having a positive effect when seen in the time construct of the present, for example, smoking being seen as a social norm, stress

Table 6.1 Types of behaviours

Type of behaviour	Examples of the behaviour
One-time/occasional behaviours A behaviour that may be carried out once or a few times in a lifespan.	Breastfeeding, sterilisation, childhood vaccinations
Routine behaviours A behaviour that is frequently undertaken with little conscious thought.	Fingernail biting, smoking, alcohol consumption
Traditional/custom-based behaviours A behaviour that is passed/shared from one generation to another in a family, a community or a population.	Formula feeding, breastfeeding, not eating certain foods, female genital mutilation
Addictive behaviours A behaviour that gives a biological or psychological reinforcement, either positive or negative; this leads to the behaviour being continued to repeat/gain further reinforcement.	Exercising, taking drugs, smoking

reliever or means to maintain weight in the present time, but it may have a negative outcome in the future, for example, facial ageing, poor pregnancy outcomes and cancer (Thompson & Almond 2014; Upton & Thirlaway 2014).

ACTIVITY

Before reading the section on factors and lifestyle behaviours:

- Identify the factors that may impact on an individual's lifestyle behaviours.
- Identify if the factors could have a positive, negative effect or both.

FACTORS AND LIFESTYLE BEHAVIOURS

Lifestyle behaviours and the factors that impact on them are multi-factorial and considered to be mainly under the control of the individual. However, how much control an individual actually has is a hotly debated area (Acheson 1998; Thompson & Almond 2014). Some factors, such as sex, age, ethnicity and genetic makeup, are considered non-negotiable factors in that they cannot be altered (Figure 6.1). However, they can impact on the way health promotion messages are accepted. Research shows that the older a person gets, the more likely they are to engage in positive health behaviours or change or moderate negative health behaviours. This is mainly due to life experiences and a better understanding of perceived risk (Hubley et al. 2013; McDade-Montez et al. 2005). This might be something a midwife might wish to consider when caring for younger women during their pregnancies, because their ability to perceive risk and change behaviours might be impaired as a result of experience, knowledge, skills and peer pressure (DoH 2011).

Evidence also identifies that women are more likely than men to take up health promotion messages. They are more likely to take care of their health, access health services earlier and adopt healthier behaviours sooner than men (Kent et al. 2014; Rongen et al. 2014). However, research also indicates that women are more likely to be 'wrapped up' in promoting the health of their families leaving their own health needs 'last on the list' (Edelman et al. 2013; Kent et al. 2014).

Pregnancy appears to act as a catalyst for health behaviour change. Concern for the well-being of the unborn child is likely to increase the woman's receptiveness to the health messages (Edvardsson et al. 2011). These alterations to her behaviour may continue and be sustained beyond childbirth and may affect her partner and other members of the family (Wilkinson et al. 2009; Wilkinson & McIntyre 2012).

Potentially, the next greatest influence on lifestyle and health behaviours is family, friends and social networks (Marmot 2007). The midwife needs to bear this in mind when encouraging healthier behaviours such as smoking cessation or healthy eating, as this will to some extent be offset by the woman's need to 'fit in'. A change that might be beneficial to the woman's health and her pregnancy may put her at odds with her social group, possibly lessening their support to her (Bowden 2006).

PRACTICE POINTS

- Younger women may perceive risk differently than older women and this may impact on their receptiveness of health promotion messages.
- Support networks might provide a positive or negative effect on the success and longevity of a health behaviour change.

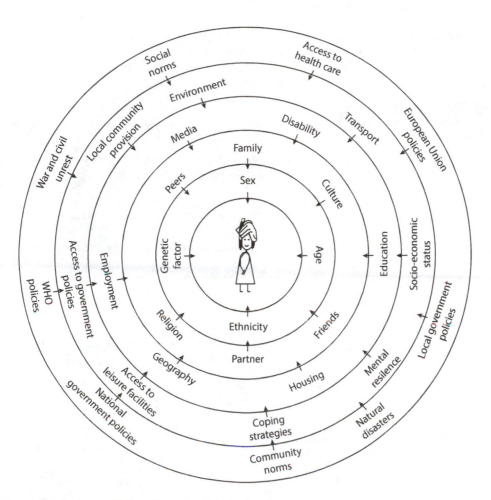

Figure 6.1 Factors and influences on health behaviours.

HEALTH BEHAVIOUR THEORY AND MODELS

The key theorem of behaviour change models is based on the following principles:

- *Biological:* this includes biological drives such as hunger, thirst, sex, genetic factors and physiological dependencies that may impact on behaviour and can be identified as out of our control.
- *Motivational:* the belief that despite the biological principle, the impact of society and culture will have some kind of mediating effect. This is the basis of the work by Maslow (1943) and his concept of the hierarchy of needs, and it postulates that the basic needs must be satiated before attempting to address the higher needs within the hierarchy.
- *Cognitive dissonance:* the concept that if you are aware that a lifestyle or behaviour is harmful you will alter it (Festinger 1957). However, this is not always a guaranteed outcome and the evidence suggested that an individual may chose to ignore anything he or she considers to be unpalatable and continue the lifestyle or behaviour (Ent & Gerend 2015; Fotulu et al. 2013).

There are a number of conceptual models of health beliefs and change. The oldest and probably the most well-known is the Health Belief Model (HBM) (Becker 1974; Rosenstock 1966). The premise is that the individual will weigh up the costs and benefits to themselves and make the decision to change based on that analysis (see Figure 6.2).

LEARNING ACTIVITY

HBM

Karlee is a 23-year-old woman who is 24 weeks into her first pregnancy. She is a smoker – approximately 18 a day – and comes to delivery suite complaining of contractions and is admitted for observation.

- Using the HBM, explore how Karlee may have made her decision to continue smoking during her pregnancy.
- Using the HBM, explore how you, as Karlee's midwife, could use this model to encourage Karlee to stop smoking.

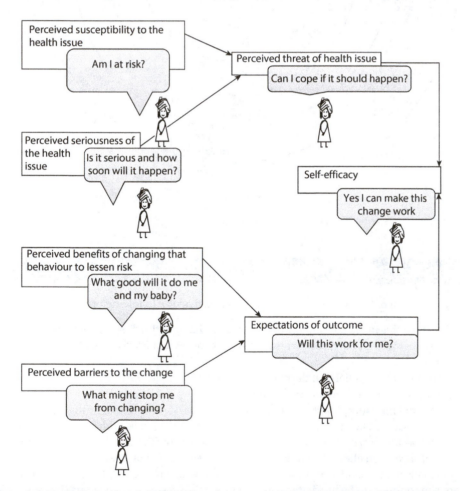

Figure 6.2 Health Belief Model. (Adapted from Rosenstock, Irwin. 1966. *Millbank Memorial Fund Quarterly*, 44: 94–121.)

REASONED ACTION AND PLANNED BEHAVIOUR

In their 'theory of reasoned action', Ajzen and Fishbein (1980) inserted the word 'intention' between attitude and behaviour. They believed that by discovering a person's intention, rather than just their attitude and their behaviour, an outcome could be more accurately predicted (Ajzen 1988; Ajzen & Fishbein 1980). They identified that the individual would weigh up his or her personal feelings along with perceived social pressure before making a decision. Therefore, the individual's behaviour was one of 'reasoned action', and its application can be shown, for example, on the predicted behaviour of a woman intending to formula feed (Figure 6.3).

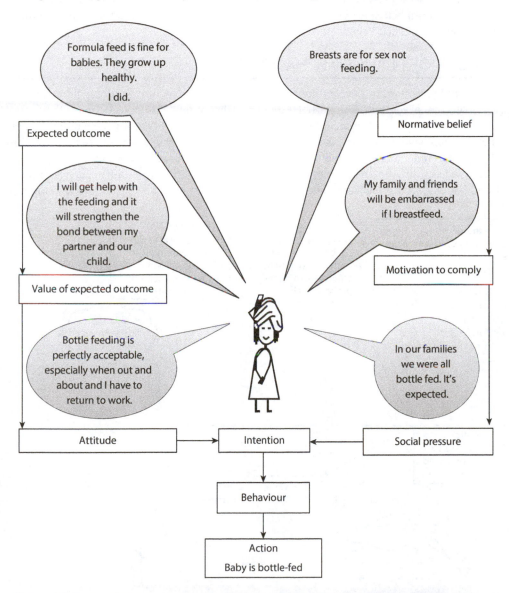

Figure 6.3 Theory of reasoned action. (Modified from Ajzen and Fishbein, 1980, by Crafter, Helen. 1997. Attitudes, values and behaviour. In Crafter H (ed.), *Health promotion in midwifery. Principles and practice*. London: Hodder, pp. 54–64.)

Within the 'theory of reasoned action', just two of the multitudes of beliefs held by an individual are identified:

- Behavioural beliefs, that is, those that make us behave in a certain way
- Normative beliefs, that is, desirable, culturally acceptable.

Ajzen and Fishbein (1980) suggest that logical psychological processes link these beliefs by way of our attitude to the behaviour, subjective norms (social pressure) and intention, each stage leading on from the preceding stage. The theory's main conviction is that individuals will weigh up their personal feelings, or attitudes, and the social pressure that they perceive (subjective norm) before arriving at and carrying out their intention to change (or not) their health behaviour. Their behaviour is then one of 'reasoned action'.

THEORY OF PLANNED BEHAVIOUR

Ajzen (1990) went on to develop the 'theory of planned behaviour' to incorporate another variable – that of control (Figure 6.4). He identified that individuals' perceptions of their control over a situation also influenced health behaviours (Ajzen 1990). It is generally thought that the more favourable an individual's attitude, subjective norm and perceived control, the stronger the individual's intention to undertake the behaviour and maintain it.

Individuals differ in the extent to which they think that they can make changes to their lives. Social learning theorists believe that this is a product of an individual's upbringing.

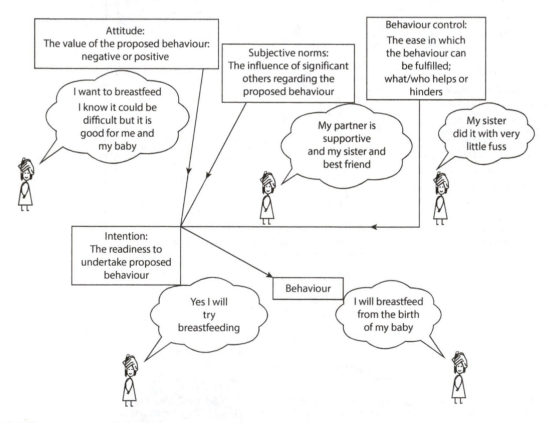

Figure 6.4 Theory of planned behaviour.

Individuals who have been rewarded for their success and have received fair punishment when they have been wrong will have a better belief in their control of their lives than those who have not been aptly rewarded and have been unfairly punished (Scriven 2010).

Although Ajzen and Fishbein (1980) suggest that their theory can be used to predict and understand attitudes and behaviour, more so than the Health Belief Model, they do not consider the impact of 'drives' that are identified in the Health Belief Model, or the issue of the locus of control nor the emotional input which is often variable and unpredictable. This is particularly so in childbirth which, by its very nature, can be a very emotional time for the woman and her partner. It is, as evidence suggests, also a time where fresh ideas and values are formulated and attitudes and beliefs changed (Edvardsson et al. 2011; Wilkinson et al. 2009).

THE TRANSTHEORETICAL APPROACH TO HEALTH BEHAVIOUR CHANGE

Although it is important to acknowledge an individual's attitudes and values in health promotion, and to respect them, it is also essential that a supportive environment be created in which an individual can challenge ideas and question beliefs. The theory of the Transtheoretical Model of Behaviour Change (TTMBHC) was designed by Proschaska and DiClemente in 1984 and followed on from an earlier work by Proschaska, who with a group of colleagues undertook a review of some 300 psychotherapeutic interventions. The model was then designed on the basis of the 10 processes identified as reoccurring in the 300 reviewed psychotherapeutic interventions, hence the term *transtheoretical* (Green et al. 2015; Figure 6.5).

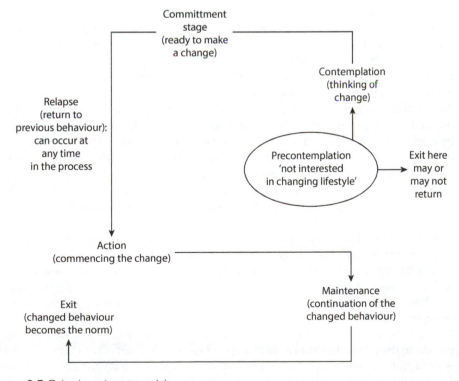

Figure 6.5 Behaviour change model.

The original use of the model was to support smoking cessation, and it very controversially indicated that relapse was a given part of the process, which could occur in any stage of the model. It has seven stages – if relapse takes place – and behaviour change is viewed as a process that unfolds over many months and is dependent on support and environment. The evidence indicated that long-term smokers took three to four attempts over a 7- to 10-year period before finally quitting (Prochaska & DiClemente 1984).

1. *The pre-contemplation stage:* This is where a woman is not anticipating change in the near future; this is because the woman may feel that there is nothing at present to change or does not see her current behaviour as having the potential to harm her. The midwife may give health education and advice to highlight a behaviour that is less healthy. It is important for the midwife to realise that the woman may be hostile to any attempt to discuss the dangers of her negative health behaviour, suggesting that she is yet to reach the pre-contemplation stage (and may indeed never do so).

   Alternatively, she may accept anti-smoking arguments but claim to feel quite powerless to stop. A time span on this is difficult because some women may remain in this stage for many years (Prochaska 2005). It is equally vital that the unhealthy behaviour is discussed by the midwife and not left as the 'elephant in the room'. The midwife should not ignore the unhealthy behaviour for fear of damaging the growing therapeutic relationship with the women (Lee et al. 2012).

2. *The contemplation stage:* This is where the woman engages in the process of wanting to change a health behaviour (Prochaska 2005). She will begin to address the health issue and its impact on herself and her child. The woman, now aware of the side effects of her negative health behaviour, is motivated to think about making the change. She now actively seeks information about the negative health behaviour and the benefits that will come by making a change to it. Empowerment is key to moving through this stage, and the midwife can use her considerable skills to facilitate this process, such as listening, assessing ambivalence and facilitating motivation, as well as assisting the woman with the collection of information (see Chapter 7). The midwife must also realise that some of her clients may never move beyond this stage.

3. *The commitment stage:* A woman entering this stage of the approach is making a serious decision to change her negative health behaviour. The midwife can help the woman by working with her to identify resources and develop action plans. The midwife can highlight coping strategies that may help when or if things get tough. Also, the midwife can help identify and develop a 'personal' support group comprising family members and friends. Towards the end of this stage, a date on which to commence the change needs to be clearly acknowledged. Prochaska (2005) identified that this stage usually lasts no more than a month.

4. *The action stage:* Here, the woman is making explicit modifications to improve her health behaviours, and this stage may take up to 6 months (Prochaska 2005). Support during this stage is vital. Midwifery support may include working with the woman and with her 'personal' support group, identifying and working with those who may block the change, knowingly or not, as well as referring her to self-help support groups or other agencies.

5. *The maintenance stage:* This stage sees the continuation of the behaviour change by the woman to the point it becomes not a change but an accepted part of her everyday life. The woman gains increasing satisfaction and confidence in herself and her coping strategies. She may notice the health benefits that the change has brought about. The midwife's

continued support reminds the woman of her success and when she begins to waver prompts the woman to re-use her action plans and her coping strategies identified in the commitment stage.

6. *The exit stage:* This is where the health behaviour has been successfully changed and maintained by the woman. At this stage, the woman is not affected by temptation and has 100% self-efficacy. Michie et al. (2011) identify that less than 20% will achieve this stage and that for the midwife and the woman it is important to recognise that for many the best they will achieve is the maintenance stage. This knowledge prevents a feeling of failure if the exit stage is not reached.

7. *The relapse stage:* It is important for both the woman and the midwife to realise that not all women will be successful at the first attempt. It is also important that relapse is seen as part of changing health behaviours, and it should not be deemed a failure on the part of the woman (Michie et al. 2011; Prochaska & DiClemente 1984). Relapse should be evaluated for its cause, and, on restarting the approach, this evaluation can be worked into an action plan, which probably can lead to the development of a more effective coping strategy. This will allow the midwife or others to offer support, particularly at the point where the relapse occurs.

PRACTICE POINTS

- There are numerous models regarding behaviours, how they are formed and how they are changed.
- No one model is a perfect fit.
- The impact of family, friends and emotions on behaviour change cannot be underestimated.
- Midwives' awareness of the different approaches to behaviour change will help develop skills and understanding to provide women with a more individualised approach to health promotion.

BEHAVIOUR CHANGE IN MIDWIFERY PRACTICE

Working with a woman to assist her in changing her behaviour is a key component of the role of a midwife (Public Health England 2013a, 2013b). It is a role that is challenging, especially when there has been a relapse or there is resistance to change. This challenge can be assisted by motivational interviewing, which is a client centred, collaborative style interaction. It focuses on the language of change, the strengthening of confidence and motivation and the identification of ambivalence (Miller & Rollnick 2013). This section will look briefly at some of the aspects of motivational interviewing that may assist midwives in the clinical area.

The key factors for a midwife supporting a woman with changing health behaviours are:

- Assessing the woman's level of knowledge
- Assessing the woman's level of motivation
- Facilitating the woman's motivation
- Identifying and managing ambivalence

GETTING STARTED

Getting started is often the most difficult part; women attending midwifery services are usually aware of the health issues that a midwife wishes to explore. The way this is addressed

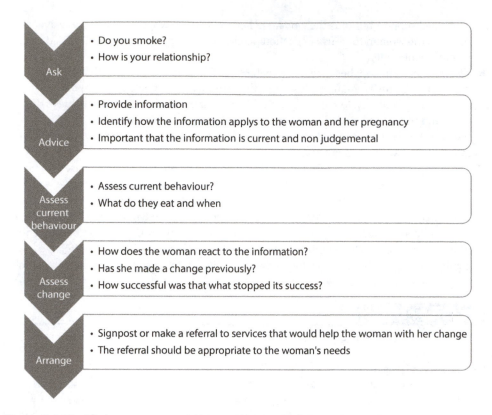

Figure 6.6 The '5As' assessment tool. (Adapted from the NHS Future Forum. 2012. *The NHS role in public health. A report from the NHS Future Forum*. London: DoH.)

by the midwife will indicate the possible success of any change of behaviour to some extent (Dosh et al. 2005). The '5As' tool has formed the foundation of the government's 'Every Contact Counts', where all health care professionals should make every contact count in terms of promoting and maintaining good health (NHS Future Forum 2012).

The '5 As' tool will help facilitate the midwife to open up the discussion (Figure 6.6):

The key to these health conversations are that they are brief and evidence based. Evidence shows that a health conversation lasting no more than 3 min can increase a person's chance of stopping smoking by up to 3% (Stead et al. 2013). This might not seem a lot but if as a midwife you consider the number of women you interact with each day and each week that percentage grows and makes a large health impact (Thompson & Almond 2014). The time restraint also stops the women from feeling as though they are being lectured at and are less likely to present barriers. Dunn and Rollnick (2003) indicate that behaviour change should be a dance and not a wrestling match where the individual is forced into submitting to the change.

CONFIDENCE AND MOTIVATION

Assessing motivation and confidence in the ability to change will allow the midwife to understand the level of support that the client might need. The use of a numbered range and back up questions can facilitate this (Miller & Rollnick 2013).

EXAMPLE

Scale of 0 to 10, with 0 indicating no change, and 10 indicating the maximum change. The question posed to the woman is, 'How confident do you feel about eating more healthy foods?'

If the woman scores less than 4, a supplementary question would be to ask why she has scored that low; if the score is above 4, then a supplementary question would be what she needs to have in place to score higher.

AMBIVALENCE

Motivational interviewing has been shown to be effective in dealing with ambivalence and developing a more effective and supportive dialogue to encourage behaviour change.

Ambivalence is when there is a level of reluctance to change; the woman appears to be of two minds as to what to do (Miller & Rollnick 2013). The reasons for this might be multifaceted; it might be due to lack of confidence in her ability to change or there may be a 'block' to the change due to family or peer pressure, for example. Evidence suggests that midwives when faced with an ambivalent client often provide information to the woman as to what they are lacking or not doing. Although this can be seen as being well intended, it could lessen the positive effect of the intervention (Miller & Rollnick 2013; Upton & Thirlaway 2010).

Motivational interviewing is not a rigid process, rather a sequential repetitive process when used with a woman whose is ambivalent to change. Miller and Rollnick (2013) and Dunn and Rollnick (2003) indicate that there are four stages in this process:

1. *Engagement:* the better the engagement, the better the outcome (Thompson & Almond 2014).
2. *Focus:* a collaborative process that focuses on the health issue and the goals to be achieved.
3. *Evoke:* allowing the woman to voice their ideas, concerns and fears about the change and what it will achieve. This is crucial to motivational interviewing (Dunn & Rollnick 2003).
4. *Plan:* the woman reaches a 'tipping point'. This moves her from focusing on why she cannot change to how she can, with the development of a plan to continue and support the change.

Miller and Rollnick (2013) indicate that motivational interviewing is designed to explore an individual's motivation and resolve to change, and the rationale for the midwife is to aim to foster a respectful and collaborative environment in which to facilitate change.

SUMMARY OF KEY POINTS

- Changing behaviours is not easy to undertake and is affected by many factors, some of which the individual may have no control over.
- Health behaviour theories and models offer the midwife an understanding of the process of change; they are not perfect exemplars.
- Pregnancy is often a time when a woman and her partner are open to new ideas and may change their attitudes as they re-evaluate their lives, learn more about themselves and join a new social group of being parents. The midwife needs to bear in mind that vulnerable women might find this difficult to achieve.
- Midwives need to be sensitive to the individual's values, the complex issues of health behaviour and the ethical dimensions of attempting to change the values and attitudes of an individual.
- Midwives also need to be aware of their own values, beliefs and attitudes, and how that may impact on the care that they give their clients.

REFERENCES

Acheson, Donald. 1998. *Independent inquiry in to inequalities in health.* London: Stationary Office.

Ajzen, Icek. 1988. *Attitudes, personality and behaviour.* Milton Keynes: Open University Press.

Ajzen, Icek. 1990. The theory of planned behaviour. *Organisational Behaviour and Human Decision Processes* 50: 179–211.

Ajzen, Icek & Martin Fishbein (eds.). 1980. *Understanding attitudes and predicting social behaviour.* Englewood Cliffs, NJ: Prentice Hall.

Barbor, Thomas, Raul Caetano, Sally Casewell, Griffith Edmonds, Norman Glebreech, Kathryn Graham, Joel Grube, Paul Gruenwald, Linda Hill, Harry Holder, Ross Homel, et al. 2010. *Alcohol: No ordinary commodity.* Research and Public Policy. Oxford: Oxford University Press.

Becker, Marshall H. (ed.). 1974. *The health belief model and personal health behaviour.* Thorofare: NJ Slack.

Bouine, Chantal, Mickey Chopra & Robert Van Der Hoeren. 2009. Trade and health 3: Trade and the social determinants of health. *Lancet* 373(9662): 502–507.

Bowden, Jan. 2006. Attitudes, values and health behaviours. In *Health promotion in midwifery principles & practice*, edited by Jan Bowden and Vicky Manning. London: Hodder Arnold.

Cherrier, Helene. 2012. Using projective techniques to consider the societal dimension of healthy practices: An exploratory study. *Health Marketing Quarterly* 29(1): 82–95.

Crafter, Helen. 1997. Attitudes, values and behaviour. In *Health promotion in midwifery: Principles and practice*, edited by H. Crafter, 54–64. London: Hodder.

DoH (Department of Health). 2010. *Delivering expectation Midwifery 2020 programme UK.* https://www.gov.uk/government/uploads/system/uploads/attachment_data/file/216029/dh_119470.pdf

DoH (Department of Health). 2010. *Our health and wellbeing today.* London: DoH.

DoH (Department of Health). 2011. *National travel survey 2010.* Statistical release. Newport: ONS.

Donaldson, Liam J. & Gabriel Scully. 2009. *Donaldson's essential public health* (3rd ed.). Padstow: Radcliffe.

Dosh, Steven, Jodi Holtrop, Trissa Torres, Anita Arnold, Jeanne Bauman & Linda White. 2005. Changing organizational constructs in to functional tools: An assessment of the 5As in primary care practices. *Annals of Family Medicine* 3(Suppl 2): s50–s52.

Dunn, Chris & Stephen Rollnick. 2003. *Lifestyle change.* London: Elsevier.

Edelman, Carole Lium, Carole Lynn Mandle & Elizabeth Kudzman. 2013. *Health promotion throughout the lifespan* (8th ed.). St. Louis, MO: Mosby.

Edvardsson, Kristina, Anneli Ivarsson, Eva Eurenius, Rickard Garvare, Monica Nystrom, Rhonda Small & Ingrid Mogren. 2011. Giving offspring a health start: Parents experiences of health promotion and lifestyle change during pregnancy and early parenthood. *BMC Public Health* 11: 936.

Ent, Michael & Mary Gerend. 2015. Cognitive dissonance and attitudes towards unpleasant medical screening. *Journal of Psychology* 25: 82–90.

Festinger, Leon. 1957. *A theory of cognitive dissonance.* Standford, CA: Standford University Press.

Fotulu, Omid, Geoffrey Fong, Mark Zanna, Ron Borland, Hua Yong & K. Michael Cummings. 2013. Patterns cognitive dissonance – Reducing beliefs among smokers, a longitudinal analysis from the International Tobacco Control: A 4 country survey. *Tobacco Control* 22(1): 52–58.

Green, Jackie, Keith Tones, Ruth Cross & James Woodall. 2015. *Health promotion planning & strategies* (3rd ed.). London: Sage.

Haslam, David. 2007. Obesity: A medical history. *Obesity Reviews* 8(Suppl): 31–36.

HM Government. 2010. *Healthy lives, healthy people: Our strategy for public health in England*. London: The Stationary Office.

Hubley, John, June Copeman & James Woodall. 2013. *Practical health promotion* (2nd ed.). Cornwall: Polity Press.

ICM (International Confederation of Midwives). 2011. *International definition of the midwife*. Netherlands, The Hague: ICM Council.

Kent, Lillian M., Darren P. Mortan, Paul M. Rankin, Bret G. Mitchell, Esther Chang & Hans Diehl. 2014. Gender differences in effectiveness of the Complete Involvement Programme Lifestyle Intervention: An Australasian study. *Health Promotion Journal of Australia* 25: 222–229.

Kerr, Jacqueline, Rolf Weitkunat & Manuel Morretti. 2005. *ABC of behaviour change: A guide to successful disease prevention and health promotion*. London: Elsevier.

Lee, Deborah J., Charlotte Haynes & Deborah Garrod. 2012. Exploring the midwife's role in health promotion practice. *British Journal of Midwifery* 20(3): 178–186.

Marmot, Michael. 2007. Achieving health equity from root causes to fair outcomes. *Lancet* 370(9593): 1153–1163.

Maslow, Abraham. 1943. A theory of human motivation. *Psychological Review* 50(4): 370–396.

McDade-Montez, Elizabeth, Cvengros James & Alan Christensen. 2005. Personality and individual differences In *ABC of behavior change. A guide to successful disease prevention and health promotion*, edited by Jacqueline Kerr, Rolf Weitkunat & Manuel Moretti, 57–71. London: Elsevier Churchill Livingstone.

Michie, Susan, Maartje M. van Stralen & Robert West. 2011. The behaviour change wheel: A new method characterising behaviour change intervention. *Implementation Science* 6: 42.

Miller, William R. & Stephen Rollnick. 2013. *Motivational interviewing helping people change* (3rd ed.). London: Elsevier.

NHS Future Forum. 2012. *The NHS role in public health. A report from the NHS Future Forum*. London: DoH. https://www.gov.uk/government/uploads/system/uploads/attachment_data/file/216423/dh_132114.pdf

NMC (Nursing and Midwifery Council). 2015. *The code*. London: NMC.

Prochaska, James O. 2005. Stages of change, readiness and motivation. In *ABC of Behavior Change. A guide to successful disease prevention and health promotion*, edited by Jacqueline Kerr, Rolf Weitkunat and Manuel Moretti, 111–127. London: Elsevier Churchill Livingstone.

Prochaska, James O. & Carlo C. DiClemente. 1984. *The transtheoretical approach: Crossing traditional boundaries of therapy*. Homewood, IL: Dow Jones/Irwin.

Public Health England. 2013a. *Nursing and midwifery contribution to public health*. London: Public Health England and DoH.

Public Health England. 2013b. *Nursing and midwifery actions at the three levels of public Health practice*. London: Public Health England and DoH.

Rosenstock, Irwin. 1966. Why people use health services. *Millbank Memorial Fund Quarterly* 44: 94–121.

Rongen, Anne, Suzan J. W. Robroek, Wouter van Ginkel, Dennis Lindeboom, Bibielle Altink & Alex Burdorf. 2014. Barriers and facilitators for participation in health promotion programmes amongst employees – A 6 months follow up study. *BMC Public Health* 14: 573.

Scriven, Angela. 2010. *Promoting health: A practical guide* (6th ed.). London: Bailliere Tindall.

Stead, Lindsay F., Diana Buitrago, Nataly Preciado, Guillermo Sanchez, Jamie Hartmann-Boyce & Tim Lancaster. 2013. Physician advice for smoking cessation. *Cochrane Database of Systematic Reviews* 2013(5): CD000165. DOI: 10.1002/14651858.CD000165.pub4. http://onlinelibrary.wiley.com/doi/10.1002/14651858.CD000165.pub4/abstract

Thompson, Susan R. & Mo Almond. 2014. Supporting people with behaviour change. In *The essential guide to public health and health promotion,* edited by Susan Thompson. Oxford: Routledge.

Upton, Dominic & Katie Thirlaway. 2014. *Promoting health behaviour: A practical guide* (2nd ed.). Oxford: Routledge.

Webber, D.E., Z. Gno & Steven Mann. 2015. The responsibilities of the healthy: A manifesto for self-care. *Self Care* 6(1): 2–9.

Wilkinson, Shelly & H. David McIntyre. 2012. Evaluation of "health start pregnancy" early antenatal health promotion workshop: A randomised controlled trial. *BMC Pregnancy & Childbirth* 12: 131.

Wilkinson, Shelly A., Yvette D. Miller & Bernadette Watson. 2009. Prevalence of health behaviours in pregnancy at service entry in the Queensland Health Service District. *Australia & New Zealand Journal of Public Health* 3: 228–233.

FURTHER READINGS

Dart, Michelle. 2010. *Motivational interviewing in nursing practice; empowering the patient.* Sudbury, MA: Jones and Bartlett Learning.

NICE. 2014. *Behaviour change: Individual approaches (PH49).* UK: NICE. http://www.nice.org.uk/guidance/ph49/resources/guidance-behaviour-change-individual-approaches-pdf

Nutbeam, Don, Elizabeth Harris & Marlene Wise. 2010. *Theory in a nutshell: A guide to health promotion theory* (3rd ed.). Sydney, Australia: Mcgraw-Hill Medical.

Information giving in health promotion

VICKY MANNING AND MARY MALONE

INTRODUCTION

Health information is central to health promotion and can be found everywhere, on television and radio, in shops, in newspapers and on high street billboards. Much of what we consume, wash with, wear or drive has a health or lifestyle message attached to it. The Internet has also made health information available to all, health professionals and the public alike, and has led to debates about the quality of health information available and how individuals and population groups have access to it (Eysenbach et al. 2004). As the Department of Health (DoH 2012, 4) says 'Information can bring enormous benefits. It is the lifeblood of good health and well-being, and is pivotal to good quality care. It allows us to understand how to improve our own and our family's health, to know what our care and treatment choices are and to assess for ourselves the quality of services and support available'. The aim of this chapter is to explore the different formats used to provide information in health promotion and how the quality of information given or received can be assessed.

COMMUNICATING HEALTH INFORMATION

Communication contributes to all aspects of disease prevention, health promotion and education for individuals, communities and whole populations. Communicating health information can be a complex process which involves the information itself, the health messages contained, the characteristics of the communicator and the person receiving the information and the environment in which the communication takes place. Health information is communicated in many different areas such as schools, home and work, and in many different formats such as the mass media, flyers, newsletters, advertising and posters. The choice of both setting and form depends on many points such as topic, target group, the health promoter, location and the amount of time planned or available. There are many aspects of good communication, and by adapting the SMART acronym these can be identified as:

- *Simple* message.
- *Meaningful*: information which has meaning for the recipient.
- *Articulated* in a non-judgmental manner.
- *Realistic*: the information relates to a change which is realistic for the recipient to make.
- *Timely*: the information is given at a time when the recipient is able and willing to use it.

Using the same SMART acronym, it is also possible to identify aspects of good health information giving.

- *Sensitive* to the unique situation of the recipient
- *Measurable*: identifies changes which are measurable
- *Achievable*: identifies changes which are achievable by the individual
- *Resources*: draws on a number of resources to give an effective health message and recognises the social, emotional and psychological resources of the recipient
- *Timely*: given at the optimum time and allows time for the recipient to digest the information and incorporate it into their lives

As stated above, communicating health information is a complex process. It is important to remember when giving any health information that it does not happen in a vacuum but is influenced by the characteristics of the information itself, the person giving it, the recipient and the external environment.

We will briefly look at each of these.

Characteristics of how the health information may be given might include:

- The format, for example, leaflet, poster, mass media, computers/Internet or apps. If the format is to use the spoken word, then using a leaflet will help enhance the message. Using more than one form of communication is more effective in increasing understanding, than using only one (Vögele 2005). However, the information giver needs to be aware of any language issues which may be present and have, for example, leaflets in different languages.
- The order in which the information is given can also influence perceptions. People tend to remember information at the beginning of the conversation, and forget the last bits; this is particularly true if it is bad news. If the topic is considered unimportant, however, the end of the message will be remembered more than the beginning (Witte 1994).

When considering who should be giving the health information, it is necessary to consider (Anderson 2012; Kourkouta & Papathanasiou 2014):

- The level of knowledge of the health care practitioners (HCPs).
- Their communication skills.
- If they have access to training, information and resources which will support them in giving the information.
- The amount of empathy they may have for the person receiving the information.
- Their own level of motivation.

When giving information, it is important to understand the possible characteristics of the person/people receiving the information.

- History: have they been seen before with regard to this issue and was health information given? Finding out will help assess if the transmission of the message had a positive or negative impact so that the format might be adjusted, if required.
- Is the recipient receptive or resistant to the health message?
- Individual resources: economic, social (support of family and friendship networks will enhance chances of success) and psychological (self-efficacy will enhance chances of success but fatalism will increase resistance to the message) (Malone et al. 2014).
- Intellectual difficulties in understanding concepts may make the health message difficult to understand. Poor literacy may mean that written messages cannot be understood. Approximately 16%, or 5.2 million, of adults in England can be described as 'functionally illiterate'. They can understand short, straightforward texts on familiar topics but reading information from unfamiliar sources, or on unfamiliar topics, could cause problems (Literacy Trust 2015).

The environment information given can affect how effectively the message is received.

- Time is the first environmental element for both the HCP and the recipient.
- Where the information is given, is there privacy, too much noise or too little space, etc.
- No matter how good the health information and communication is, people may not be ready to hear it because it may not be a good time in their lives; they may not want to be told how to live their lives or for others to make decisions for them (Miller & Rollnick 2012).

PRACTICE POINTS

- Using more than one form of communication is more effective in increasing understanding than using only one.
- Communication is affected by many elements such as the information format, the willingness of the recipient to receive the message to where the information is being given.

HCPs, such as midwives and health visitors, have the advantage of regular face-to-face contact with women and families when a baby is either expected or just born. All families want the best for their children and so are more likely to be receptive to health messages. In order to maximise the health-promoting potential of their role, midwives need to understand how the women and families they work with are assessing risk and how those women view the health promotion options available both for themselves and their families. The Health Belief Model by Becker (1974) helps to explain how health messages may be received and acted upon. It examines the roles of risk and benefit analysis in health (see Chapter 6).

The Health Belief Model (Becker 1974) assumes that people assess both the risk of acting, or not acting, in relation to a particular behaviour and the potential benefit to be gained through altering their behaviour. The following example illustrates how this might work:

- A young woman, who is 12 weeks post-partum, receives an invitation for cervical screening. If she is in good general health and has no immediate experience of cancer, she may decide that the risk to her is minimal and decline the invitation.
- However, if she begins to experience symptoms, such as post-coital bleeding, and knows that these symptoms are not normal and might be associated with cervical cancer, she may perceive an increased risk and take action, that is, have a cervical smear test.

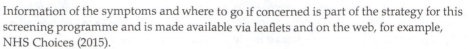

Information of the symptoms and where to go if concerned is part of the strategy for this screening programme and is made available via leaflets and on the web, for example, NHS Choices (2015).

- Her perception of risk may also increase if a family member, a friend or a media personality of a similar age (such as Jade Goody*) is identified as having cervical cancer.

ENSURING QUALITY OF INFORMATION

In 2000, the Bristol Royal Infirmary Inquiry from the DoH (2000) provided guidance on the quality of health.

Although old, many of the recommendations made in the report were related to information giving and still have poignancy.

- Information which should be provided for patients and carers. Information on treatment should be given in a variety of forms and in stages and reinforced over time (Recommendation 4).
- Information should be tailored to individual needs, circumstances and wishes (Recommendation 5).
- Information is to be based on currently available evidence with a summary, which is comprehensible to the client (Recommendation 6).
- Modes of providing information, whether leaflets, video/DVDs, tapes or CDs, should be regularly updated and developed with the help of patients (Recommendation 6).
- Clients should receive guidance on sources of information available on the Internet that are reliable and of good quality (Recommendation 9).

While not specifically developed for health promotion, these concepts are fundamental to public health and health promotion (DoH 2002, 29–30).

LEARNING ACTIVITY

Think about your communication with women and their families. Reflect on how you feel your communication measures up to the requirements suggested above.

There are several tools available to assess the quality of patient information, mainly looking at written and online sources (Moult et al. 2004; NHS 2011; National Cancer Institute 2015). The three key elements for written material identified are accuracy, clarity and relevance.

Accuracy:

- *Consistency:* Not contradicting itself, consistent layout and brand identifiable, for example, logos.
- *Continuity:* Information presented in the context of other resources, for example, Is it part of a series? Are other resources clearly signposted?
- *Current:* Is the information up to date? Is the date clearly presented? Are references or sources of information dated?
- *Reliability:* Is the information evidence based?

---

* Jade Goody was a reality TV celebrity, who at the age of 27 died from cervical cancer. Within the UK we saw a 12% increase across the UK in the number of women attending for the routine cervical smear screening, the majority encouraged by Jade and her story and also her linking (in the terminal stages of her disease) to Jo's Trust – a cervical cancer charity in the UK. Please see the links: https://en.wikipedia.org/wiki/Jade_Goody; https://www.jostrust.org.uk/

Clarity:

- *Appearance of text:* One font used throughout, no over-use of bold font.
- *Presentation:* Information summarised, bullet pointed, good line spacing, clearly labelled diagrams and images, style maintained throughout.
- *Content:* Sentences of not more than 20 words, jargon avoided, specialist terms or abbreviations explained.

Relevance:

- *Accessible:* Does the information meet the needs of the patient? Is it available in other languages and formats and is this information provided?
- *Appropriate:* Does it meet the needs of the target group?
- *Patient involvement:* Has the information been designed with input from patients and the public?

For Internet sources, the authors above and Breckons et al. (2008) also identify who runs/pays for the site? Is the site free of bias and how up to date is the information?

LEARNING ACTIVITY

- Acquire some leaflets or look at a website on a health topic that interests you and that the women in your area may access.
- Using the quality attributes, compare them for the aspects mentioned above.
- How easy was this to do?
- How much time did it take to achieve a good review of the leaflets you chose?
- Do you think that you could do this regularly to ensure that your clients are receiving high-quality information?

JUDGING THE ADEQUACY OF COMMUNICATION

Fischhoff et al. (2011) provides some guidance as to how to assess if the communication is adequate.

A communication is adequate if:

- It contains the information needed for effective decision making.
- Users can access that information.
- Users can comprehend what they access.

A materiality standard for communication content:

- A communication is adequate if it contains any information that might affect a significant fraction of users' choices.

A proximity standard for information accessibility:

- A communication is adequate if it puts most users within close proximity of the needed information, given their normal search patterns.

A comprehensibility standard user understanding:

- A communication is adequate if most users can extract enough information to make sound choices.

All of these quality tools require time and effort to use and are intended for the professional appraiser. When women read leaflets, they may need to discuss them, which can also take time. You may need to review the quality of information provided by your department so that you can discuss the issues with the woman with confidence. Face-to-face discussion is not especially easy to achieve and requires a variety of skills. Below are some suggestions for midwives using and reviewing different modes of communication.

FACE-TO-FACE COMMUNICATION

Pregnant women and new parents learn about childbirth and parenthood in different ways. One main source of information will be from midwives who are in an ideal position to provide health information (McNeill et al. 2012). Midwives spend a great deal of their time in face-to-face communication with women, couples and families, so they require effective communication skills. Effective communication underpins health information; it reduces anxiety and improves understanding which, in turn, helps clients to make informed choices (Hamilton & Martin 2007) (Box 7.1).

For verbal communication, four key elements are vital for quality (Hamilton & Martin 2007):

1. To listen carefully: Find out what information individual women want. Communication is not all one way and should involve finding out what the needs of the client or the community are (Wigens 2006). Some clients may require help from the midwife to articulate their needs, because this may be a new concept for them. Midwives need to be prepared to 'listen' to women. Listening is a skill often underestimated and is more important than the ability to hear, as it involves interpretation of the verbal and non-verbal communication that is taking place. The listener is required to give the person speaking time to express his or her opinions and needs. For some, voicing their own needs is not easy and the listener can help by paying attention, being encouraging, paraphrasing what is being said, reflecting feelings and meanings and then summing up to ensure that what has been said has been understood properly (Scriven 2010; England & Morgan 2012; Kourkouta & Papathanasiou 2014).
2. Explain things clearly, think carefully about what message is to be given and give it in an easily understandable manner. It may require the use of written material or DVD and so on to reinforce the information.
3. Show respect for what the client or the family has to say. Communication is rarely effective without respect being overtly shown. This entails acceptance of the woman and her family without judgment of who they are or their lifestyle.
4. Spend enough time with the client.

BOX 7.1: A framework for effective communication

1. INTERACT with the patient
2. Establish the INTENTION of the interaction
3. Decide on the INTERVENTION to be used
4. Assess the IMPACT of the intervention(s)
5. Evaluate the IMPLICATIONS of the subsequent information obtained and then act accordingly

Source: From Hamilton, Stephen J. & David J. Martin. 2007. Clinical development: A framework for effective communication skills. *Nursing Times* 103(48): 30–31.

Crafter (1997), England and Morgan (2012) and Davis and Day (2010) have given a few suggestions on how to facilitate face-to-face communication.

GENUINENESS

The woman knows that she is dealing with a 'real' person, so games or ploys are not necessary.

EMPATHY

Empathy means taking seriously the ideas, beliefs and concerns of the other party. It is the ability to put oneself in another person's position and see things from his or her perspective.

KINDNESS

Small acts of kindness are often remembered for a long time, as are perceived acts of unkindness.

HONESTY

Most people value honesty because it engenders trust. Dishonesty or concealment of information is usually discovered fairly quickly, and this can have long-term serious consequences for the woman in her dealings with all health professionals who she comes into contact with in the future.

DIPLOMACY

Diplomacy is necessary for skilled communication, especially when there is bad news to impart. It is a skill that develops with experience, often of previously poorly managed situations, and practice.

REFLECTION

Reflect on personal biases and prejudices that may affect the way you communicate with some women and their families. Also, reflection on practice can transform knowledge and experience into personal learning.

BALANCING SKILLS

Part of effective communication is being able to balance when to listen and when to provide information. Sometimes women will desire information, or they may need support for a decision that they have made about their care.

STANDING BACK

Standing back from a situation is a skill developed through self-awareness and experience. It allows the woman to make her choice and live with it, and respects her for her right to choose. For the midwife, it means not being personally affronted if a woman chooses to continue to smoke, or partake in health-damaging behaviour, but continuing to provide support that is non-judgmental of the person.

NON-ENGLISH SPEAKING

People with limited command of English often find it difficult to gain adequate information about health and may not be aware of how to access health care (Phul et al. 2003). For this population, it has been found that a one-to-one meeting is useful, although translators can make the information stilted. The use of verbal presentations, video/telephone translation and/or leaflets in the relevant language has all been found to be very useful to improve communication (Downing & Roat 2002).

All of the above-mentioned modes of communication can contribute to the development of a trusting relationship between the individual and the health promoter which, in turn, helps to promote acceptance of the message for health.

USING INFORMATION FROM THE MEDIA

Each format for providing information is influential, with the most influential being the mass media. Getting health messages across via the media has grown to a great extent in the past 30 years. The public now receives a vast amount of health messages through this mode, through watching television; listening to the radio; reading magazines, newspapers and leaflets; and viewing billboards and posters.

Messages about health are also provided as entertainment on the television and are considered to be a powerful tool for reaching a wide audience. Many soap operas have health messages within them and can portray healthy behaviours as normal (Verma et al. 2007). Television programmes can also portray risky behaviour such as heavy drinking or smoking but do not show the possible consequences of that behaviour (BBC 2008). Mass media can provide information to a wide population quickly, giving (or not giving) reminders of the effects of health-damaging behaviours and the benefits of adopting healthy behaviours (Naidoo & Wills 2009).

Raising awareness on its own is unlikely to lead to long-term changes in the health behaviour of individuals (Scriven 2010). The value of the acquisition of such knowledge is therefore debatable. However, as health becomes more prominent in the media, the subsequent widespread public awareness may make people discuss health more. What is recognised is the enormous potential that the media has to convey messages to large audiences (Green et al. 2015).

The use of mass media to convey health messages has had mixed success (Slater 2005). An example is the 'Change for Life' campaign which was started in 2009 by the DoH. It is a complex initiative using mass media to convey health messages. In one evaluation, the study group recognised the logo and were aware of the campaign, but the campaign had little impact on attitudes or behaviour (Croker et al. 2012). In 2003, the government launched the '5-A-DAY' campaign. This uses many different modes of communication to convey this health message to a wide spectrum of the public. A YouGov survey of 2,000 people for the World Cancer Research Fund found that, on average, 17% of lower income households eat at least five portions per day, compared with 27% for those in higher income groups (BBC 2012), which suggests partial success (BBC 2013).

Health is used as entertainment, but it is often the 'bad news' messages that generate some increased awareness of health issues which are often highlighted with shocking headlines. This can provide a distorted message to the public of the issue being discussed (Scriven 2010).

In addition, viewers may misinterpret or misunderstand the message being provided, whether positive or negative, which can be quite difficult to counteract, because viewers may think that the information is correct, especially if provided by an 'expert'. Midwives need to take time to listen to the perceived message and then to provide an alternative view, which may need to be backed up with written material.

PRACTICE POINTS

- There are many health messages being given by mass media. Be prepared to talk about them.
- Do not make the assumption that the targeted group for the health message will decide to take up the message and change behaviours.

USING LEAFLETS AND THE WRITTEN WORD

Clients have been shown to remember only about 20% of what they are told during a medical consultation. Up to 50% of what is discussed will be retained if written information is also provided (Moult et al. 2004). As mentioned above, there is approximately 5.2 million adults in England who are 'functionally illiterate' (Literacy Trust 2015). This means that some women may not be able to read a leaflet (or the information from a recommended web page).

Leaflets are considered expert opinion, but there is some evidence to show that different leaflets on the same topic are not always consistent in the information they provide, for example, use of different terminologies and different risk factors may cause confusion and distress (Jones 2003). There is a constant tension about what information should be provided – general advice or specific information – and how much (Payne 2002). The answer to these questions depends on the target audience and the aim of the circulation of the leaflet. When giving out a leaflet, the midwife should be aware of its content and be equipped to talk to the woman or her family about the content. Also, the midwife should be able to give information of where to go for further information.

LEARNING ACTIVITY

- Look again at the leaflets or web page you reviewed for quality.
- What information do they present: general or specific?
- Have you used them to give health information to women?
- If so, reflect on how you did this and if there is anything you might change in the future.

The manufacturers of health products advertise their goods in many different formats and this can include 'health promotion' leaflets that may be available to women at chemists, doctor's surgeries, health centres and antenatal clinics. Ensuring that the information is not misleading is important as they do have a vested interest to sell their product(s).

Leaflets are not a substitute for discussing issues with women and families, although they can be used effectively to introduce topics before discussion, such as HIV screening during the antenatal period, or as a memory aid for subjects such as postnatal exercises.

PRACTICE POINTS

- Health professionals have a responsibility to have read the leaflets they are giving out or to have looked at any website(s) suggested.
- By knowing what the content is, the HCP can discuss the topic with more confidence and answer questions.

USING INFORMATION TECHNOLOGY

Information technology (IT) has transformed communication with clients. IT has grown so much in recent years not only because of the great leap forward in the development of technology but also because there is a great hunger for information and a need to store and retrieve it efficiently. Books, DVDs, television and newspapers provide excellent everyday modes of mass communication, but computers, mobile phones and other handheld devices allow for ever more efficient communication. One in three people use their smart phones to access health information (Aungst 2012).

The Internet is one form of interactive mass media that has advanced rapidly in a very short span of time. Eighty-six per cent of the adult population has broadband access (ONS 2015) with 78% of adults accessing the Internet every day. Forty-nine per cent of people use computers to access health information (ONS 2015). The Internet does have advantages such as access to information that is specific and personal, access to information on demand, being distributed widely and updated easily. It also provides more choice, access to support from health care providers and communication with others with similar problems to exchange and share information (Office of Disease Prevention and Health Promotion 2014). In one small study, women were observed using the web to gain health information. The women felt that the Internet influenced their decision-making and improved their communication with their doctors. Their doctors were however considered the main source of information (Sillence et al. 2007). Care needs to be taken in relation to the reliability and accuracy of information (NHS Choices 2014; Eisenberg et al. 2015). Midwives need to be able to support clients accessing information on the web so that they can do so safely and feel confident to talk about what they have found out (Rogers & Mead 2004; Bernstam et al. 2005).

PRACTICE POINTS

- Leaflets and information sheets do not replace a discussion about the health topic.
- Leaflets and information sheets are to back up what has been discussed and act as a memory aid for the woman when she returns home.
- Remember there is a substantial number of women who may find it difficult to comprehend what is presented to them in the form of leaflets or on the web.
- Always check their understanding.

The use of leaflets and also the Internet are invaluable resources for the women and midwives, but the quality of the information is to be ensured. If leaflets are given out or web pages are being recommended, make sure that they are checked because they are subject to frequent change. Suggesting the use of the Internet for acquiring information comes with the responsibility to remind the users that the information provided in chat rooms and on some websites may be of a poor quality or inaccurate. Information comes in so many formats and midwives should make themselves available to discuss issues that may be raised from the information found and to review the quality of the information retrieved.

SUMMARY

- When giving health information, think about using more than one format; it may help to make the message more understandable, for example, verbal, written, use of DVDs or CDs and web pages.
- Before providing information to women or their families, consider carefully what you want to convey, where the information is being given and the amount of time that you have.
- Midwives need to listen to women to find out their personal attitudes and opinions on health. Information may need to be repeated several times because, depending on the circumstances of the woman, she may or may not be ready to accept or use the information at a certain point in time.
- The quality of the information is an important factor. Quality assurance is a time-consuming practice but worth doing to ensure that clients have the best available information on which to base any health choices.
- Quality applies to all modes of information provision. It is particularly relevant in mass media and the Internet. Midwives need to evaluate the quality of information that they may be given by women under their care.
- The mass media are a very powerful tool for providing information to a wide audience but misinterpretations or misunderstandings can, and do, arise.
- Spending time with women who gather information from the Internet or who want to discuss something that they saw on television can be time-consuming but will help women to make more informed choices.

REFERENCES

Anderson, Lanette. 2012. *How effective is our nursing communication? Nurse together.com.* http://www.nursetogether.com/how-effective-our-nursing-communication (accessed September 2015).

Aungst, Timothy. 2012. *Smartphones and access to health information, results of a Pew Internet Research Project.* http://www.imedicalapps.com/2012/11/smartphones-health-information-results-pew-research/ (accessed September 2015).

BBC. 2008. *Soaps 'miss out health messages'.* http://news.bbc.co.uk/1/hi/health/7802985.stm (accessed September 2015).

BBC. 2012. *Only one in five eats five a day, poll suggests.* http://www.bbc.co.uk/news/health-18032209 (accessed September 2015).

BBC. 2013. *Five-a-day campaign: A partial success.* http://www.bbc.co.uk/news/health-20858809 (accessed September 2015).

Becker, Marshall H. (ed.). 1974. *The health belief model and personal health behaviour.* Thorofare, NJ: Slack.

Bernstam, Elmer, Dawn Shelton, Muhammad Walji & Funda Meric-Berstam. 2005. Instruments to assess the quality of health information on the World Wide Web: What can our patients actually use? *International Journal of Medical Informatics* 74: 13–19.

Breckons, Matthew, Ray Jones, Jenny Morris & Janet Richardson. 2008. What do evaluation instruments tell us about the quality of complementary medicine information on the Internet? *Journal of Medical Internet Research* 10(1): e3.

Crafter, Helen (ed.). 1997. Midwives and communication. In *Health promotion in midwifery: Principles and practice,* Crafter Helen (Ed.), pp. 105–124. London: Arnold.

Croker, Helen, Rebecca Lucas & Jane Wardle. 2012. Cluster-randomised trial to evaluate the 'Change for Life' mass media/social marketing campaign in the UK. *BMC Public Health* 12: 404.

Davis, Hilton & Crispin Day. 2010. *The family partnership model.* London: The Psychology Trust.

DoH (Department of Health). 2000. *Final report of the Bristol Royal Infirmary inquiry.* http://webarchive.nationalarchives.gov.uk/20090811143745/; http://www.bristol-inquiry.org.uk/final_report/report/index.htm (accessed September 2015).

DoH (Department of Health). 2002. *Learning from Bristol; The Department of Health's Response to the Report of the Public Inquiry into children's heart surgery at the Bristol Royal Infirmary 1984–1995.* London: TSO. http://webarchive.nationalarchives.gov.uk/20130107105354/; http://www.dh.gov.uk/prod_consum_dh/groups/dh_digitalassets/@dh/@en/documents/digitalasset/dh_4059479.pdf (accessed September 2015).

DoH (Department of Health). 2012. *The power of information: Putting all of us in control of the health and care information we need.* DoH. https://www.gov.uk/government/uploads/system/uploads/attachment_data/file/213689/dh_134205.pdf (accessed 21 September 2015).

Downing, Bruce & Cynthia E. Roat. 2002. *Models for the provision of language access in health care settings.* Hablamos Juntos and the National Council on Interpreting in Health Care. http://hablamosjuntos.org/pdf_files/Models_for_the_Provision_of_Language_Access_final_.pdf (accessed September 2015).

England, Carole & Ransolina Morgan. 2012. *Communication skills for midwives.* Maidenhead: Open University Press.

Eisenberg, Staci, Megan H. Bair-Merritt, Eve R. Colson, Timothy C. Heeren, Nicole L. Geller & Michael J. Corwin. 2015. Maternal report of advice received for infant care. *Pediatrics* 136(2): e315–e322.

Eysenbach, Gunther, John Powell, Marina Englesakis, Carlos Rizo & Anita Stern. 2004. Health related virtual communities and electronic support groups: Systematic review of the effects of online peer to peer interactions. *BMJ* 328: 1166.

Fischhoff, Baruch, Noel T. Brewer & Julie S. Downs. 2011. *Communicating risks and benefits: an evidence based users guide.* Silver Spring, MD, FDA. http://www.fda.gov/downloads/AboutFDA/ReportsManualsForms/Reports/UCM268069.pdf (accessed September 2015).

Hamilton, Stephen J. & David J. Martin. 2007. Clinical development: A framework for effective communication skills. *Nursing Times* 103(48): 30–31.

Green, Jackie, Keith Tones, Ruth Cross & James Woodall. 2015. *Health promotion planning & strategies* (3rd ed.). London: Sage.

Jones, Sandra. 2003. A review of the consistency of breast cancer screening pamphlets produced by health authorities in Australia. *Health Education* 103: 166–176.

Kourkouta, Lambrini & Ioanna V. Papathanasiou. 2014. Communication in nursing practice. *Materia Sociomed* 26(1): 65–67.

Literacy Trust. 2015. *Literacy rates in UK.* http://www.literacytrust.org.uk/adult_literacy/illiterate_adults_in_england (accessed September 2015).

Malone, Mary, Alison E. While & Julia Roberts. 2014. Parental health information seeking and re-exploration of the 'digital divide'. *Primary Health Care Research & Development. Primary Health Care Research and Development* 15(2): 202–212.

McNeill, Jenny, Jackie Doran, Fiona Lynn, Gail Anderson & Fiona Alderdice. 2012. Public health education for midwives and midwifery students: A mixed methods study. *BMC Pregnancy and Childbirth* 2012(12): 142. http://www.biomedcentral.com/1471-2393/12/142 (accessed September 2015).

Miller, William & Stephen Rollnick. 2012. *Motivational interviewing, helping people change.* New York: Guilford Press.

Moult, Beki, Linda Frank & Helen Brady. 2004. Ensuring quality information for patients: Development and preliminary validation of a new instrument to improve the quality of written health care information. *Health Expectations* 7: 165–175.

Naidoo, Jeanie & Jane Wills. 2009. *Health promotion foundations for practice* (3rd ed.). Edinburgh: Baillière Tindall.

National Cancer Institute. 2015. *Using trusted resources.* http://www.cancer.gov/about-cancer/managing-care/using-trusted-resources (accessed September 2015).

NHS. 2011. *NHS brand guidelines.* NHS. http://www.nhsidentity.nhs.uk/tools-and-resources/patient-information/written-information%3a-general-guidance (accessed September 2015).

NHS Choices. 2014. *Staying safe on line.* http://www.nhs.uk/aboutNHSChoices/aboutnhschoices/staying-safe-online/Pages/find-health-information-online.aspx (accessed September 2015).

NHS Choices. 2015. *Cervical cancer—Symptoms.* http://www.nhs.uk/Conditions/Cancer-of-the-cervix/Pages/Symptoms.aspx (accessed September 2015).

Office of Disease Prevention and Health Promotion. 2014. *Health communication and health information technology.* Washington, DC: US Department of Health and Human Services. https://www.healthypeople.gov/2020/topics-objectives/topic/health-communication-and-health-information-technology (accessed September 2015).

ONS (Office of National Statistics). 2015. *Statistics bulletin Internet access—Households and individuals 2015.* http://www.ons.gov.uk/ons/dcp171778_412758.pdf (accessed September 2015).

Payne, Sheila. 2002. Balancing information needs: Dilemmas in producing patient leaflets. *Health Informatics Journal* 8: 174–179.

Phul, Ashley, Peter Bath & M. Jackson. 2003. The provision of information by health promotion units to people of Asian origin living in the UK. *Health Informatics Journal* 9: 39–56.

Rogers, Anne & Nicola Mead. 2004. More than technology and access: Primary care patients' views on the use and non-use of health information in the Internet age. *Health and Social Care in the Community* 12: 102–110.

Scriven, Angela. 2010. *Promoting health: A practical guide* (6th ed.). Edinburgh: Baillière Tindall.

Sillence, Elizabeth, Pam Briggs, Peter Harris & Lesley Fishwick. 2007. How do patients evaluate and make use of online health information? *Social Science & Medicine* 64(9): 1853–1862.

Slater, Michael. 2005. Mediated communication. In *ABC of health behavior: A guide to successful disease prevention and health promotion,* edited by Jacqueline Kerr, Rolf Weitkunat & Manuel Moretti, 303–314. Edinburgh: Elsevier.

Verma, T., Jean Adams & Martin White. 2007. Portrayal of health-related behaviours in popular UK television soap operas. *Journal of Epidemiology and Community Health* 61(7): 575–577.

Vögele, Claus. 2005. Education. In *ABC of health behavior: A guide to successful disease prevention and health promotion,* edited by Jacqueline Kerr, Rolf Weitkunat and Manuel Morretti. Edinburgh: Elsevier.

Wigens, Lynne. 2006. *Communication in clinical settings.* Cheltenham: Nelson Thornes.

Witte, Kim. 1994. The manipulative nature of health communication research: Ethical issues and guideline. *American Behavioral Scientist* 38: 385–393.

FURTHER READINGS

Medline guide to healthy web surfing. 2015. https://www.nlm.nih.gov/medlineplus/healthywebsurfing.html

Medline Plus. 2014. *Evaluating health information.* https://www.nlm.nih.gov/medlineplus/evaluatinghealthinformation.html

U.S. Department of Health and Human Services, Office of Disease Prevention and Health Promotion. 2010. *Health literacy online: A guide to writing and designing easy-to-use health Web sites.* Washington, DC: U.S. Department of Health and Human Services, Office of Disease Prevention and Health Promotion. http://health.gov/healthliteracyonline/Web_Guide_Health_Lit_Online.pdf

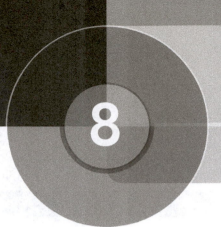

8

Partnership working and midwifery: Interprofessional, interagency and intersectoral

EDDIE WEST-BURNHAM

INTRODUCTION

Better is possible. It does not take genius. It takes diligence. It takes moral clarity. It takes ingenuity. And above all, it takes a willingness to try.

Gawande (2007, 246)

Much has been written on the links of poor health status, inequalities and material deprivation. As part of the present government's attempt to address this issue, considerable focus has been placed on the benefits of partnership working; indeed, it has become one of the 'fundamental principles' in delivering on the health inequalities agenda. With a key role in public health, the midwife needs to develop an understanding of the concept of partnership working and the midwife's role within it.

This concept of partnership working is not a new one, but as far as current policy development is concerned, it has emerged from being taken for granted and largely in the background to taking centre stage. So although it may be considered de rigueur by those writing public health policies, strategies and guidelines, what it means, how it works and how successful it could be can provide a considerable challenge to those health professionals, including midwives, who are charged with working with the concept.

This chapter will consider the importance and relevance of partnership working in midwifery practice. It cannot provide a one-size-fits-all template detailing how the perfect partnership will be achieved. It will, however, offer a range of options enabling the practitioners to pick and choose the key elements to fit their own particular public health scenario.

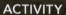
BACKGROUND

Public health is anticipatory, focusing on the prevention of illness rather than the provision of treatment and care. It is entrenched in the positive theory of health and is concerned with the promotion of health and social well-being in its widest sense (Donaldson & Scully 2009). This need to improve and protect the health of a population has existed for millennia – the Romans' approach to sanitation is an example. The development of public health in the United Kingdom truly started in the nineteenth century following the Chadwick report after the cholera epidemics in 1842. This raised the issue of health problems being linked to poor housing and insanitary conditions (Scriven 2010). Although progress in this concept was slow for the next 100 years or so, it was the creation of the National Health Service (NHS) in 1948 and its subsequent numerous reorganisations that led to a revival in public health strategies from the 1970s onwards.

This revival was influenced by a number of documents published by the World Health Organization (WHO) during the 1970s and 1980s, which were influential in the development and thinking about health promotion and public health, the most significant being the Ottawa Charter (WHO 1986). This charter identified three broad strategies for working to promote health:

1. *Advocacy:* to ensure the creation of conditions favourable to health.
2. *Enabling:* through creating a supportive environment but also giving people the information and skills that they need to make healthy choices.
3. *Mediation:* between different groups to ensure the pursuit of health.

The opportunities for the midwife to use her public health knowledge and health promotion skills within the first two strategies are clear. However, the focus of this chapter is on the third point – partnership working. It is here that there is a danger that midwives will be excluded as most partnership working is driven through primary care and public health networks, where there is little formal contact with midwives (West-Burnham 2006).

It is however important to remember that midwives work in partnership every day they practice; each delivery, consultation and examination is done in partnership with women, their partners and families as well as other members of the multidisciplinary team to achieve a positive outcome (Miller & Wilkes 2015). This is especially so when working with women who may be particularly vulnerable or at risk. In these instances, midwives will work with a range of different agents to achieve a positive experience and outcome (Miller & Wilkes 2015; PHE 2013a).

As part of the commitment to *Health for All by the Year 2000* (WHO 1985), the WHO outlined a set of guiding principles with which to orientate health promotion work, including:

- Equity
- Empowerment
- Community participation
- Multi-sectoral collaboration
- Emphasis on primary health

The suppression and the eventual publication of the Black Report in 1981, and the emergence of the international agenda for health promotion, brought to the fore the need for closer working relationships to meet the growing emphasis being placed on public health.

The white paper 'Healthy lives, healthy people: Our strategy for public health in England' (DoH 2010) is the latest in a long line of government white papers on health and its promotion, and it offers a great opportunity to make a profound and sustained approach to improve the public health of the population. Indeed, even though it was written over a decade ago, the statement from Dowling et al. (2004, 309) is as pertinent today as it was then: 'it is difficult to find a contemporary policy document or set of good practice guidelines that does not have collaboration as the central strategy for the delivery of welfare'.

Equally there have been a number of recent publications that have identified the important role that midwives have within public health. In 2013, a series of documents, that were developed by the DoH and Public Health England (PHE) in partnership with the Royal College of Midwives (RCM) and the Royal College of Nursing (RCN), were published.

The 'Midwifery Public Health Contribution' (PHE 2013a), 'Nursing and Midwifery Contribution to Public Health' (PHE 2013b) and the 'Evidence Base of the Public Health Contribution of Nurses and Midwives' (PHE 2013c) clearly show the role of the midwives in public health and how their actions can be maximised to impact at multiple levels and within the approaches that require partnership to best succeed.

The Midwifery 2020 report (Midwifery 2020 Programme 2010) scoped the role of the midwife in terms of public health and identified a ground-level role, which all midwives meet, and a strategic role in the form of consultant midwife, with public health specialism incorporating the skills of collaboration and partnership working.

Partnership working is not a new area for midwives to work. The success of midwifery partnership projects within the Sure-Start and Sure-Start Plus programmes (Lewis 2004), weight management interventions and perinatal domestic abuse programmes offers strong practical examples of all these policy recommendations regarding the midwife's role in public health (NICE 2010; Williams et al. 2013). However, it is an area that needs continued strengthening.

DEFINING PARTNERSHIP WORKING

Partnership working takes many forms and the terminology used to describe it varies enormously; to start with, there are numerous different terms, including

- Working together
- Integration
- Interdisciplinary partnership working
- Joined up thinking/working
- Cooperative working
- Collaboration
- Multidisciplinary working
- Strategic alliance
- Multi-agency
- Intersectoral
- Coalition
- Transdisciplinary working
- Synergistic working

With a plethora of terms, it is no surprise that there is a multitude of definitions as to what partnership working is. Within the commercial world where partnership working has a long history, the World Bank Partnership group (1998) indicated that it is a collaborative relationship which works towards shared objectives via an agreed division of labour.

Others have chosen to define partnership with regard to the extent that partnership could work. Percy-Smith (2005, 28–29) used this approach by devising a ladder definition of partnership:

- *Information exchange:* Involving mutual learning, knowledge of what each partner does and could do, openness about decision-making processes, new methods of access to information.
- *Planning action:* Involving identifying local and service needs where cross boundary working is needed and could be effective. Debate of local needs and priorities, agree different partners' contributions, and decide actions and processes. Identify (the need for) new partners.
- *Implementing projects and service plans:* Joint or separate action taken on agreed plan, identify monitoring methods and review processes, mutual feedback on success/failure.
- *Coordination and cooperation in practice:* Involving active coordination process; coordinator knows what's going on, draws on each (autonomous) partner as appropriate, and helps to nurture developmental and cooperative culture and involve and support new partners.
- *Collaboration and full partnership:* Involving separate and distinct roles but shared values and agenda. Pooled resources, blurred boundaries, continuously developing to meet changing needs. Less powerful partners supported to play a full role.

Within in health and social care definitions have also been set have been within the concept of compassion in practice (PHE 2013b) which can be best seen in the following definition (Tunnard 1991, cited in Jackson & Morris 1994, 1):

> The essence of partnership is sharing. It is marked by respect for one another, role divisions, rights to information, accountability, competence, and value accorded to individual input.
> In short, each partner is seen as having something to contribute, power is shared, decisions are made jointly and roles are not only respected but are also backed by legal and moral rights.

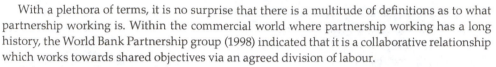

WHY IS PARTNERSHIP IMPORTANT AND WHAT WORKS?

What are the benefits of partnership working? More significantly, are there any benefits to partnership working (Ross et al. 2015) or is it, as many who have tried and failed to get a partnership up and running would suggest, a bureaucratic nightmare and an unnecessary distraction from getting the work done?

Despite the anxieties felt by many, there is an emerging evidence base testifying for the benefits for both service users and service providers of working in partnership with other services (Hogg et al. 2013; Williams et al. 2013). A partnership approach founded on cooperation and collaboration between all relevant providers will have a number of benefits for service users. The Department of Health provides a very strong critique of agencies that fail to work in partnership, setting out a clear rationale why services must work together more effectively (DoH 1998, 3):

> All too often when people have complex needs spanning both health and social care good quality services are sacrificed for sterile arguments about boundaries. When this happens, people, often the most vulnerable in our society … and those who care for

them find themselves in the no man's land between health and social services. This is not what people want or need. It places the needs of the organisation above the needs of the people they are there to serve. It is poor organisation, poor practice, poor use of taxpayers' money – it is unacceptable.

To achieve a successful partnership, that being an arrangement between two or more groups, organisations or individuals to work together to achieve common aim(s), there needs to be a number of key principles in place. Hudson (2000) defines a number of key principles for strengthening strategic approaches to collaboration:

- *Shared vision:* Specifying what is to be achieved in terms of user-centred goals, clarifying the purpose of collaboration as a mechanism for achieving such goals, and mobilising commitment around goals, outcomes and mechanisms.
- *Clarity of roles and responsibilities:* Specifying and agreeing 'who does what', and designing organisational arrangements by which roles and responsibilities are to be fulfilled.
- *Appropriate incentives and rewards:* Promoting organisational behaviour consistent with agreed goals and responsibilities, and harnessing organisational self-interest to collective goals.
- *Accountability for joint working:* Monitoring achievements in relation to the stated vision, holding individuals and agencies accountable for the fulfilment of pre-determined roles and responsibilities, and providing feedback and review of vision, responsibilities, incentives, and their inter-relationship.

The current economic climate has placed unprecedented pressure on the public purse, most significantly health and social care. In the eyes of many, partnership working offers an opportunity to provide financial benefit and achieve better use of scarce resources by innovation and the creative use of existing resources, the elimination of duplication, the creation of cost-effective pathways and the delivery of seamless services.

Added to this, partnerships usually have the following characteristics:

All stakeholders must

- Have a degree of personal investment in the partnership
- Trust each other
- Have respect for what each partner brings to the relationship
- Have similar value systems
- Agree that a partnership is necessary
- Understand what each stakeholder can contribute and place a degree of value on his or her uniqueness

LEARNING ACTIVITY

Review the characteristics in the box above and apply them to a public health intervention you are involved in such as a breastfeeding café or perinatal mental health support group.

Does this partnership have these characteristics? Are there barriers to these characteristics being achieved?

Partnerships can work in different ways and there is no one model that can be considered to be the 'best'. There are, however, a number of ingredients which – if present – will facilitate successful partnership working.

The Partnership Readiness Framework (Greig & Poxton 2001) is one particularly useful approach to consider how best to mix the key ingredients of effective partnership working. If used effectively, it can gauge different partners' perspectives of how well the different dimensions and aspects of a partnership are functioning and developing at any given time.

This information can be used to:

- Identify priorities for aligning goals and outcomes.
- Identify and share available skills and resources across the partnership or local system.
- Identify priorities and actions to improve local service delivery and the nature of local partnership working.

The framework can also be used over a period of time to see how the partnership evolves and develops in response to its environment and the needs/priorities of local communities it is serving.

The quality of the information that is gathered will form a positive foundation on which to build a plan that all parties can sign up to with a vision that is agreed and understood; however, it does not matter how much quantitative or qualitative data are available if other key elements are not in place.

- The partnership has clear, effective leadership.
- The role of each partner is identified and is clear to others in the partnership.
- There is shared ownership of the partnership and the partners feel there is 'something in it for them'.
- There are dedicated resources and time for the administration and operation of the partnership.

Added to this is the need to recognise the impact of culture and the significant differences organisational cultures within the partnership can have. As Kruse and Louis (2009) highlight, culture describes 'how things are' and 'how things operate' and reflects how we view the world. In order to change a culture, it is necessary first to understand the current model in action and understand the priorities for all parties involved.

If there is sufficient understanding of the cultural needs (both organisational and across the area of operation), it will help develop trust and create a supportive atmosphere where suggestions and ideas can be developed and conflicts addressed. The strength of a combined approach to resolving a particular issue is often lost because the demands of the few (often larger) stakeholders can overwhelm the collective desire of the many – such is the short-sighted nature of UK policy.

> The power of collective capacity is that it enables ordinary people to accomplish extraordinary things – for two reasons. One is that knowledge about effective practice becomes more widely available and accessible on a daily basis. The second reason is more powerful still – working together generates commitment. Moral purpose when it stares you in the face through students and your peers working together to make lives and society better, is palpable, indeed virtually irresistible. The collective motivational well seems bottomless.
>
> Fullan (2010, 72)

Anyone working in health and social care will be aware of the term 'silo thinking' and how pervasive it is in certain organisational cultures. A *silo mentality* has been defined as 'an attitude found in some organisations that occurs when several departments or groups do not want to share information or knowledge with other individuals in the same company' (www.investopedia.com/terms/s/silo-mentality.asp). A silo mentality reduces efficiency and actively contributes to failing partnership opportunities. Silo working persists across the NHS and within the current system of partnership working.

LEARNING ACTIVITY

Reflect on the term silo mentality and identify how it could impact on setting up a health intervention that requires a partnership approach.

STAKEHOLDER ENGAGEMENT AND SERVICE USER BENEFIT

The choice of partner and level of engagement from stakeholders is hugely important. Partnerships are formed for many different reasons; the Audit Commission offers five main reasons as to why agencies might want to develop partnerships (Dickenson & Glasby 2008).

- To deliver coordinated packages of care to people
- To tackle so-called wicked issues (i.e. cross-cutting, complex problems where we do not really know the best way of responding to the issue at stake)
- To reduce the impact of organisational fragmentation and minimise the impact of any perverse incentives that arise from it
- To bid for, or gain access to, new resources
- To meet a statutory requirement

Another reason often cited is the somewhat woolly notion of *added value*. This is one of the more challenging phrases that many in public health face. It is clear, however, that when it works well, partnership working does create added value and enable something to be achieved that would not be realised individually.

Many partnerships evolve from existing networks or where there is a history of collaborative work between potential partners. This is not always healthy and very often there are circumstances where it is important to invite new partners to the table.

Very often the question has to be asked as to which is more important for practitioners and the organisation they work for; to stand alone and look after their own interests or to work as part of a bigger entity. This is especially true for 'third sector' partners – the voluntary organisations and charities but is becoming more significant for NHS organisations. But, what of the needs and benefits to service users?

Research would suggest that one of the key advantages for service users is improvements of services. Kennedy et al. (2001), researching good practice in multi-agency working on homelessness, found that services were improved for those clients who were accessing more than one service or organisation – especially those using jointly provided services or those within multi-agency case review meetings. Two particular aspects of improved services for service users were reported: better access to services and services having a more preventative/early intervention focus.

Within midwifery, works by Power (2015) and Garrod (2012) have highlighted the importance of engaging with service users, their partners and families to look at care provision and the development of partnership working that includes women, their partners and families as an equal partner, besides strengthening social capital and the health benefits that it brings

(West-Burnham 2006). Midwives are well placed to develop social health gain by encouraging and sustaining the promotion of social networks and social capital, aided by their experiences of working within communities (Piper 2005).

It is important to identify that it is not always plain sailing; the role of the voluntary and community sector and of service users and carers is often unclear in partnerships and integrated teams. There is rarely clarity about whether this is expected to be an advocacy, operational, representative or strategic role (Marks 2007).

BARRIERS TO PARTNERSHIP WORKING

For all the positive statements and opportunities relating to partnership working, the ever changing face of health, social care and education in the United Kingdom often results in partnerships being destabilised by the constant reforms in policy. This is especially true in public health where changes in national agenda have significantly disrupted the delivery of services. The public health white paper, 'Healthy lives, healthy people' (DoH 2010), outlined major changes in the way in which public health services have been commissioned and delivered.

There are many obstacles thrown in the way for potential collaborators to overcome at individual, organisational and structural level – even when it appears that all the key elements are in place. Barriers can be of a practical nature, such as policy dictates, or softer, such as attitudes of particular stakeholders. For example, even where there may be pockets of high trust among like-minded midwives in a maternity unit, there may be weak relational trust within the larger organisation or distrust between the management hierarchies.

In their research looking at partnerships and public health, Taylor-Robinson et al. (2012) highlight the complexity of decision making as particularly challenging, especially the perception of limited influence at the local level. Decisions were felt to be taken at a national (government) or international (European Union or World Health Organisation) level, with population-wide primary prevention thought only to be effectively tackled through national or international efforts. There was the sense that this could lead to a feeling of being overwhelmed by the complexity of the task.

With the focus on joint working and current demands to integrate, there is often an expectation that voluntary organisations and public sector agencies will work together and form partnerships. In research looking at power, conflicts and resolutions, Pettigrew (2003) found from the experience of managers from both the voluntary and public sectors, who are involved in a wide range of partnerships, a variety of reasons for failure, including

- Gaps in the organisational membership required for the purpose of the partnership (often private businesses in partnerships led by the public sector)
- Unwilling participant organisations and senior managers 'just turning up' because of a sense of duty rather than being actively involved
- Conflicting and sometimes hidden agendas, goals and targets between participant organisations and the partnership
- Conflicting allocation of resources/funding between partnerships where one organisation or agency is a member of each (or several) partnership(s) competing for resources/funding
- Hostility or suspicion about knowledge sharing between agencies
- Conflicting professional cultures and practices in the participating agencies (e.g. between health and social care)

- Inadequate resources available to support and sustain the work of the partnership
- Power struggles between member organisations within the partnership
- A history of previous difficult relationships between partners

This multisectoral approach requires strong leadership and a shared vision which articulates an approach to political, economic, social and technological analysis as well as financial, moral and ethical dimensions. To achieve this, a mutually agreed framework which encompasses the competing needs of diverse stakeholders often with conflicting priorities is required. The development of collaborative leadership will better enable managers to resolve conflicts and navigate through the complex policy framework and the ever present financial challenges.

LEARNING ACTIVITY

Review the reasons why partnership working fails and apply these points to a multi-agency health intervention within your practice area. Identify in what ways these could be prevented.

The economic downturn has also had an impact on the appetite for partnership working. There are significant costs to partnership working which can result in tensions, not least the arguments about who will provide what and where does the accountability lie. There are also obstacles to overcome in trying to identify whether the outcomes justify the costs and the necessary investment.

The right attitude is hugely important, both externally to key stakeholders and internally to own operations. As with any relationship, transparency and honesty is key to establishing a successful rapport. Always treat others as you would expect to be treated yourself. As Herold and Fedor (2008, 10) suggest, 'People do not *"naturally"* resist change; they resist change they do not understand, the value of which they do not see, or the demands of which they cannot meet'.

Another issue is language. How midwives communicate and build relationships is central to achieving successful outcomes at an individual as well as a strategic level. The core skills of communication and developing and establishing partnerships with women and their families, especially in relation to issues of inclusion, inequality, empowerment, participation and power dynamics, are vital. At a strategic level, establishing a positive partnership with colleagues (paid and unpaid) can help to overcome perceived boundaries between services and organisations, and support the development of working that will be of benefit to patients and people who use our services. Developing a shared language and common understanding of terms used locally to describe ways of working together can make a significant impact on this partnership.

The same could be said of the NHS, the organisations delivering social care and service users. It would be important to ensure a common understanding of the words to be used to prevent language being used as a barrier and a divisive tool between the partner groups.

In summary, Hudson (2000) condenses these into five key barriers to achieving effective partnership working, which include:

- Structural (the fragmentation of service responsibilities across and within agency boundaries)
- Procedural (differences in planning and budget cycles)
- Financial (differences in funding mechanisms and resource flows)
- Professional (differences in ideologies, values and professional interests)
- Perceived threats to status, autonomy and legitimacy

It is worth remembering that a failed partnership can have a significant domino effect, often leaving a long-term legacy of mistrust or conflict between different individuals or organisations. Egos can get in the way, and sabotage good working relationships leaving individuals compromised in their organisation and community.

BENEFITS TO PARTNERSHIP WORKING

As Ballach and Taylor (2001, 1) observe, 'Superficially, partnership working makes a lot of sense'. Partnerships are a dynamic entity and as such the expectations and relationships are constantly evolving in a manner similar to that of the group. Establishing and maintaining a partnership is a complex, challenging process requiring commitment, patience, tolerance, trust, respect, a healthy dose of pragmatism and practical understanding. The success, or otherwise, of a partnership depends as much on the investment, commitment skills and attitude of the individual as on the engagement of the individual's host agency and the structure/environment in which the relationship exists.

This opportunity for successful collaboration needs to be built, as Nutbeam and Harris (2010) acknowledge, on the foundations of necessity and opportunity. As highlighted earlier, the recent documents identifying the contribution midwives make to public health fully recognise the skills and knowledge they have (PHE 2013a, 2013b, 2013c). These skills are often used on a one-to-one or small group basis, such as supporting a newly delivered mother to breastfeed her baby or undertaking antenatal education classes. These policy documents now highlight the impact midwives could have at community and population levels as well as maximise and strengthen their public health skills, such as developing social health gains with social capital building and social networking.

Effective public health must be based on the WHO principles promoting upstream health interventions to prevent the development of avoidable ill health rather than the traditional focus on downstream medical intervention that often treats preventable diseases. Public health requires action at all levels of the policy continuum, and any health care or social care professional working to a public health 'brief' has to engage in partnership working.

Working across a health economy, public health practitioners (i.e. any individual working to improve the health of the general public) need to join with other key stakeholders in housing, education, police, youth services and environmental health. The role of the midwife offers a unique opportunity to identify some of those individuals who are experiencing health inequalities and who are most vulnerable to any number of physical, social or psychological problems (West-Burnham 2006).

Numerous opportunities exist in the health-promoting role of the midwife to develop partnership working. Two particular areas are highlighted here – promoting breastfeeding and reducing the prevalence of smoking in pregnancy and beyond.

Promoting breastfeeding has many physical and psychosocial benefits for both mother and child, including lowering the incidence and severity of many infections and protection from many adverse health outcomes such as reduction in the risk of type 2 diabetes and cardiovascular problems later in life for the infant and a reduction in the risk of breast and ovarian cancer and hip fractures for the mother. Evidence shows that these health improvements are both short term and long term, benefitting individuals as well as whole populations (UNICEF 2012 and see chapter 9 on breastfeeding).

There are numerous opportunities to promote breastfeeding that go beyond the normal interaction that the midwife will have with the mother. By taking a partnership approach to offering continuous psychosocial and emotional support before childbirth, during labour and in the months after, both professionals and appropriately trained and supported laypeople could assist the mother and promote the benefits of breastfeeding.

It has been well documented that smoking has many potential problems for the woman, the fetus and the neonate, including raised blood pressure, reduced birth weight and increased risk of sudden infant death syndrome (see Chapter 16, Smoking, Pregnancy and The Midwife). Evidence as with breastfeeding indicates both short- and long-term health benefits to the woman, her baby and family as well as the wider community and the general population.

Good partnership working is critical for building an economic, effective and efficient health and social care system across the United Kingdom and within it a series of strong, effective relationships within and across organisations.

SUMMARY

- The essence of partnership is sharing.
- It is marked by respect for one another, role divisions, rights to information, accountability, competence, and value accorded to individual input.
- For effective partnerships to achieve success, it requires open, transparent communication, efficient transmission of information and social and professional interaction within and across networks.
- Many people make assumptions about the role of the midwife and get it wrong. It is the role of the midwife to communicate and clarify how specialised their role is and what they will bring to the partnership.
- There needs to be an acknowledgement of differences in power. Many partnerships will/ should include service user representation of some kind. It is important that non-professionals feel included and are encouraged to contribute to discussions and that all views are taken on board – including those of a parent, child or lay person.
- Communication (both vertical and horizontal) is key, not just with families and outside agencies but within the midwife's host organisation.
- Effective partnership working is not easy – it takes time, commitment, resources and a range of other elements.
- Consequently, no partnership should be entered into lightly; it has to have a strong rationale and ultimately result in good-quality care and support for women and their needs relating to pregnancy, childbirth and the newborn.
- It is vital for midwives to realise their full potential in partnership working and public health, and it is important for them to engage fully with those involved at all levels of strategic development and to get involved at the community level and the population level.

REFERENCES

Ballach, Susan & Marilyn Taylor. 2001. *Partnership working: Policy and practice.* Bristol: The Policy Press.

Dickenson, Helen & Jon Glasby. 2008. Getting the measure of partnerships. *Community Care,* 30–31 September.

DoH (Department of Health). 1998. *Partnership in action: New opportunities for joint working between health and social services – A discussion document.* London: Department of Health.

DoH (Department of Health). 2010. *Healthy lives, healthy people: Our strategy for public health in England*. https://www.gov.uk/government/publications/healthy-lives-healthy-people-our-strategy-for-public-health-in-england

Donaldson, Liam J. & Gabriel Scully. 2009. *Donaldson's essential public health* (3rd ed.). Padstow: Radcliffe.

Dowling, Bernard, Martin Powell & Caroline Glendinning. 2004. Conceptualising successful partnerships. *Health and Social Care in the Community* 12(4): 309–317.

Fullan, Michael. 2010. *All systems go: The change imperative for whole-system reform*. London: Sage.

Garrod, Debbie. 2012. TALKBACK: A strategic approach to working with maternity service users. *The Practicing Midwife* 15(4): 18–20.

Gawande, Atul. 2007. *Better: A surgeon's notes on performance*. New York: Picador.

Greig, Rob & Richard Poxton. 2001. From joint commission to partnership working: Will the New Policy Framework make a difference. *International Journal of Integrated Care* 9(4): 32–38.

Herold, David & Donald Fedor. 2008. *Change the way you lead change: Leadership strategies that really work*. Stanford, CA: Stanford University Press.

Hogg, Rhona, Deborah Ritchie, Bregje deKok, Cathy Wood & Huby Guro. 2013. Parenting support for families with young children: A public health, user focus study undertaken in a semi-rural area of Scotland. *Journal of Clinical Nursing* 22: 1140–1150.

Hudson, Bob. 2000. Interacgency collaboration – A skeptical view. In *Critical Practice in health and social care,* edited by Brechin Ann, Brown Hilary and Maureen A. Eby. London: Sage.

Kennedy, Catherine, Lynch Emily & Robina Goodlad. 2001. *Good practice in joint/multiagency working on homelessness (Homelessness Task Force Research Series)*. Edinburgh: Scottish Executive.

Kruse, Sharon & Karen Louis. 2009. *Building strong school cultures: A guide to leading change*. Thousand Oaks, CA: Corwin.

Lewis, Marie. 2004. Working together to make a difference. *Midwives* 7: 422–423.

Marks, Linda. 2007. Fault-lines between policy and practice in local partnerships. *Journal of Health Organization and Management* 21(2): 136–148.

Midwifery 2020 Programme. 2010. *Midwifery 2020 delivering expectations*. London: Midwifery.

Miller, Suzanne & Liz Wilkes. 2015. Working in partnership. In *Midwifery: Preparation for practice* (3rd ed.), edited by Sally Pairman, Jan Pincombe, Carol Thorogood & Sally Tracy. St Louis: Mosby.

NICE (National Institute for Health and Care Excellence). 2010. *Weight management before, during and after pregnancy NICE guidelines* (PH27). London: NICE.

Nutbeam, Don & Elizabeth Harris. 2010. *Theory in a nutshell: A practical guide to health promotion theories* (3rd ed.). Sydney: McGraw-Hill.

Percy-Smith, Janie. 2005. *Definitions and models: What works in strategic partnerships for children*. Ilford: Barnado's.

Pettigrew, Paul. 2003. Power, conflicts and resolutions: A change agent's perspective on conducting action research within a multi-organizational partnership. *Systemic Practice and Action Research* 16: 375–391.

PHE (Public Health England). 2013a. *Nursing and midwifery contribution to public health*. London: Public Health England and DoH.

PHE (Public Health England). 2013b. *Nursing and midwifery actions at the three levels of public Health practice*. London: Public Health England and DoH.

PHE (Public Health England). 2013c. *The evidence base of the public health contribution of nurses and midwives*. London: Public Health England and DoH.

Piper, Stewart. 2005. Health promotion: A framework for midwives. *British Journal of Midwifery* 13: 284–288.

Power, Alison. 2015. What do service users want and who care? *British Journal of Midwifery* 23(8): 594–596.

Ross, Graham, Sibbald Shannon & Pooja Patel. 2015. Public health partnership: Does the evidence justify the enthusiasm. *Healthcare Management Forum* 28(2): 79–81.

Scriven, Angela. 2010. *Ewels and Simnett's promoting health: A practical guide* (6th ed.). London: Bailliere Tindall.

Taylor-Robinson, David, Ffion Lloyd-Williams, Lois Orton, May Moonan, Martin O'Flaherty & Simon Capewell. 2012. *Barriers to partnership working in public health: A qualitative study*, edited by Ross JS. *PLoS One* 2012; 7(1): e29536. doi: 10.1371/journal.pone.0029536.

Tunnard, Jo. 1991. As cited in Jackson Shirley, Morris Kate, *1994 looking at partnership teaching in social work qualifying programmes*. London: CCETSW.

UNICEF. 2012. *Health benefits of breastfeeding.* http://www.babyfreindly.org.uk/health.asp

West-Burnham, Eddie. 2006. Partnership working and the midwife. In *Health promotion in midwifery: Principles and practice* (2nd ed.), edited by Jan Bowden and Vicky Manning. London: Hodder Arnold.

Williams Helen, Foster David & Pauline Watts. 2013. Perinatal domestic abuse: Midwives making a difference through effective public health practice. *British Journal of Midwifery* 21(2): 852–858.

World Bank. 1998. *World Bank Partnerships Group, Strategy and Resource Management, "Partnership for Development: Proposed Actions for the World Bank"* (discussion paper, 20 May 1998). Washington, DC: World Bank.

WHO (World Health Organization). 1985. *Health for all by the year 2000*. Geneva: WHO.

WHO (World Health Organization). 1986. *The Ottawa Charter for health promotion*. Geneva: WHO.

FURTHER READINGS

Ham, C. 2010. Working Together for Health: Achievements and Challenges in the Kaiser NHS Beacon Sites Programme, Health Services Management Centre, University of Birmingham.

Putnam, Robert. 2000. *Bowling alone: The collapse and revival of American community*. New York, Simon Schuster.

Williams, P. & H. Sullivan. 2010. Despite all we know about collaborative working, why do we still get it wrong? *Journal of Integrated Care* 18(4): 4–15.

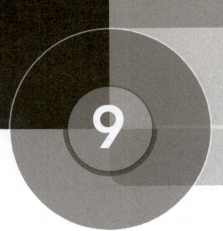

Breasts, bottles and health promotion

9

LOUISE ARMSTRONG

INTRODUCTION

The topic of infant feeding in the United Kingdom today provokes much discussion among mothers and midwives alike. There is irrefutable evidence that breastfeeding provides the healthiest start for babies and over the last two decades, it would appear that this message is being successfully communicated.

The initiation, prevalence and duration of breastfeeding have all increased since 1990. At first sight, this is good news and shows that successful health promotion strategies have been employed. Despite this, however, there can be no room for complacency as there are many babies not receiving any breast milk at all. Not being breastfed as a baby is a major contributing factor to health inequality. There are also many aspects of our culture which do not embrace breastfeeding as 'normal', along with distortion in the media and advertising in the way in which breasts and breastfeeding are presented.

This chapter will explore the latest breastfeeding initiative, prevalence and duration rates; present factors which have and are contributing to a 'bottle feeding' culture within the United Kingdom; outline why breastfeeding matters; examine health promotion initiatives and interventions shown to be successful in breastfeeding promotion; and finally identify gaps in our knowledge and suggest future direction.

These successful initiatives include the 'Baby Friendly' Initiative (BFI), antenatal education, peer support, best clinical practices and proactive support from knowledgeable midwives. It concludes with suggestions for future health promotion.

INITIATION, PREVALENCE AND DURATION OF BREASTFEEDING

The most recent infant survey, McAndrew et al. (2012), presents a full picture of infant feeding data and shows the successful increase in breastfeeding rates in the past two decades. Over the whole of the United Kingdom, 81% of mothers initiate breastfeeding (this is babies ever put to the breast, even if this is only once). This is an increase of 5% from 76% in 2010. The mothers in England showed the greatest increase (5%) and highest rates of incidence of breastfeeding (78% in 2005 and 83% in 2010) (see Table 9.1).

Similar to the 2005 data, the figures at 1 week after childbirth reveal 69% of mothers are still breastfeeding (a loss of 12%) and by 6 weeks the figure goes down to 55% (a loss of 26%). By 6 months, the figure is further down to only 34% (a loss of 47%; see Table 9.2). It should be noted that these figures refer to any breastfeeding and not exclusive breastfeeding. Therefore, many of the babies are being 'mixed' fed. The evidence supports that for optimal infant health, exclusive breastfeeding needs to continue until the infant is 6 months old (WHO 2011). At 6 months (although some researchers argue even later), weaning can be commenced whilst breastfeeding continues. Ideally, babies should continue being breastfed as well as receiving solids until they are 2 years of age (WHO 2011). There would be considerable cultural change needed before becomes commonplace in the United Kingdom.

McAndrew et al. (2012) also identifies that the 'typical breast feeder' has particular characteristics (see Box 9.1)

Table 9.1 Incidence of breastfeeding (that is any breastfeeding from birth, even if this is only one breastfeed)

	2005 (%)	2010 (%)
England	78	83
Scotland	70	74
Wales	67	71
Northern Ireland	63	64
United Kingdom	76	81

Source: From McAndrew, Fiona, et al. 2012. *Infant Feeding Survey 2010*. London, UK: National Statistics.

Table 9.2 Duration of breastfeeding (that is any breastfeeding occurring, even if alongside bottle feeding)

Time	UK total in 2010 (%)	UK total in 2005 (%)
Birth	81	76
One week	69 (loss of 12%)	63 (loss of 13%)
Six weeks	55 (loss of 26%)	48 (loss of 28%)
Six months	34 (loss of 47%)	25 (loss of 51%)

Note: Babies exclusively breastfed for the DoH recommended 6 months are 1 in a 100.
Source: From McAndrew, Fiona, et al. 2012. *Infant Feeding Survey 2010*. London, UK: National Statistics.

Another important point to be noted from the 2010 infant feeding survey is that the majority of mothers who discontinue breastfeeding during the first 2 weeks would have liked to carry on longer. Interestingly, this has been the same in all previous infant feeding surveys which would indicate that this remains an area of health promotion focus. Mothers said that 'more support and guidance from hospital staff' (McAndrew et al. 2012, 82) could have helped. This supports health promotion strategies which educate health professionals and peer supporters.

This means that even the 'well motivated' mother who intends to exclusively breastfeed can be let down by the current maternity system, discontinuing breastfeeding and joining the 'lost 12%' at just 1 week into the experience. A typical story is detailed (see Figure 9.1) as an attempt to incorporate the data from the infant survey along with some cultural perspectives.

What follows is an all too typical story (see Figure 9.1):

Well-motivated Chloe becomes pregnant for the first time and has hospital antenatal care from a midwife. She does not see the same midwife at every appointment. Chloe attends hospital antenatal classes and one of those is devoted to breastfeeding. The message is clear – breastfeeding is the 'best' and Chloe has already decided to breastfeed. Chloe is likely to have seen adverts for 'follow-on' formula, is likely to have been breastfed herself and has her own body image issues (or not). Her husband equally has his story and is not likely to have been included in the antenatal education sessions. He may or may not be supportive of the decision to breastfeed. Chloe gives birth in hospital narrowly escaping a caesarean section. Attempts are made to initiate breastfeeding during a period of skin-to-skin contact soon after birth. The baby boy is sleepy and a 'slow starter' with breastfeeding. Chloe is transferred to the postnatal ward. She makes various attempts and asks the midwives for help with attachment which is not easily achieved. The day wears on and eventually Chloe becomes concerned that her baby has not really had a breastfeed yet and starts to lose confidence in breastfeeding. Chloe considers bottle feeding as a solution. At this stage, the midwife's response becomes critical – if she (the midwife) sees bottle feeding as the solution and/or Chloe asks for a bottle, then mother and baby risk becoming part of the lost 12% cascade. If the midwife proactively offers help with breastfeeding, this can be prevented. The proactive help from the midwife ideally should have come soon after birth or early on the postnatal ward.

There are several places during the cascade in Figure 9.1 where both proactive help and effective health promotion intervention were possible to prevent the 'lost 12%' cascade occurring. The ideal scenario, with the appropriate intervention, is shown in Figure 9.2.

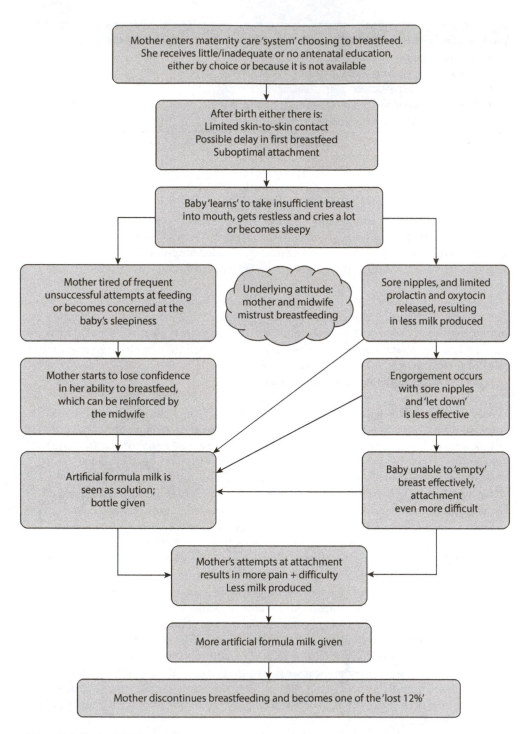

Figure 9.1 The lost 12% cascade.

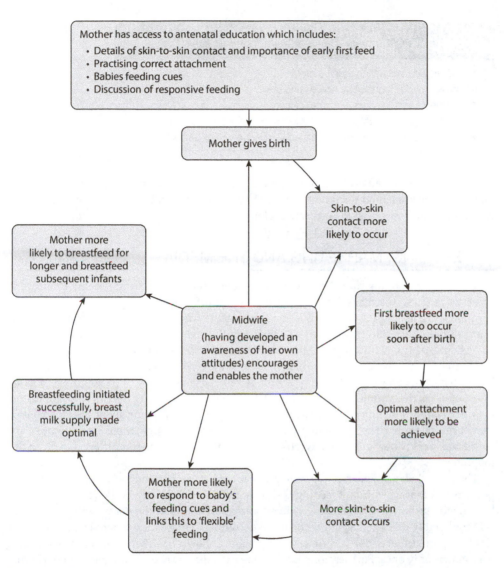

Figure 9.2 Preventing the lost 12% cascade.

THE BOTTLE FEEDING CULTURE IN THE UNITED KINGDOM

In order to understand how and why we are and where we are in the United Kingdom with infant feeding, it is helpful to consider the historical perspective and how that has shaped our situation. How have we become a culture that values 'bottle feeding'?

Breastfeeding babies have been a normal part of human history from its very beginning. It is only as recently as the twentieth century that the incidence has sharply decreased. Although breastfeeding is physiologically normal, easy and natural, it has now often become difficult for mothers to achieve. Therefore, infant formula 'milk' given via a feeding bottle (bottle feeding)

> **BOX 9.2: Factors that have shaped the United Kingdom into a bottle feeding culture**
>
> - Advertising, marketing and the media
> - The ability to manufacture bottles and teats
> - Women's emancipation and employment
> - Medical control of childbirth and making infant feeding 'scientific'
> - Family 'norms', 'My mother bottle fed us and we turned out OK'

has gained wide spread acceptance in the United Kingdom and has become the most commonly employed method for infant feeding. Key contributory factors that have combined to cause this shift from breast to bottle are explored in Box 9.2.

ADVERTISING, MARKETING AND THE MEDIA

Advertising, marketing and the media have shaped the current bottle feeding culture in three ways. First, the marketing and advertising of infant formula is a powerful tool that is influencing us to use formula milk as an acceptable substitute for breast milk. Although the International Code of Marketing of breast milk substitutes (WHO 1981) prohibits the advertising of infant formula for newborn babies on television and in health care settings, the companies get around this by advertising 'follow-on' infant formula (given to babies 6 months onwards). By using techniques such as continuity of packaging and labelling between the various stages of infant formula, manufacturers create an association between 'follow-on' formula and the earlier newborn formula. This shapes the perception that formula from birth has actually been advertised. Although there is awareness and concern over this new genre of advertising, the code is yet to be strengthened to close this loophole.

The second way in which popular media shape the current culture, and perhaps the most powerful, is that when infant feeding is shown, it is almost entirely bottle feeding. Rarely is breastfeeding shown. Bottle feeding is therefore demonstrated as 'the norm' within family life. It is confidently displayed as if it is the usual or 'normal' choice for women. Henderson et al. (2000) reported that of the 235 times infant feeding shown on UK television, breastfeeding was shown only once. Furthermore, if/when breastfeeding is shown, it is presented as problematic, comical or extreme (as in documentaries showing women breastfeeding children over 5 years old).

The third aspect of media influence is the portrayal of the female body, and breasts in particular. The sexualisation of breasts is both acceptable and widespread within society. Materials with pornographic or erotic content, usually featuring women, emphasise breasts as being 'for sex' and to please men. This causes confusion in women (and men) as to the function and role of breasts (Palmer 2009). If it is more acceptable within our society to show breasts for erotic purposes than to feed an infant, this can cause a barrier against breastfeeding. A woman's own perception of her breasts may influence her choice in infant feeding and furthermore may lead her to be concerned that breastfeeding may remove or lower her sex appeal (Jackson 2000).

Does the media shape or merely reflect culture? This is an important question to answer. Henderson et al. (2000) suggest that at the very least it reinforces ideas about what is normal within society. It would be difficult to believe this did not shape culture.

FAMILY 'NORMS' – 'MY MOTHER BOTTLE FED US AND WE TURNED OUT OK'

Women can powerfully influence other women. The influence of a new mother's family and friends should not be underestimated. If her own mother breastfed or her peer group are breastfeeding, a woman is likely to breastfeed. The same is true of bottle feeding. Choosing breastfeeding when your own mother did not and neither are your peer group is a bold step to take. Should this mother get to the point of initiating breastfeeding, unless all goes well immediately, there may well be pressure from others to discontinue and do what they did, indeed what is 'normal'.

Women who either bottle-feed their babies from the start or who struggled to breastfeed, and then bottle fed, who then go on to see no particular health detriment in any of their children are unlikely to seriously question the 'safety' of bottle feeding as an alternative to breastfeeding. Indeed, some will become powerful advocates of bottle feeding vocalising their own experience as sure evidence or 'proof' of all is well.

MIDWIVES AND THEIR OWN EXPERIENCES

The vast majority of midwives are women and therefore are not isolated from any of these influences themselves. They enter midwifery with their own infant feeding history, their own body image and their own values and beliefs. These will not necessarily be conducive to promoting or supporting women to breastfeed despite this being part of the role of the midwife.

It is important to understand that changes in attitudes or values cannot be forced on anyone. Therefore, it is imperative that, at the outset of the pre-registration programme, student midwives are given the opportunity, in the safety of the educational environment, to examine their own attitudes. This takes skill on the part of the facilitator – if not, well facilitated, unfavourable, entrenched attitudes could result.

REFLECTION

A mother, who has just given birth to her first baby in hospital, tells the midwife she wants to breast-feed. The baby is wide awake.

Consider the following possible responses:

- 'Let's see if we can get her on.........'
- 'I'll just weigh her, clean her up a bit and then we'll have a go'
- 'How confident are you feeling about that? What help would you like?'

Which response is closest to your own?
What do you think the different responses might say about the midwife's own attitude to breastfeeding?

WHY BREASTFEEDING MATTERS

Breastfeeding matters simply because of the overwhelming, indisputable evidence of the damage *not* breastfeeding can have on the health of mothers and infants and on health care. Never before has such a large part of human civilisation chosen to ignore such a basic part of its physiology. Many researchers believe we have only just begun to discover the true extent of what we are putting at risk. The science of epigenetics, currently in its infancy, already has evidence that the first nutrition outside the womb has a potentially expansive effect on the epigenome which in turn affects DNA (Wilson 2014). The effects of this are far reaching and can last several generations.

THE DIFFERENCES BETWEEN FORMULA AND BREAST MILK

Formula composition differs substantially from breast milk. It does not confer or develop immunity or promote neurological development (Michaelsen et al. 2009). Infant formula 'milk' is chemically modified cow's milk, and although babies have been fed alternatives to breast milk before, this is the first time in human history that one mammal species has been fed another mammal's milk on such a worldwide scale. Each mammalian species produces its own species-specific milk which its female feeds her newborn. The composition, particularly the protein content of the milk, is physiologically designed for the development of that particular species. Therefore, to risk feeding one species' milk to another on the current scale is a worldwide human experiment. The results are as yet not fully understood, but we are gaining evidence of the adverse effects. There is a possibility it could be catastrophic.

THE DANGERS ASSOCIATED WITH BOTTLE FEEDING

The health dangers associated with bottle feeding are now well known and well evidenced among the midwifery scientific community. There is good-quality evidence that the short- and long-term health risks for babies *not* receiving breast milk and of their mothers *not* breast-feeding are considerable. Importantly, these health risks are irrespective of income and

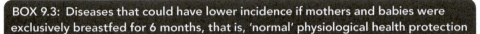

BOX 9.3: Diseases that could have lower incidence if mothers and babies were exclusively breastfed for 6 months, that is, 'normal' physiological health protection

'Normal' health includes protection against the following for the *mother*:

- Breast cancer
- Ovarian cancer
- Diabetes

'Normal' health includes protection against the following for the *baby*:

- Gastrointestinal infection
- Lower respiratory tract infection
- Acute otitis media (middle ear infection)
- Necrotising enterocolitis
- Sudden infant death syndrome
- Asthma
- Leukaemia
- Diabetes
- Coeliac disease
- Cardiovascular disease
- Sepsis
- Obesity
- Cognitive outcomes (lower IQ)

Source: From Renfrew, Mary, et al. 2012. *Preventing disease and saving resources: The potential contribution of increasing breastfeeding rates in the UK*. London: Baby Friendly Initiative.

social class (Renfrew et al. 2012). This makes the extent of the issue very significant. Besides being sicker, particularly with chronic health conditions, and becoming ever more so as a society, the economic cost in terms of health care is forecast to be unsustainable.

A list of diseases that affects mothers and babies that can be significantly reduced if babies are exclusively breastfed for the recommended 6 months can be found in Box 9.3. This could be described as 'normal' physiological health protection.

Unfortunately, the differences between formula and breast milk, along with the knowledge of the dangers associated with bottle feeding, are not common knowledge among health care professionals, women and the wider society. Where health care professionals have some understanding, they do not always accept or recognise the gravity of the situation. This can result in little urgency or emphasis in the need for health promotion.

In 2012, Renfrew et al. published a comprehensive study into the costs of *not* breastfeeding. They calculated the decrease in incidence of the diseases presented in Box 9.3 and the financial savings this might make to the UK health service. It provides strong evidence to support breastfeeding being not 'best' but normal.

HEALTH PROMOTION: BREAST IS NOT BEST, IT'S NORMAL

All efforts towards developing effective health promotion take place against this unfavourable backdrop of our current UK bottle feeding culture. It is clear that the promotion of breastfeeding goes far beyond what happens (or does not happen) in maternity services. Attitudes, values and beliefs cannot easily be changed. At best, they need to be sensitively and appropriately challenged with re-examination and change being encouraged. It is also true that health promotion needs to seek wider influence in media, popular culture, policy makers and government.

The more ingrained into our present culture bottle feeding becomes and the less visible breastfeeding becomes (particularly in public), the more bottle feeding is perceived as a 'safe' alternative to breastfeeding and breast milk. The more it is perceived as a 'safe' alternative, the wider the acceptance becomes and so it goes on. Although breastfeeding incidence is increasing in the United Kingdom (McAndrew et al. 2012), there is still much health promotion to be done to change the current cultural climate.

The factors that have contributed to the decline in breastfeeding and rise in the acceptance of bottle feeding during the twentieth century are much discussed both among health professionals and mothers themselves. Most agree that the decline is multi-factorial. Some of the factors can be seen in Box 9.2. This has had serious health, financial and economic implications both for babies and women and hence is of major health promotion concern.

In order to deploy health promotion resources effectively, it is important to identify which health promotion strategies are successful. Once the evidence is established, those successful can be appropriately implemented.

HEALTH PROMOTION INITIATIVES AND PRACTICES WHICH HAVE BEEN SHOWN TO WORK

'BABY FRIENDLY' INITIATIVE

The 'Baby Friendly' Initiative is perhaps the single most effective infant feeding health promotion initiative ever introduced. It has been well evaluated and evidence has shown that in accredited facilities, breastfeeding initiation, duration and prevalence increase (Cattaneo and Buzzetti 2001). Introducing BFI and working towards accreditation effectively incorporates nearly all of the other health promotion initiatives and practices shown to work.

HOSPITAL AND COMMUNITY TRUSTS

The latest updated award for hospitals and community trusts was devised and launched in 2012 (BFI 2012a). It replaced the former 'Ten Steps' and '7 Point Plan' with new standards that are detailed in Box 9.4.

BOX 9.4: BFI standards for hospital and community trusts

The new standards have three stages and have also encompassed neonatal units and public health nursing services:

Stage 1   Building a firm foundation – this involves having written policies and guidelines; planning an education programme for the staff; having processes in place for auditing standards and ensuring there is no promotion of breast milk substitutes, teats or dummies.

Stage 2   An educated workforce – this involves implementing education to all staff in line with their role.

Stage 3   Parents' experiences of maternity services (this is further broken down into parents experiences of neonatal units, health visiting and public health nursing services as well as children's centres or equivalent).

BOX 9.5: BFI university educational standards

Standard 1   Make a written commitment to adhere to the BFI standards

Standard 2   Ensure all students are equipped with the knowledge and skills to implement the BFI learning outcomes in the relevant clinical setting

Standard 3   Provide teaching without involvement, sponsorship or promotional materials from companies covered by the international code

---

As a result, the BFI has become a well-known and respected initiative which incorporates the current best evidence available. BFI standards are considered the 'gold standard' for maternity services.

UNIVERSITY UNDERGRADUATE EDUCATIONAL STANDARDS

The BFI introduced Educational Standards for Universities in 2002 and updated them in line with the 2012 revised BFI standards (BFI 2012b). These were aimed at setting standards for the content of infant feeding education for university undergraduate programmes. This results in newly qualified midwives (and health visitors) acquiring knowledge, skills and favourable attitudes at the point of registration and thereby entering clinical practice well educated. The university standards can be seen in Box 9.5.

Although these standards are yet to be formally evaluated, they have been well received by lecturers, students and trust employers. Again, these standards have become the benchmark for infant feeding education. It stands to reason that if infant feeding education during pre-registration education is strengthened by BFI accreditation, there is a positive knock-on effect in maternity services that benefits mothers and babies.

ANTENATAL EDUCATION AND PEER SUPPORT

Some type of antenatal education, usually taking the form of a series of classes, is offered by most maternity units. The content, programme, delivery and facilitation of the sessions can vary greatly from one place to another making the overall provision (and therefore the education) haphazard. The other important issue is that attendance at antenatal classes is voluntary. Generally it is the more highly motivated and educated socio-economic groups who choose to attend so the classes do not necessarily reach the demographic of women who may well benefit from them. Some initiatives have tried to overcome this by customising classes to target specific groups, for example, teenage women.

The evidence, for which antenatal interventions may increase breastfeeding initiation and duration, is small and only involves evaluation from the women attending. In order to make the sessions as effective as possible, various educational approaches, styles and methods have been tried. They include:

- Information giving (verbal and leaflets)
- Discussion sessions (facilitated by professionals or peers)
- Experiential learning 'workshop' style sessions (facilitated by professionals or peers)
- Involving male partners specifically in some way
- Any combination of the above

> **BOX 9.6: Factors shown to be ineffective in antenatal and postnatal education**
>
> - Antenatal education by a paediatrician
> - Written educational materials used alone
> - Single home visit by community nurse following early discharge
> - The training of health professionals alone
>
> *Source:* Winterburn, Susan. 2007. Primary Health Care 17(2):43–47; Department of Health. 2004. *Good Practice and Innovation in Breastfeeding.* London: DoH.

There appears to be a consensus that there is no one way that increases breastfeeding duration. A combination of approaches can produce significant increases in breastfeeding duration (Renfrew et al. 2005). The Cochrane review (Lumbiganon et al. 2012) summary concludes that it is not possible to recommend one specific type of antenatal education, although there are some approaches that are ineffective (see Box 9.6).

There have been some creative attempts to develop experiential workshops applying sound educational theory that moves well away from limited passive listening by women to more fully involving them during the session. Noel-Weiss et al. (2006) developed a 'prenatal breastfeeding workshop to support maternal breastfeeding self-efficacy'. A controlled trial compared attendees with a matched cohort who had received routine care. They showed that attendees had higher self-efficacy scores and a higher proportion was exclusively breastfeeding. However, the overall breastfeeding duration rate was the same as the control group.

Another very interesting and unique study (Reeve et al. 2004) used an antenatal experiential learning session aimed at supporting women's choices to breastfeed. This was unusual because it was targeting all women (not just those who wanted to breastfeed) and was designed to help them make an informed choice about their method of feeding.

Attendees were compared with a non-attending group. The results showed a significant difference in that the number of attendees breastfeeding at 4 months was double the number of non-attendees. Reeves et al (2004) suggest this may be because the women had greater confidence in their decision to breastfeed and had been better equipped by more fully considering the influences they may get on their decision.

All authors suggest much larger randomised controlled trials being undertaken before any real conclusions can be drawn. It is important that these approaches are not dismissed on the basis of further studies being needed.

Other antenatal initiatives have been tried with either unknown or varying effectiveness:

- Antenatal home visits by Health Visitors (HVs) (Winterburn 2007)
- Follow-up phone calls post workshops (Renfrew et al. 2005)
- Professionals being offered 'informal' teaching sessions (Abbott et al. 2006)
- Antenatal workshops aimed at reducing nipple pain (Duffy et al. 1997)
- Male partner influence

In recent years, there has also been a move away from face-to-face delivery to Internet-based sessions (Giglia & Binns 2014).

It is too early to say what women think of these changes, but it is difficult to believe that this provision has not been done simply to save money rather than catering for women's needs as the social side, often so well evaluated by women is missing.

USING PEER SUPPORTERS

The Cochrane review (Lumbiganon et al. 2012) concludes that involving peer supporters during the antenatal period – not just in antenatal classes setting, but in other ways such as counselling and visiting – is effective with increasing breastfeeding initiation. This is important as peer supporters can therefore make a contribution to the multidisciplinary team. As it has been identified, often a combination of approaches is more effective than any one single approach (Lumbiganon et al. 2012); involving trained peer supporters throughout the childbirth continuum is good, effective practice. Peer supporters are often locals and therefore know the local demographics and can identify with the women. Using peer-led postnatal support groups and/or home visits can increase breastfeeding duration. They also contribute to a supportive environment which nurtures breastfeeding women (Oakley et al. 2014). This has been found to be a necessary factor, especially with young women (Brown et al. 2011).

MALE PARTNER INFLUENCE – OF UNKNOWN EFFECT

This is important in the breastfeeding agenda. Actively involving the male partner during antenatal education is of unknown effectiveness. To what extent men (the husband, the father of the baby, the partner) influence both the initial decision to breastfeed and breastfeeding duration is unknown. There is discussion that their influence is underestimated and that they should be included in health promotion interventions to a much greater extent than at present (Kenosi et al. 2011). Overlooking the influence of men in the breastfeeding debate could be to potentially overlook an effective strategy (Sharma & Petosa 1997). One American study (Sciacca et al. 1995) found that involving men in antenatal classes and offering them an incentive to attend resulted in a two- to three-fold increase in breastfeeding rates. It is not known whether these results could be generalised in the UK population.

It has been suggested that the perceptions of breastfeeding, gender roles, women's sexuality and initial decision to breastfeed are all factors in which men have real influence (Jackson 2000). The language that men use can greatly impact their partner's ability to feel confident about breastfeeding (Okon 2004). It can potentially be disempowering if it is defeatist or nonchalant. How a man views the female body, that is, for his sexual gratification or otherwise (Palmer 2009), his own social class, childhood experiences of seeing breastfeeding and his relationship with his own mother (Jackson 2000) have also been suggested as significant. Sharma and Petosa (1997) suggests that 'negative attitudes' about what breastfeeding might do to women's breasts and a perceived delay in developing a relationship with the baby are very real and could be detrimental in decision making.

Authors agree that much more research into the contribution and influence men have needs to be undertaken. Meanwhile, it would seem appropriate to involve men in some way perhaps tailor making antenatal education to actively involve them rather than to treat them as an 'add on'. These could either be with women or for men alone. Opportunity to enhance self-efficacy and discussion to set realistic expectations could prove effective. Sessions to potentially consider strategies such as enhancing father–infant relationship by creating a special 'father–infant' time (Sears 1992), discussing the 'changing sexuality' of women after they become mothers (Jackson 2000) and greater knowledge of health outcomes (Sharma & Petosa 1997) have been suggested. Discussion about breastfeeding in public could also be included.

PRACTICE POINTS

Consider what antenatal education is currently offered for women at your workplace.

Does the provision include:

1. Choice of times and venues (hospital or community)?
2. Are there any 'private' classes available, if so, what do they include?
3. What is included in the content and what educational approaches are used?
4. Are male partners actively included?
5. Could you influence changes to any of these aspects?

CLINICAL PRACTICE WHICH SUPPORTS BREASTFEEDING

The following practices bear a weight of evidence demonstrating their effectiveness. They should be embedded into any maternity services policy or guideline and be standard care. All of these are reflected within the BFI accreditation standards and hence form part of the culture within a unit.

- Timing of the first breastfeed (i.e. early, soon after birth)
- Skin-to-skin (or kangaroo care) contact between mother and baby
- Unrestricted feeding/contact between mother and baby from birth onwards
- Proactive support from knowledgeable professionals or peers
- Avoidance of supplementary fluids (formula, dextrose or water) unless there is clear medical indication

TIMING OF FIRST FEED AND SKIN-TO-SKIN CONTACT

Timing of the first breastfeed, skin-to-skin contact and unrestricted contact between mother and baby are linked. Although hospitals may prescribe a set time after birth in which the baby should have its first feed such as 30 min or an hour, for example, evidence shows us that even with a normal healthy baby, there can be considerable variation in the baby's behaviour and readiness to feed immediately after birth (Widström et al. 1990). It can also be affected by pethidine during labour (Righard & Alade 1990).

There is also evidence to suggest that this period after birth between mother and baby, if left uninterrupted by 'routine' care such as weighing, wrapping the baby, etc., encourages instinctive interaction between the two of them. Given time, babies often attach themselves to their mother's breast and initiate breastfeeding. However, it is also important to note that there is no evidence to support the criticality of this time – should these practices not occur immediately after birth, it does not mean that a mother's breastfeeding will not be successful. Mothers with a delay to the initiation of breastfeeding need to be reassured that close and intimate contact with their baby at a later stage is also normal.

UNRESTRICTED FEEDING/CONTACT BETWEEN MOTHER AND BABY FROM BIRTH ONWARDS

Unrestricted feeding relates to both the frequency (how often the baby goes to the breast) and the duration (how long the baby remains attached to the breast) that occurs with breastfeeding.

This is now often called 'responsive' feeding instead of 'demand' or 'baby-led' feeding.

The length of a breastfeed is directly related to the rate of milk transfer (Howie et al. 1981). Therefore, some babies can take all they need in feeds as short as 3–4 min and others will need 45–60 min. However, there is a note of caution here. If a baby is sub-optimally attached, the milk transfer rate would be adversely affected and prolonged feeding could just make the mother's nipples sore.

The frequency of feeding is also very variable, although an individual baby will eventually show some pattern. Some babies revisit the breast after a very short interval, perhaps as short as 15–20 min and others anything from 1.5 to 4 h (Renfrew et al. 2000). Therefore, imposing some sort of regime is generally unhelpful.

PROACTIVE SUPPORT FROM KNOWLEDGEABLE PROFESSIONALS OR PEERS

Professional assistance should be made available after childbirth and during the stay in hospital. Mothers themselves have identified this as key to them not discontinuing breastfeeding before they want to (McAndrew et al. 2012). Help should be appropriately proactively given whilst respecting the natural mother–baby interaction (Renfrew et al. 2000).

This help should include the ability to help the mother achieve optimal attachment and positioning of her baby at the breast which she describes as 'pain-free' (Renfrew et al. 2000). As such, this forms a key professional skill which is a 'cornerstone' of the BFI accreditation for both trusts and universities.

It cannot be overemphasized that help and support need to be proactively offered. This is so important and has the power to change the culture on a postnatal ward in favour of lengthening breastfeeding duration and preventing the 'lost 12%' cascade in Table 9.2. If professionals and/or peers simply wait until a mother asks for help (which she may be reluctant to do perceiving the staff to be busy), many opportunities to prevent and avoid common problems such as sore nipples will be lost.

> ### PRACTICE POINT
> Consider what is meant by 'proactive' support and help with breastfeeding.
>
> Do you consider there is a culture of offering support and help with breastfeeding at your workplace? If not, how could the culture be changed or further encouraged?

AVOIDANCE OF SUPPLEMENTARY FLUIDS (FORMULA, DEXTROSE OR WATER) UNLESS THERE IS CLEAR MEDICAL INDICATION

Avoiding supplementing the baby with formula, dextrose and/or water is another fundamental practice which prevents the 'lost 12%' cascade (Table 9.2 and Figure 9.2). If the midwife suggests bottle feeding as a solution two things occur: the mother's confidence is lowered and the physiology of milk production is adversely affected. The perception of there being 'not enough milk' is reinforced. Figure 9.2 demonstrates this scenario.

It is also important here to realise the importance of the professional's own values and attitudes to infant feeding, as discussed earlier in this chapter. Some professionals, usually those with poor knowledge and skill, will suggest bottle feeding as a solution more readily than others.

These aspects of best practice, along with others such as audit, are largely encompassed by the BFI accreditation. It is therefore unsurprising that the BFI accreditation status is shown to work.

HEALTH PROMOTION WITHIN THE CONTEXT OF CONTINUITY OF CARER

Health promotion undertaken within the context of continuity of carer appears to be effective (Bonuck et al. 2002). This is perhaps because greater satisfaction is gained on both sides in the relationship. The sense of 'task'-focused care takes a back seat and the well-being of the woman stands a much greater chance of taking centre stage. This is true of most health care interventions including breastfeeding.

Should all these measures be put in place in every maternity unit and the necessary educational standards in universities, then the outcome of Chloe and many others might look more like the successful outcome shown in Figure 9.2.

HEALTH PROMOTION AND INFANT FEEDING: FUTURE DIRECTION

To move further forward and increase the rates of initiation, duration and prevalence of breastfeeding, there are some clear messages. In maternity units, the initiatives that have been shown to be effective need to become more widespread. All maternity units need to become 'Baby Friendly'; all universities offering pre-registration programmes need to incorporate the BFI educational standards; and there is a need to make antenatal education much more of a focus using a combination of educational approaches which are then evaluated. The involvement of the male partner and his influence on breastfeeding requires more research. The prevailing 'bottle feeding culture', and in particular the media aspects of it, needs much further discussion with midwives and others who may have much greater influence.

SUMMARY OF KEY POINTS

- Although the breastfeeding initiation rate in the United Kingdom has shown a steady increase since 1990, there is still much to be achieved, particularly with the exclusive breastfeeding rate at 6 months. This is only 1 in 100 babies (McAndrews et al. 2012).
- The current culture in the United Kingdom is one of 'bottle feeding'. Several factors have combined to cause this influence – advertising, marketing, the media and family 'norms' ('my mother bottle fed us and we turned out OK').
- Midwives are part of the culture and come into the profession with their own values, beliefs and attitudes. This affects the care and support they give. Raising awareness of these attitudes, ideally during pre-registration, could improve care.
- Breastfeeding matters because the costs of *not* breastfeeding in terms of health, finance and economics are considerable and unsustainable.
- Breastfeeding is not best; it is normal.
- Health promotion initiatives that have been shown to be effective at increasing breastfeeding rates need to become more widely adopted.
- Much more evidence needs to be generated in the area of antenatal education – different educational approaches and how male partners could be involved in particular.
- Creative ways of influencing the media need to be explored.

REFERENCES

Abbott, Stephen, Mary J. Renfrew & Alison McFadden. 2006. 'Informal' learning to support breastfeeding: Local problems and opportunities. *Maternal & Child Nutrition* 2(4):232.

BFI (Baby Friendly Initiative). 2012a. *Guide to Baby Friendly Initiative standards*. UK: UNICEF. http://www.unicef.org.uk/Documents/Baby_Friendly/Guidance/Baby_Friendly_guidance_2012.pdf (accessed September 2015).

BFI (Baby Friendly Initiative). 2012b. *Implementing the UNICEF UK Baby Friendly standards in universities: Learning outcomes and topic areas*. London: UNICEF. http://www.unicef.org.uk/Documents/Baby_Friendly/Going%20Baby%20Friendly/University_learning_outcomes.pdf (accessed September 2015).

Bonuck, Karen, Peter S. Arno, Margaret M. Memmott, Kathy Freeman, Marji Gold & Diane McKee. 2002. Breastfeeding promotion interventions: Good public health and economic sense. *Journal of Perinatology* 22:78–81.

Brown, Amy, Peter Raynor & Michelle Lee. 2011. Young mothers who choose to breast feed: The importance of being part of a supportive breast-feeding community. *Midwifery* 27(1):53–59.

Cattaneo, Adriano & Roberto Buzzetti. 2001. Effect on rates of breastfeeding of training for the Baby Friendly Hospital Initiative. *BMJ* 323:1358–1362.

Department of Health. 2004. *Good Practice and Innovation in Breastfeeding*. London: DoH.

Duffy, Elizabeth, Patricia Percival & Esma Kershaw. 1997. Positive effects of an antenatal group teaching session on postnatal nipple pain, nipple trauma and breastfeeding rates. *Midwifery* 13:189–196.

Giglia, Roslyn C. & Colin W. Binns. 2014. The effectiveness of the Internet in improving breastfeeding outcomes. *Journal of Human Lactation* 30(2):156–160.

Henderson, Lisa, Jenny Kitzinger & Jo Grenn. 2000. Representing infant feeding: Content analysis of British media portrayals of bottle feeding and breast feeding. *British Medical Journal* 321:1196.

Howie, P.W., M.J. Houston, A. Cook, L. Smart, T. McArdle & A.S. McNeilly. 1981. How long should a breastfeed last? *Early Human Development* 5(1):71–77.

Jackson, Karen B. 2000. Women, men, breastfeeding and sexuality. *British Journal of Midwifery* 8(2):83–86.

Kenosi, Mmoloki, Collin Hawkes, Eugene Dempsey & C. Anthony Ryan. 2011. Are fathers underused advocates for breastfeeding? *Irish Medical Journal* 104(10):313.

Lumbiganon, Pisake, Ruth Martis, Malinee Laopaiboon, Mario Festin, Jacqueline J. Ho & Mohammad Hakimi. 2012. Antenatal breastfeeding education for increasing breastfeeding duration (review). *The Cochrane Library* 9(11):CD006425.

McAndrew, Fiona, Jane Thompson, Lydia Fellows, Alice Large, Mark Speed & Mary J. Renfrew. 2012. *Infant Feeding Survey 2010*. London, UK: National Statistics.

Michaelsen, K.F., L. Lauritzen & E.L. Mortensen. 2009. Effects of breastfeeding on cognitive function. Edited by G. Golderg et al., *Breastfeeding: Early influences on later health, advances in experimental medicine and biology*. Dordrecht: Springer Sciences.

Noel-Weiss, Joy, Andre Rupp & Betty Cragg. 2006. Randomized controlled trial to determine effects of prenatal breastfeeding workshop on maternal breastfeeding self-efficacy and breastfeeding duration. *Journal of Obstetric, Gynecologic, and Neonatal Nursing* 35(5):616–624.

Oakley, Laura L., Jane Henderson, Maggie Redshaw & Maria A. Quigley. 2014. The role of support and other factors in early breastfeeding cessation: An analysis of data from a maternity survey in England. *BMC Pregnancy and Childbirth* 14:88.

Okon, Miranda. 2004. Health promotion: Partners' perceptions of breastfeeding. *British Journal of Midwifery* 12(6):387–393.

Palmer, Gabrielle. 2009. *The politics of breastfeeding*. London: Pinter and Martin.

Reeve, Jacquie R., Sarah E. Gull, Martin H. Johnson, Sally Hunter & Michael Streather. 2004. A preliminary study on the use of experiential learning to support women's choices about infant feeding. *European Journal of Obstetrics Gynecology and Reproductive Biology* 113(2):199–203.

Renfrew, Mary, Lisa Dyson, Louise Wallace Liz D'Souza, Felicia McCormick & Helen Spiby. 2005. *The effectiveness of health interventions to promote the duration of breastfeeding: Systematic review*. London: National Institute for Health and Clinical Excellence.

Renfrew, Mary, Subhash Pokhrel, Maria A. Quigley, Felicia McCormick & Julia Fox-Rushby. 2012. *Preventing disease and saving resources: The potential contribution of increasing breastfeeding rates in the UK*. London: Baby Friendly Initiative.

Renfrew, Mary, Mike Woolridge & Helen Ross McGill. 2000. *Enabling women to breastfeed*. Norwich, UK: The Stationery Office.

Righard, L & M.O. Alade. 1990. Effect of delivery room routines on success of first breastfeed. *The Lancet* 336(8723):1105–1107.

Sciacca, John P., Brenda L. Phipps, David A. Dube & Michae I. Ratliff. 1995. Influences on breastfeeding by lower-income women: An incentive-based approach, partner-supported educational program. *Journal of American Diet Association* 95:323–328.

Sears, W. 1992. The father's role in breastfeeding. *Clinical Issues, Nurses Association of the American College of Obstetricians and Gynecologists* 3:713–716.

Sharma, Manoj & Rick Petosa. 1997. Impact of expectant fathers in breastfeeding decisions. *Journal of the American Dietetic Association* 97(11):1312.

WHO (World Health Organization). 1981. *International code of marketing of breast-milk substitutes*. Geneva: WHO.

WHO (World Health Organization). 2011. *Exclusive breastfeeding for six months best for babies everywhere*. Statement, January. http://www.who.int/mediacentre/news/statements/2011/breastfeeding_20110115/en/index.html

Widström, A., V. Wahlberg, A.S. Matthiesen & P. Eneroth. 1990. Short-term effects of early suckling and touch of the nipple on maternal behaviour. *Early Human Development* 21(3):153–163.

Wilson, Laurel. 2014. Epigenetics and breastfeeding—The potential long-term impact of breast milk. In *Baby Friendly Initiative Annual Conference*, Newcastle, UK. http://www.unicef.org.uk/BabyFriendly/News-and-Research/News/Hear-Laurel-Wilsons-conference-talk-in-full/

Winterburn, Susan. 2007. Does antenatal home visiting by health visitors influence breastfeeding rates? *Primary Health Care* 17(2):43–47.

FURTHER READINGS

WHO. 2003. Global strategy for infant and young child feeding. http://apps.who.int/iris/bitstream/10665/42590/1/9241562218.pdf?ua=1&ua=1

WHO. 2015. Breastfeeding resources. http://www.who.int/topics/breastfeeding/en/

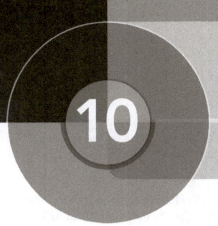

The role of complementary and alternative medicine in health promotion

10

PENNY CHARLES

This chapter explores the role of complementary and alternative medicine (CAM) in health promotion and how these therapies are used by midwives and women in maternity care. The health care professionals (HCPs) who use CAM the most in clinical practice are midwives and nurses. A wide range of self-help CAM therapies are chosen by women during the childbearing period and for the family use at home. These therapies may be provided by a midwife who is suitably qualified or a complementary practitioner trained in her or his own specialty. Both CAM and midwifery follow the same philosophy of care of holism. The use of case studies explores this concept, working in partnership with women and the role of psychoneuroimmunology or mind–body medicine. The integration of CAM and its philosophy and how this could help to provide positive health promotion in midwifery is discussed.

DEFINITIONS OF COMPLEMENTARY AND ALTERNATIVE MEDICINE

The World Health Organization (WHO) definition of CAM is:

> Health practices, approaches, knowledge and beliefs incorporating plant, animal and mineral based medicines, spiritual therapies, manual techniques and exercises, applied singularly or in combination to treat, diagnose and prevent illnesses or maintain well-being. (2003, 1)

It refers to practices which are rooted in the culture and beliefs of societies, such as in developing countries, where there is an absence of biomedical practice. This is useful to understand the role of CAM as the sole provider of health care.

In the Western world, complementary therapies are seen as complementary to conventional medicine. Ernst and Watson's (2012, 772) research into midwives' use of complementary and alternative treatments (CATs) cites the Cochrane Collaboration's theoretical definition (Wieland et al. 2011, 8) of CAM as:

> a broad domain of healing resources that encompass all health systems, modalities, and practices and their accompanying theories and beliefs, other than those intrinsic to the politically dominant health systems of a particular society or culture in a given historical period.

In maternity care, midwives and women appear to be drawn to the fact that 'many of the modalities embedded under the CAM rubric are denoted by a philosophical approach which promotes the body's natural healing ability and acknowledges the role of lifestyle choices on well-being' (Hall et al. 2012, 4). Midwives are encouraged to promote women's health and to work with women facilitating choice and control as a priority in childbirth (DoH 2007). Women using CAM before pregnancy may simply choose to continue with the use or turn to using CAM as an added support for coping with the changes or problems that pregnancy may bring about. We will familiarise ourselves with CAMs and then look more deeply into the reasons why both midwives and women choose to promote health in this way.

DIFFERENT CATEGORISATIONS OF CAM

Some forms of CAM originate from Eastern or Western philosophies of care. Within the Eastern philosophy are practices such as acupuncture, acupressure or shiatsu, and within the Western philosophy are osteopathy, chiropractic, homeopathy and naturopathy. All these traditions look at the person seeking help holistically and may use diagnostic methods specific to their therapy and then work towards bringing the body into alignment. CAM therapies usually do not solely concentrate on the presenting problem but take time to explore other issues of the client's life such as diet, emotional well-being, exercise, work/life balance and try to support improvement where possible, as highlighted in the WHO (2003) definition. In this way, they are very much like any health professional trying to give health promotion.

Many women promote their own health by using different forms of CAM. They may use techniques such as breathing and relaxation or use easily bought over the counter remedies such as homeopathy, herbs, flower remedies and essential oils. The list of complementary therapies that may be used by women is extensive.

ACTIVITY

Think of the CAMs you have seen used in pregnancy and in other areas of health care (or have you used yourself). Now list all the different modalities that can be used to support the body to get back into harmony. (Check your answers in Box 10.1.)

BOX 10.1: Different types of complementary therapies used by women

- Acupuncture
- Alexander technique
- Aromatherapy
- Ayurvedic medicine
- Baby massage
- Bach flower remedies
- Bowen technique
- Breathing
- Buteyko
- Chiropractic
- Craniosacral therapy
- Crystal healing
- Dietary supplements
- Dowsing
- Hair analysis
- Herbal medicine
- Homeopathy
- Hydrotherapy
- Hypnotherapy
- Imagery

- Iridology
- Kinesiology
- Massage
- Meditation (including mindfulness)
- Music
- Naturopathy
- Nutritional medicine
- Osteopathy
- Radionics
- Reflexology/reflex zone therapy
- Reiki
- Relaxation techniques
- Shiatsu
- Spiritual healing
- Tai Chi
- Therapeutic touch
- Traditional Chinese medicine
- Visualisation
- Yoga

USE OF CAM IN THE UNITED KINGDOM AND MATERNITY CARE

In 2000, the House of Lords commissioned a report (2000) to investigate why the public turns to CAM for treatments and are prepared to pay for sessions when there is a National Health Service (NHS) in place which treats and cares for patients for free. The reasons from Thompson and Feder (2005) included:

- People suffering from persistent symptoms that were not cured and subsequently feeling that orthodox medicine had failed them.
- People having real or perceived adverse effects of conventional treatments.
- People believing in the philosophy of the CAM, concerning the body's natural healing ability, and being respected for making their own lifestyle choices.

Warriner et al. (2014) found women valued the CAM practitioner viewing and treating them 'as a whole' and not through the 'fragmenting lens' of the time-pressured environment of primary care. The women in the study talked about the medicalisation of conventional care, and how they felt like that they were on a 'conveyor belt' instead of being treated as an individual, that they were an 'unimportant number' and that care was generally a 'tick box' exercise.

Women were the most frequent users of CAM for eliciting support with their lives, to help with anxiety, depression and eating a healthy diet. Forty-four per cent of the UK population uses CAM at some point in their lives and 26% of the population has used some form of CAM in the past 12 months (Hunt et al. 2010). Yoga and prayer were not included as therapies, but if they had been included, the statistics may have increased significantly.

The above research shows CAM is popular within the general population in the United Kingdom, but its use in midwifery is less clear. Hall and Jolly (2014) found that 33% of women did not disclose their use of CAM to an HCP and 81.3% of women were not asked by an HCP about their use of CAM. Mitchell (2010) found that where CAM has been successfully introduced into the NHS, it is often only maintained by a few enthusiastic and courageous individuals and the service discontinued once these individuals leave. With policy changes and funding issues, midwives are less interested in using CAM and it is becoming 'invisible' in hospitals (Cant et al. 2011). Midwives who were dual trained (in both a complementary therapy and as a midwife) often used their skills covertly as admitting to using CAMs may be considered taboo in hospitals. This was attributed to the fear of being a scapegoat if anything went wrong, blaming the problem on the CAM or the individual using it. Tiran (2012) points out that being with a midwife who has 'dual knowledge' offers benefits for women. The midwife trained in a complementary therapy is an expert in two fields and can relate how best the CAM can be used to support the woman, rather than a CAM specialist who may be unfamiliar with the process of childbirth. The midwife may integrate her CAM knowledge and skills into her midwifery field of practice and the woman would benefit from receiving it as a client of the NHS.

The most commonly used CAM techniques in maternity care are aromatherapy, reflexology, herbal remedies, homeopathy, acupuncture and different types of massage (Hall et al. 2012). Marc et al. (2011) in a Cochrane Review found some evidence that mind–body interventions helped anxiety in pregnancy, and Ernst and Watson (2012) found some encouraging findings for relaxation and hypnotherapy. It has also been shown that mindfulness meditation (for mental health promotion) in antenatal classes had significant positive impacts on women suffering from anxiety, fear of birth and stress in pregnancy (Byrne et al. 2014).

Explicit CAM use is probably dependent on the acceptance of CATs by the midwifery leaders in positions of power. Williams and Mitchell (2007) found that midwifery managers cited promoting normal birth, encouraging less medical intervention and achieving a greater satisfaction with service for women as the reasons for using CAM in maternity units. Hall et al. (2012) maintain that midwives who support the use of CAM do it for both the woman's and their own professional autonomy.

SAFETY

The midwife practicing CAMs is obliged by the Code (NMC 2015) to ensure its safe use and that it is in the best interests of the women in her care. The NMC (2007, 2015), The Royal College of Nurses (RCN 2003) and The National Institute for Health and Care Excellence (NICE 2008) propose the parameters of good care for childbearing women and provide guidelines on how to use CAM for midwives. NICE (2008) guidelines on antenatal care state that few complementary therapies have been established as safe and effective, so women should be advised to use them sparingly. The NICE (2008) guidelines do however support massage and aromatherapy for anxiety, acupuncture to relieve back and pelvic pain and ginger and vitamin B6 to alleviate nausea.

Mitchell (2010) cites that there are a variety of herbal remedies and products which women may prefer to use instead of what they consider to be possibly teratogenic, and therefore possibly harmful, pharmaceuticals. Using complementary therapies safely should be paramount for midwives. As an example, Tiran (2012) discusses the use of ginger in pregnancy for nausea and vomiting. She highlights how inappropriate it is for HCPs to advise that ginger is a safe remedy

> ## BOX 10.2: Resources for information about CAMs
>
> - Yourself! Reflect on the experience you have had or seen with CAMs so that you may understand how and why it may be a health-promoting experience for women and families in your care.
> - Go on a complementary therapy study day for midwives.
> - Be familiar with the NMC Code and DoH publications regarding CAM use in midwifery.
>
> Use websites which have information on recent research on complementary therapies to keep up to date and safe in your practice such as:
>
> www.evidence.nhs.uk
>
> www.rccm.org.uk (research council for complementary medicine)
>
> www.cochranelibrary.com

for *all* women since this depends on the woman's individual obstetric and medical history. A ginger biscuit or stem ginger would probably not contain enough ginger to be harmful but ginger capsules bought over the counter may have a detrimental effect on some women. Tiran explains that ginger has been found to be an anticoagulant and may have effects on the cardiovascular system and other body systems. Tiran's message is that there is robust research showing that ginger is very effective for nausea and vomiting but advises due care and attention and good history taking to ensure that it does no harm for that particular woman. Nevertheless, confusingly, ginger is one of the stated NICE (2008) recommendations for midwives to use to alleviate nausea and vomiting. In order for midwives to be able to provide excellent care for women, an open dialogue regarding women's CAM use would be beneficial.

> ## PRACTICE POINT
>
> Make a point of asking women if they are using CAM therapies, as they can react adversely when taken with conventional medicine.

> ## ACTIVITY
>
> Think what resources you could use to find out about complementary therapies, so that you are safe in your practice and so that you can give informed choice to women.

See Box 10.2 for some suggestions.

EFFECTIVENESS

Ernst and Watson (2012) explored midwives' use of CAM treatments and found that although few studies showed effectiveness, none reported any harm. The effectiveness of CAM is a contentious issue. By its very nature, it is a difficult topic to research due to the way it is practiced. A therapist may be treating a particular condition, such as back ache, but for each client, the approach might be different as each treatment is based on an individualised holistic approach.

The effect of the therapeutic relationship and an element of placebo effect can make interpretation of data complex. This may be caused by the differences in each individual being treated, the method and duration of treatment needed for the individual, the outcome measurement employed and the control intervention used. It is very difficult to know if positive results in the research process are the result of the effects of the therapy, the practitioner–client therapeutic relationship or other possibilities such as a placebo effect (this may be explained as the clients' expectations having an effect on the treatment outcome). In the world of CAMs, the placebo effect can be seen not as a derogatory judgement on a human's sense of well-being but a very powerful tool capable of creating feelings of well-being and instigating the healing process (Kaptchuk & Miller 2015).

Hunt et al. (2010) state that limited evidence does not mean a lack of effect. This is a specialised area and there are complex factors to be considered. There are often no explanations that satisfy orthodox science (at present) as to how some of these CAM methods work. Orthodox medicine can struggle to comprehend CAM as in some therapies there is no apparent treatment given such as in spiritual healing or it seems impossible that the treatment could do anything because of such minimal amounts of medicine such as in homeopathy.

HEALTH PROMOTION AND ITS RELATIONSHIP WITH CAM

The first part of the WHO definition of health promotion is 'Health promotion is the process of enabling people to increase control over, and to improve, their health' (WHO 1986). Using CAM during the period of childbirth can help women to feel empowered and involved in the birth process and their care. Both midwives and CAM practitioners approach care holistically, and health promotion is an integral part of how they both practice as can be seen from the definition above. CAM can, for example, support women to counteract stress, fear and feel more in control of their circumstances and hopefully improve their health.

HOLISM

The holistic philosophy was one of the main reasons cited as to why women use CAM (Hall et al. 2012). The aim of this concept is to 'make whole', by helping the body heal itself or maintain a balance and thereby understanding the connection between the physical, mental, emotional and spiritual levels. Gaining information about the client is essential and includes a detailed history of physical, emotional, spiritual, social and lifestyle information, with an emphasis on what is important for a particular woman at a particular point in time. The CAM practitioner may work on one or several levels depending on the therapy used, with the knowledge, or expectation, that this will positively affect the whole person. In terms of health promotion, for example, it is acknowledged that working on promoting mental health will promote general well-being as will be illustrated in the first case study. In the second case study, working on a spiritual level illustrates this holistic effect by positively facilitating the woman and baby.

At the start of a CAM consultation, information needs to be gathered. This takes time, which may be at a premium in midwifery care. Sometimes, the woman does not have adequate time to recount her 'story' and express any concerns, especially if they are of a sensitive nature. When bookings occur without such a strict time allocation, such as at home, women can feel valued and listened to. Midwives work hard with their communication skills to build rapport but are often curtailed by time limits. Women who visit CAM practitioners (outside the realm of midwifery) are not restricted to the same tight schedules, although there are necessary boundaries in place.

Rose's case study, illustrating how aromatherapy helped with physical and mental health issues, follows.

Case study: Rose

Rose attended nine aromatherapy sessions throughout her pregnancy with an aromatherapist (who was dual trained as a midwife and aromatherapist).

Rose's main concern was worrying about the impending birth of her baby. This caused her to feel anxious which affected her mood and her sleep. Rose attributed this concern to two previous traumatic childbirth experiences. Rose also experienced stress caused by the uncertainty surrounding her partner's employment and the addition of a large extension to their house. Mandarin essential oil (*Citrus reticulata*) was used as part of the treatment in regular massages to good effect. Mandarin essential oil relaxes and uplifts.

Rose's medical history highlighted asthma as a problem. Rose ensured her own health by using an inhaler daily to prevent an attack. On arrival at her appointment, Rose often suffered from some slight breathlessness which was noticed by the aromatherapist. On these occasions, Frankincense (*Boswellia thurifera*) essential oil was used in her massage to very good effect. Frankincense can help to slow and steady the breathing, thus calming anxiety (Battaglia 2004). After aromatherapy massage treatment, Rose could often reduce the inhaler use for the next 48–72 h.

Rose remained well throughout her pregnancy and this may have been aided by working with a holistic approach. Rose's mental well-being seemed to be supported by her CAM as she worked seamlessly through her anxieties and concerns simply by sharing them with the CAM practitioner. It helped that the aromatherapist had enough time to hear Rose's concerns. One example of how her mental health was supported was with an enquiry into iron-rich foods. Rose had received the information that her haemoglobin levels were low. Unfortunately, midwifery-staffing levels were very poor and she had not been able to discuss this issue with her midwife who would normally have been the professional to deal with this concern. Consequently, she was left confused and anxious about the meaning of this test, whether she could actively change the levels herself or whether she had no choice but to take the iron supplements prescribed for her. Together the client and CAM practitioner explored the foods and drinks that would increase and decrease iron levels plus alternatives to conventional iron supplements. Rose facilitated her own health promotion by sharing her concerns and educating herself in partnership with her CAM practitioner, who had the time to explore her worries and considered this time and exploration part of the holistic process. Rose consequently gained confirmation of the knowledge that she already had about iron-rich foods, gained some new information and subsequently felt more in control of her own health. This health education would also benefit her family in the future.

Another factor was having her physical health promoted by massage, which created deep relaxation for Rose. The essential oils were chosen to work on whatever areas needed attention at that moment. The oils worked synergistically on different areas (physical, mental and emotional) at the same time, which further complemented the care for Rose.

In the last month of her pregnancy, Rose's partner was taught some very simple massage moves for the hands and arms (which could be transferred to other parts of the body) and a massage oil was prepared for use in labour. Her partner could carry on supporting Rose and also be happily occupied with a useful job and benefit from smelling and receiving the oil through his skin. The advice was to massage for approximately 15 min every hour or as requested by Rose.

Many midwifery units in the United Kingdom train qualified midwives in the use of a few essential oils with women in labour. The aim is to keep birth as normal as possible. The oils can facilitate pain relief, dispel anxiety and relax women. Some of them enhance contractions which can help augment labour. Midwives can suggest women to use them in the bath, as an inhalation or as a massage. The oils can have a positive effect on not only the woman but also her partner and the midwives working on the ward who smell them.

THE ROLE OF TOUCH

Rose took responsibility for promoting her own health by choosing regular aromatherapy massage. In this way, she gained support for the impending birth. Research into massage demonstrates how an individual's self-esteem may be increased with caring touch (Field 2014). This can provide necessary confirmation and affirmation which positively affect the person's mental and emotional health. In the case of Rose, she may not have been aware that by choosing massage she was not only treating herself to an enjoyable experience (important in itself) but also helping herself to feel more confident about the workings of her own body. Massage can promote positive belief in one's own body, enabling and empowering women to cope in labour. A letting go or surrendering to the labour process may occur because of an innate confidence in one's body and its capabilities.

ACTIVITY

List the ways of promoting health that were illustrated in Rose's case study.

See Box 10.3 for suggested ways.

WORKING IN PARTNERSHIP WITH WOMEN

Another reason cited as to why women choose to see a complementary therapist is that clients want equal partnership in their health care. Many midwives would argue that, as autonomous practitioners, who care for women, there is little room for the reductionist approach, which is

---

BOX 10.3: Health promotion activities for Rose

Prevention of physical problems
1. Chest infection prevented or ameliorated as a result of provision of essential oils.
2. Reduction of the need for daily inhaler use.

Prevention of mental health problems
3. Listening to Rose's story before the massage.
4. Giving Rose time to talk over her concerns.
5. Using touch in massage to increase self-esteem.

General overall prevention of stress
6. Stress release as a result of regular, sensitive massage and relaxed atmosphere.
7. Possible prevention of distress of partner by teaching him massage moves before labour.
8. Taught strategies for helping to cope during labour, if needed.

often a criticism of the doctor–patient relationship (Davis-Floyd & St John 1998). This approach is criticised for defining the woman by any problem that she may have, be it a minor pregnancy disorder or a more serious complication. There may be a distinct feeling of hierarchy with the woman feeling intimidated and subjected to a patriarchal approach to care, which can be detrimental to health promotion. This style of care could probably make the woman feel that the people in authority have the information and all she needs to do is follow orders. This can leave a woman feeling disempowered and without the necessary knowledge to exercise control and choice.

THE THERAPEUTIC RELATIONSHIP, COMPASSION AND KINDNESS

There are many factors of the CAM encounter which resemble holistic midwifery care which contributes to a therapeutic relationship. This therapeutic relationship involves value and support with the aim of empowerment and enabling the woman simply 'to be'. One part of the process of 'being' was found in the compassion shown by the health care practitioner. Rose evaluated the aromatherapy sessions positively saying that the aromatherapist 'managed my changing shape and massage positions with delicacy and above all *kindness*'. In the event Rose had a normal birth and did not have the time or need for any extra support from her partner because she had a supportive midwife whom she also described as *very kind*. Rose evidently valued this element of care in both the midwife and the CAM practitioner. The compassion that she experienced promoted mental health as the HCP practiced in an unconditional and accepting manner. This kindness and compassion gave no room for any judgement and allowed Rose truly to be herself, which positively reinforced Rose's sense of self. This increased self-empowerment may have contributed to enabling her to cope better with the childbearing process. The connection between the mind and the body is well known and is often seen clearly in midwifery. The science of mind–body medicine or psychoneuroimmunology (PNI) is well respected in CAM (Fenwick 2001).

PSYCHONEUROIMMUNOLOGY

PNI is 'the study of the intricate interaction of consciousness (psycho) brain and central nervous system (neuro) and the body's defence against infection and abnormal cell division (immunology)' (Fenwick 2001, 216). Studies have shown that a positive affective response to circumstances, loving supportive relationships, optimism for the future and learning how to cope with psychological stress may all keep our immune system healthy.

PNI appears to work at a level which cannot be seen or felt. Midwives see this, for example, when the midwife is in a position to practise her skills and let a woman freely express her anxieties, emotions and fears. This may be all that is needed to promote normal childbearing. However, sometimes there is an unanswered situation when there is no obvious reason for delay in the birthing process. Several types of CAM may be utilised to promote health in this situation, which means bringing the body back into balance and harmony (PNI). Some examples of this are reflexology, homeopathy and spiritual healing. In spiritual healing, it is recognised that there is meaning in giving birth and that it may be a mystical experience for some women.

In the case of Lily, PNI may have played a role in the outcome. Lily had support from her midwives, partner and friends and was at ease with the midwives, feeling comfortable discussing anxieties with them. Lily was confident she was looking after herself and promoting her own health.

Case study: Lily

Lily was 41 weeks pregnant and had planned a home birth. Since the pregnancy was now overdue there was concern from the professionals caring for Lily regarding the continuing health of the baby. The necessary tests to monitor the baby's well-being and the function of the placenta were booked for the following day. Lily was worried that she would end up giving birth in hospital. She talked to her friends who recommended that she contact a healer who had experience in end of pregnancy issues. The healer listened to Lily's concerns and took a history. Lily confirmed that although she was delighted to be pregnant, she had some concerns about whether she would love her baby which she had already openly discussed with the midwives and her partner. Healing was undertaken by the healer. This involved the healer tuning into Lily and her baby and revealed the need to think positively about welcoming the arrival of the baby. Lily practiced some positive affirmations concentrating on visualising her baby being born and being open to any issues or feelings arising for her. This process seemed to stir up and encourage feelings of love and excitement. A few hours later that night Lily's membranes broke and she went into spontaneous labour. Her baby was born at home.

The healer worked with the aim of providing what Lily and her baby needed from a spiritual perspective. This type of healing may have identified an issue at a physical, mental or emotional level (PNI) and was working holistically. The healer's perspective was of promoting balance and achieving harmony for mother and child through the modality of healing. The practice of using positive affirmations promoted the health and interconnectedness of baby and mother. Although this episode cannot be identified as proof that the healing actually worked (as Lily may have achieved a normal birth at home going into spontaneous labour without this intervention). Lily found the process of healing relaxing and so felt it was helpful. In addition, she achieved her choice and goal of a home birth. Lily reported feeling so supported that she would not want to undergo any subsequent pregnancies without a healer caring for her in a complementary fashion to her midwifery care. The healing identified an area that was a subconscious concern to Lily and the positive affirmation created harmony and wholeness (PNI).

Many different forms of CAM may find areas of imbalance of which the client is not aware and therefore over which she has no conscious control. These forms of CAM often look at the body in a very different way to orthodox medicine and so may be difficult to explain within a medical reductionist framework.

The case of Lily highlights the spiritual area of health promotion, which illustrates a belief that we are all interconnected at some level. When we can truly be with a woman as a midwife and truly be with a client as a CAM practitioner, this has been shown to promote health positively. This entails believing that women's bodies can work as they are meant to and that, unless there is a mechanical problem, women can birth their babies normally. The focus that a midwife or CAM practitioner has on the woman is vitally important to promote health.

In physical terms, this *may* mean maintaining eye contact, tuning into the woman's needs, using or not using touch as necessary or as requested. Conversely, Odent (2009) stipulates the importance of *not* having eye contact with the woman. He states that even this eye contact may inadvertently pull the woman out of her own successful way of coping. This of course depends on the individual woman. The midwife can be with-woman in many different ways. One way is concentrating her thoughts fully on the woman, not 'letting her thoughts run away with her' by, for example, compiling a list of what to buy for tea tonight, but keeping her awareness open positively to the woman's birthing process. The intention of the practitioner in CAM would be to treat the whole woman (and this would be the same for the midwife practising holistically). Often this would explicitly mean being there for the woman, being her advocate, and the woman knowing that she can trust the midwife/CAM practitioner.

> **PRACTICE POINT**
>
> Midwives and CAM practitioners are both trained to work holistically, considering the woman as a whole person and working with women and their families in partnership.

INTEGRATION OF CAM

Women may choose not to disclose the use of CAM to a midwife for fear of receiving a negative attitude (Hall & Jolly 2014; Mitchell 2010). Thomson et al. (2014) found that people may begin to use CAM before they seek help from conventional medicine or as a last resort maybe after an unsatisfactory outcome with medical treatment or in the search for a clearer understanding of the problem or issue (Hall et al. 2012).

Netherwood and Derham (2014) propose a more integrated health care system, that is, to bring homeopaths and other complementary therapists together with adult nurses and midwives as part of an inter-professional education programme. This could help break down prejudices, gain a better awareness of self and others and realise organisational limitations regarding the use of CAM in medical settings. Ideally, a CAM therapist interested in promoting health would communicate with the appropriate health professional with the woman's consent. It is important that health professionals broach the subject of CAM with their clients in order to give them informed choice (Hunt et al. 2010).

CONCLUSION

CAMs are being integrated into midwifery to help promote normal birth, and this push for integrated health care is coming from women and like-minded CAM-trained midwives. It is recognised that CAM is becoming more popular but we may not have a true indication of the number of women who use CAM because women often do not disclose their use of CAMs to HCPs or midwives. Then also HCPs and midwives do not enquire if women are using any CAMs.

Two different case studies have illustrated how the promotion of mental and spiritual health achieved holistic care and may have facilitated normal childbirth. The role of CAM therapies in health promotion is specifically through the empowerment of women to be themselves. CAM practitioners work with women using compassion and support. A therapeutic partnership with the woman is created, and this has been shown to increase control and choice which then can successfully promote health in childbearing.

SUMMARY OF KEY POINTS

- Knowledge about CAM is important so that midwives can offer informed choice to women and women can feel empowered, in control and keep birth as normal as possible.
- Women use CAM in pregnancy and childbirth but often do not inform health practitioners. Health care professionals need to ask women about their use of CAM in pregnancy to ensure safety, to facilitate good team working and integration of CAM.
- It is important to fully understand the meaning of holism, because it is this philosophy of care that women seem interested in pursuing in childbirth.
- Midwives can be dual trained, which means that CAM therapies can be offered on the NHS and therefore be available to all women.
- Working with CAM therapies can lead to an improvement in self-esteem, mental and physical well-being, foster partnership working and be therapeutic increasing the experience of kindness and compassion.

REFERENCES

Battaglia, Salvatore. 2004. *The complete guide to aromatherapy* (2nd ed.). Australia: The Perfect Potion.

Byrne, Jean, Yvonne Hauck, Colleen Fisher, Sara Bayes & Robert Schultze. 2014. Effectiveness of a Mindfulness-Based Childbirth Education pilot study on maternal self-efficacy and fear of childbirth. *Journal of Midwifery & Women's Health* 59(2): 192–197.

Cant, Sarah, Peter Watts & Annemarie Ruston. 2011. Negotiating competency: Professionalism and risk. The integration of complementary and alternative medicine by nurses and midwives. *Social Science and Medicine* 72(4): 529–536.

Davis-Floyd, Robbie & Gloria St. John. 1998. *From doctor to healer. The transformative journey.* London: Rutgers University Press.

DoH (Department of Health). 2007. *Maternity matters. Choice, access and continuity of care in a safe service.* London: DoH.

Ernst, Edzard & Leala K. Watson. 2012. Midwives' use of complementary/alternative treatments. *Midwifery* 28: 772–777.

Fenwick, Peter. 2001. Psychoneuroimmunology: The mind–brain connection. In: Peters David (ed.), *Understanding the placebo effect in complementary medicine.* London: Churchill Livingstone, pp. 215–226.

Field, Tiffany. 2014. Massage therapy research review. *Complementary Therapies in Clinical Practice* 20(4): 224–229.

Hall, Hannah & Kate Jolly. 2014. Women's use of complementary and alternative medicine during pregnancy. A cross sectional study. *Midwifery* 30(1): 499–505.

Hall, Helen, Lisa McKenna & Debra Griffiths. 2012. Midwife's support for complementary and alternative medicine. A literature review. *Women and Birth* 25(1): 4–12.

House of Lords Select Committee on Science and Technology. 2000. *Complementary and alternative medicine.* London: The Stationery Office.

Hunt, Katherine, Helen Coelho, Barbara Wider, Rachel Perry, S. Hung, Rohini Terry & E. Ernst. 2010. Complementary and alternative medicine use in England: Results from a national survey. *International Journal of Clinical Practice* 64(11): 1496–1502.

Kaptchuk, Ted & Franklin Miller. 2015. Placebo effects in medicine. *New England Journal of Medicine* 373: 8–9.

Marc, Isabelle, Narimane Toureche, Edzard Ernst, Ellen Hodnett, Claudine Blanchet, Sylvia Dodin & Merlin Njoya. 2011. Mind-body interventions during pregnancy for preventing or treating women's anxiety. *Cochrane Database Systematic Review* 7. http://onlinelibrary.wiley.com/doi/10.1002/14651858.CD007559.pub2/epdf

Mitchell, Mary. 2010. Risk, pregnancy and complementary and alternative medicine. *Complementary Therapies in Clinical Practice* 16(2): 109–113.

Netherwood, Maggie & Ruth Derham. 2014. Interprofessional education: Merging nursing midwifery and CAM. *British Journal of Nursing* 23(13): 740–743.

NICE (National Institute for Health and Clinical Excellence). 2008. *Antenatal care*. London: NICE.

NMC (Nursing and Midwifery Council). 2007. *Standards for medicines management*. London: NMC.

NMC (Nursing and Midwifery Council). 2015. *The code for nurses and midwives: Professional standards of practice and behaviour for nurses and midwives*. London: NMC.

Odent, Michel. 2009. *The function of the orgasms: The highways to transcendence*. London: Pinter & Martin.

RCN (Royal College of Nursing). 2003. *Complementary therapies in nursing, midwifery and health visiting practice*. London: RCN.

Tiran, Denise. 2012. Ginger to reduce nausea and vomiting during pregnancy. Evidence of its effectiveness is not the same as proof of safety. *Complementary Therapies in Clinical Practice* 18(1): 22–25.

Thompson, Trevor & Gene Feder. 2005. Complementary therapies and the NHS. *British Medical Journal* 331(7521): 856–857.

Thomson, Patricia, Jenny Jones, Mathew Browne & Stephen Leslie. 2014. Why people seek complementary and alternative medicine before conventional medical treatment. A population based study. *Complementary Therapies in Clinical Practice* 20(4): 339–346.

Warriner, Sian, Karen Bryan & Anna Maria Brown. 2014. Women's attitudes towards the use of CAM in pregnancy. *Midwifery* 30(1): 138–143.

WHO (World Health Organization). 1986. *The Ottawa Charter for health promotion*. Geneva: WHO.

WHO (World Health Organization). 2003. WHO traditional medicine. Fact Sheet No. 134 http://www.who.int/mediacentre/factsheets/2003/fs134/en/

Wieland, Susan, Manheimer Eric & Berman Brian. 2011. Development and classification of an operational definition of complementary and alternative medicine for the Cochrane Collaboration. *Alternative Therapies in Health and Medicine* 17(2): 50–59.

Williams, Julie & Mary Mitchell. 2007. Midwifery managers' views about the use of complementary therapies in the maternity services. *Complementary Therapies in Clinical Practice* 13(2): 129–135.

FURTHER READINGS

NHS choices. 2014. All about complementary and alternative medicine. http://www.nhs.uk/Livewell/complementary-alternative-medicine/Pages/complementary-alternative-medicines.aspx

Complementary Therapies in Clinical Practice journal

WHO. 2015. Traditional and complementary medicines. http://www.who.int/medicines/areas/traditional/en/

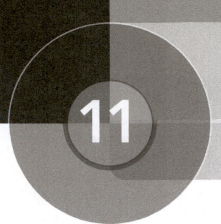

Mental health promotion in midwifery practice

IAN P S NOONAN

INTRODUCTION

This chapter aims to explore how midwives can promote the mental health of all women in their care. This includes women who have or who are at risk of mental illnesses as well as women who are mentally fit and well and who we want to help maintain or improve their psychological well-being throughout their pregnancy and labour.

In order to achieve this, we first need to explore and define mental health and mental illness to know what they are and consider how pregnancy might impact on them. The chapter will then identify the specific risks to mental health associated with pregnancy, childbirth and the postnatal period, before exploring interventions to promote maintenance of well-being and to prevent relapse in pregnant women with mental health problems. These different approaches will be broadly framed within a model of primary, secondary and tertiary illness prevention as defined by Boyce et al. (2010) in their exploration of health promotion in public health, and by an exploration of the model of mental health promotion and demotion proposed by MacDonald and O'Hara (1998) known as the *Ten Elements of Mental Health*.

Examples applied to practice will be used to illustrate the concepts and approaches and learning activities identified to help explore how the mental health of women in our care may be promoted or demoted. The learning outcomes for this chapter are:

- For midwives to be able to promote the mental health of all women in their care through primary, secondary and tertiary illness prevention interventions.
- For midwives to understand what bio-psycho-social factors might put a woman's mental health at risk during pregnancy.
- For midwives to consider what sociological and organisational factors, impacting both on the women in their care and on the exercise of their practice, might risk demoting women's mental health.

MENTAL HEALTH

If we are aiming to promote something, we need to know what it is. However, both mental health and mental illness are difficult concepts to define. The World Health Organization (WHO 2014) defines mental health as follows:

> Mental health is defined as a state of well-being in which every individual realizes his or her own potential, can cope with the normal stresses of life, can work productively and fruitfully, and is able to make a contribution to her or his community.

This is a positive definition and is meant to be inclusive and applicable globally. However, the concept of mental health is defined not as a discrete phenomenon but in relation to someone's social role, ability to cope, work and contribute to their community. Inevitably, this means that what appears to others as mentally healthy differs throughout our lives and in different cultures. It immediately illustrates one of the dilemmas faced by women who have children and chose to, or feel obliged to, return to work and for those who are able to, or chose to stay at home to, raise their children. What is considered fruitful, productive or a contribution may represent a judgement by others rather than solely the women's own values, ideas and hopes. It is perhaps this very tension between one's own desires and the expectations and values of others that is most keenly felt in pregnancy when everyone seems to have an opinion about what is the right thing to do. This tension could be viewed as a stressor in the stress–vulnerability model discussed later and illustrated in Figure 11.2.

If we compare this definition with what Keith Tudor (1996) describes as the eight elements of mental health, it is clear that there are further possible tensions. Tudor (1996) suggests that mental health is dynamic and responsive to our ability to cope; ability to manage tension and stress; self-concept or identity; self-esteem; self-development; ability to exercise autonomy; ability to adapt to change; and ability to harness support available. This flexible and fluid definition seems at odds with the WHO (2015) definition that mental health is a 'state' – something fixed and permanent in some way. For many, pregnancy and childbirth are among the biggest and most dramatic changes in their lives. It therefore has the ability to affect women's mental health both positively and negatively.

ACTIVITY

Think about women you have cared for and identify the ways in which their experience of pregnancy and childbirth may have impacted on each of Tudor's eight elements of mental health.

Try to consider how they might be affected positively and negatively.

For example, in terms of autonomy, a woman may find the choices offered to her while booking an appointment and whilst agreeing to her birth plan positive, as she gets to consider, express and agree the type of labour she would like to have and rule out things she would like to avoid. However, if these are compromised in an emergency situation and she and her partner are involved in making quick decisions that go against her values, her autonomy may feel undermined.

As with the autonomy example, there are no concrete right or wrong answers to this. In your reflection, it may be helpful to think of things on a continuum: Was the woman's experience or my practice more likely to be in the direction of promoting or demoting each of the eight elements of Tudor (1996)?

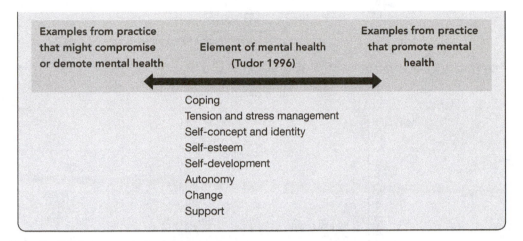

Examples from practice that might compromise or demote mental health	Element of mental health (Tudor 1996)	Examples from practice that promote mental health
	Coping	
	Tension and stress management	
	Self-concept and identity	
	Self-esteem	
	Self-development	
	Autonomy	
	Change	
	Support	

MacDonald and O'Hara (1998, 10) conclude that there is no single definition of mental health that includes the human needs and psychological constructs as well as the 'social conditions, structures, contexts and processes in which the individual's experiences are grounded'. Broadly speaking, any definition needs to include the recognition that health in any context is a balance of self, others and the environment (WHO 2004) and that mental health is more than merely the absence of mental illness. In this way, the mental health of all women in our care should be prioritised. This is both an ideal value and a professional requirement in midwifery practice.

The Nursing & Midwifery Council, in Section 3 of *Prioritising People* in The Code (NMC 2015), requires us to make sure that people's physical, social and psychological needs are assessed and responded to, for which one must:

3.1 pay special attention to promoting well-being, preventing ill health and meeting the changing health and care needs of people during all life stages…

3.3 act in partnership with those receiving care, helping them to access relevant health and social care, information and support when they need it, and

3.4 act as an advocate for the vulnerable, challenging poor practice and discriminatory attitudes and behaviour relating to their care.

Part 3.1 of the code relates to primary prevention of mental illness and parts 3.3 and 3.4 to both secondary and tertiary prevention as outlined below.

MENTAL ILLNESS

Some models explain mental illness as the deficit or outcome of an interaction between our stressors and ability to cope with them. Albee and Ryan-Finn (1993) proposed a formula for mental illness in order to identify where there might be opportunities for mental health promotion, explaining that mental illness resulted when stress, exploitation and organic factors outweighed or exceeded our ability to cope, self-esteem and social support (Figure 11.1).

Similarly, Zubin and Spring (1977), in an attempt to explain why some people get schizophrenia and others do not, devised the stress–vulnerability model, which can in turn be used to explain other mental illnesses. They suggested that individual vulnerability to, or ability to cope with, either internal or external stressors determined whether someone was able to tolerate the stress and integrate the experience or were vulnerable to an episode of mental illness. This is illustrated in Figure 11.2.

$$\text{Mental illness} = \frac{\text{Organic factors} + \text{stress} + \text{exploitation}}{\text{Coping skills} + \text{self-esteem} + \text{social support}}$$

Figure 11.1 A formula explaining mental illness.

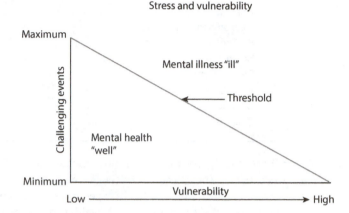

Figure 11.2 The stress–vulnerability model. (From Zubin, Joseph and Bonnie Spring. 1977. *Journal of Abnormal Psychology* 86(2):103–126.)

Zubin and Spring (1977) suggest that we all have an innate vulnerability to mental illness that could be considered low or high depending on a number of factors (Figure 11.2). Honig (1993), specifically in relation to hearing voices, identifies six factors that combine to form our vulnerability: personality traits, important life events, social isolation, physical disease, genetic disposition and early experiences. These could be considered as our 'fixed assets' that form who we are and how we respond to most situations from late adolescence onwards.

For example, someone who has parents with acute mental illnesses may have a genetic predisposition and have had an insecure attachment to their primary carer (particularly if their mother was ill postnatally), impacting on some negative early life experiences and social isolation in adulthood. For this person, with a high vulnerability, it may only take what others might perceive as a relatively small challenging or stressful event to become mentally ill. For another person, without any family history of illness, a secure attachment and happy upbringing, who is physically well and socially engaged, their vulnerability might be low, but exposed to a high level of stress, they could still become ill.

There are limitations to this model. Many of us experience symptoms of stress that exceed either our ability to cope or the limits of our vulnerability: for example, anxiety about an observed assessment in practice or a sleepless night thinking about someone in our care. In noticing and doing something about these symptoms, we might be at, but not crossing, the imaginary threshold into illness. It is more like a zone in which the interaction of our vulnerability and stress causes concern but not necessarily mental illness.

ACTIVITY

Think about your own vulnerabilities: how might your early life experiences, physical health, social life, etc. influence the ways in which you respond to stress.

Recall a time when you have experienced the sort of stress that has challenged your ability to cope. What did you notice that might suggest your individual vulnerability risked being exceeded?

It is important to consider these models before introducing a definition of mental illness in order to try and avoid any sense that mental illness is something that happens to 'other people'. By considering what impacts on a continuum of mental health and what interactions impact on our potential to experience mental illness, it is hoped that this will convince you that it is relevant to all of us and all of the women in our care. We all have some vulnerabilities and are all exposed to stress.

The mental health charity, MIND, uses the broader term 'mental health problems' and gives an excellent plain language summary of what these might be from the point of view of the person experiencing them:

> Mental health problems can affect the way you think, feel and behave. Some mental health problems are described using words that are in everyday use, for example 'depression' or 'anxiety'. This can make them seem easier to understand, but can also mean people underestimate how serious they can be.
>
> A mental health problem feels just as bad, or worse, than any other illness – only you cannot see it. Although mental health problems are very common – affecting around one in four people in Britain – there is still stigma and discrimination towards people with mental health problems, as well as many myths about what different diagnoses mean.
>
> There are also a lot of different ideas about the way mental health problems are diagnosed, what causes them and which treatments are most effective.
>
> However, despite these challenges, it is possible to recover from a mental health problem and live a productive and fulfilling life. It is important to remember that, if you have a mental health problem, it is not a sign of weakness.
>
> MIND (2015)

One of the difficulties in defining mental illness is whether to describe it from the personal, subjective experience of living with the illness; from the perspective of the clinician in terms of which diagnostic criteria it meets; or from the point of view of the family, carers or wider society on whom the illness impacts. The WHO (2014) definition focusses on a symptomatic approach:

> Mental disorders comprise a broad range of problems, with different symptoms. However, they are generally characterized by some combination of abnormal thoughts, emotions, behaviour and relationships with others. Examples are schizophrenia, depression, intellectual disabilities and disorders due to drug abuse. Most of these disorders can be successfully treated.

Both of these definitions overlook to some degree the social process and the impact of environment and culture. MacDonald and O'Mara incorporated these into their 10 elements of mental health, each of which offers a continuum of factors that promote or demote mental health. Mental health and illness are often described as polar opposites on a continuum, and sometimes on dual continua of mental illness and mental well-being (e.g. Westerhof & Keyes 2010). However, as Tudor (1996) points out, these continua are mistakenly described on a plane, whereas he views the continuum more as a slide:

This suggests that it is easier to maintain than to regain mental health (Figure 11.3). Whilst many people make a full recovery, learn from it and integrate their experience of mental illness, others find it has a profound impact on their relationships, social function, employment, housing, all putting them at risk of social exclusion (Repper & Perkins 2003) which is why mental health promotion and mental illness prevention are so important.

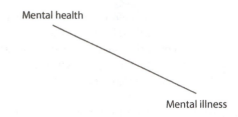

Figure 11.3 Continuum of mental health and mental illness as a slide.

PERINATAL MENTAL ILLNESS PREVENTION AND MANAGEMENT

In midwifery, perinatal mental health problems affect up to 20% of women, and only 50% of those experiencing perinatal anxiety or depression are identified in spite of regular contact and screening (Khan 2015) (Figure 11.4). The NICE guidelines are clear that many mental illnesses present in the same way during pregnancy as at any other time, but that there are also specific risks to women's mental health in the perinatal period (NICE 2014):

- Increased rate of relapse of bipolar affective disorder (postnatal)
- Increased rate of first presentation of bipolar affective disorder (postnatal)
- Normal changes in appetite during pregnancy might mask changes that are a symptom of mental illness

Furthermore, treatment during and after pregnancy often has to differ because of possible impacts of the treatment on the mother and the baby:

- Taking psychotropic medications during pregnancy and whilst breastfeeding is problematic. None is safe or licenced for use during pregnancy, but there are also risks to the mother's mental health of stopping medication treating an existing mental illness.
- Women who stop their psychotropic medication during pregnancy have an increased risk of post-partum psychosis.
- Depression and anxiety are the most common mental health problems during pregnancy, with around 12% of women experiencing depression and 13% experiencing anxiety at some point; many women will experience both. Depression and anxiety also affect 15%–20% of women in the first year after childbirth.
- During pregnancy and the postnatal period, anxiety disorders, including panic disorder, generalised anxiety disorder (GAD), obsessive–compulsive disorder (OCD), post-traumatic stress disorder (PTSD) and tokophobia (an extreme fear of childbirth), can occur on their own or can coexist with depression.
- Psychosis can re-emerge or be exacerbated during pregnancy and the postnatal period. Post-partum psychosis affects between 1 and 2 in 1,000 women who have given birth. Women with bipolar I disorder are at particular risk, but post-partum psychosis can occur in women with no previous psychiatric history.
- Changes to body shape, including weight gain, in pregnancy and after childbirth may be a concern for women with an eating disorder. Although the prevalence of anorexia nervosa and bulimia nervosa is lower in pregnant women, the prevalence of binge eating disorder is higher.

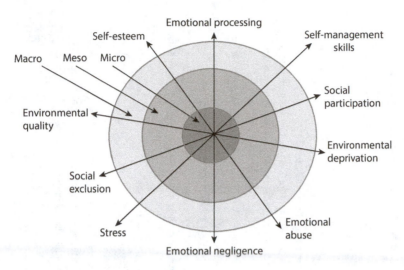

Figure 11.4 The 10 elements of mental health promotion and demotion. (From MacDonald, Glenn, and Kate O'Hara. 1998. *Ten Elements of Mental Health, Its Promotion and Demotion: Implications for Practice.* London: Society of Health Education & Health Promotion Specialists.)

- Smoking and the use of illicit drugs and alcohol in pregnancy are common, and prematurity, intrauterine growth restriction and fetal compromise are more common in women who use these substances, particularly women who smoke (NICE 2014).

In terms of management of mental illness, the NICE guidelines outline core principles that have to be applied to the care of all women (Table 11.1). The recommendations are structured over time from women of childbearing potential, those planning pregnancy, through pregnancy and the postnatal period, and consider interventions for traumatic experiences or stillbirths and organisational responses to the management of mental illness in pregnancy (NICE 2014).

MENTAL HEALTH PROMOTION IN MIDWIFERY

All of the NICE guideline recommendations focus on tertiary prevention strategies. They are meant to minimise the risk of relapse and reduce the incapacity or injury caused in the group of women who have mental health problems. However, The Royal College of Midwives (RCM) is clear that all women should have their emotional well-being assessed and that screening for post partum depression should be routine (RCM 2014). These are primary and secondary prevention strategies aimed at promoting the mental health of all.

The different types of prevention are defined and illustrated with examples in Table 11.2.

As a minimum standard for postnatal care, the RCM (2014) state that all women should have their emotional well-being and emotional attachment to the child assessed at each postnatal visit, that transient low mood or anxiety that does not resolve within 10–14 days should be formally assessed for mental health problems and that parents and primary carers who are identified as having attachment problems should receive services and support to improve their relationship with the baby.

Table 11.1 Summary of the NICE guidelines for antenatal and postnatal mental health

NICE core recommendation	Detail	Examples in practice
Considerations for women of childbearing potential	Discuss with all women of childbearing potential who have a new, existing or past mental health problem: • The use of contraception and any plans for a pregnancy; how pregnancy and childbirth might affect a mental health problem, including the risk of relapse; how a mental health problem and its treatment might affect the woman, the fetus and the baby; how a mental health problem and its treatment might affect parenting. • Do not offer valproate for acute or long-term treatment of a mental health problem in women of childbearing potential.	Community midwife liaison with: • Mental health services • GP practices • Primary care • Health education for women of childbearing potential • Mental health service-user and advocacy groups

Principles of care in pregnancy and the postnatal period	Develop an integrated care plan for a woman with a mental health problem in pregnancy and the postnatal period.	Integrated care plans should set out:
		• The care and treatment for the mental health problem
		• The roles of all health care professionals, including who is responsible for:
		  • Coordinating the integrated care plan, the schedule of monitoring
		  • Providing the interventions and agreeing on the outcomes with the woman

Treatment decisions, advice and monitoring for women who are planning a pregnancy, pregnant or in the postnatal period	Mental health professionals providing detailed advice about the possible risks of mental health problems or the benefits and harms of treatment in pregnancy and the postnatal period should include discussion of the following, depending on individual circumstances: • The uncertainty about the benefits, risks and harms of treatments for mental health problems in pregnancy and the postnatal period and the likely benefits of each treatment, taking into account; • The severity of the mental health problem • The woman's response to any previous treatment • The background risk of harm to the woman and the fetus or the baby associated with the mental health problem	Providing information and advice and liaising with specialists, for example: • Mental health pharmacists • Obstetricians • Psychiatrists • Specialist mental health midwives Acting as an advocate for women to ensure their voice is heard in the multi-disciplinary discussions

(Continued)

Table 11.1 (Continued) Summary of the NICE guidelines for antenatal and postnatal mental health

NICE core recommendation	Detail	Examples in practice
	• The risk to mental health and parenting associated with no treatment • The possibility of the sudden onset of symptoms of mental health problems in pregnancy and the postnatal period • The risks or harms to the woman and the fetus or the baby associated with each treatment option • The need for prompt treatment because of the potential effect of an untreated mental health problem on the fetus or the baby • The risk or harms to the woman and the fetus or the baby associated with stopping or changing a treatment	
Recognising mental health problems in pregnancy and the postnatal period and referral	At a woman's first contact with primary care or her booking visit, and during the early postnatal period, consider asking the depression identification questions in the column on the right as part of a general discussion about a woman's mental health and well-being	Ask the following screening questions: • During the past month, have you often been bothered by feeling down, depressed or hopeless? • During the past month, have you often been bothered by having little interest or pleasure in doing things? Also, consider asking about anxiety using the 2-item Generalised Anxiety Disorder (GAD-2) scale: • Over the past 2 weeks, how often have you been bothered by feeling nervous, anxious or on edge? • Over the past 2 weeks, how often have you been bothered by not being able to stop or control worrying?
Providing interventions in pregnancy and the postnatal period	All health care professionals providing assessment and interventions for mental health problems in pregnancy and the postnatal period should understand the variations in their presentation and course at these times, how these variations affect treatment, and the context in which they are assessed and treated	Organise inter-professional education and professional development with maternity services, health visiting and mental health services

(Continued)

Table 11.1 (*Continued*) Summary of the NICE guidelines for antenatal and postnatal mental health

NICE core recommendation	Detail	Examples in practice
Considerations for women and their babies in the postnatal period	Discuss with a woman whose baby is stillborn or dies soon after birth, and her partner and family, the option of one or more of the following: • Seeing a photograph of the baby • Having mementos of the baby • Seeing the baby • Holding the baby	This should be facilitated by an experienced practitioner and the woman and her partner and family should be offered a follow-up appointment in primary or secondary care If it is known that the baby has died in utero, this discussion should take place before the delivery, and continue after delivery, if needed
The organisation of services	Clinical networks should be established for perinatal mental health services, managed by a coordinating board of health care professionals, commissioners, managers, and service users and carers	A specialist multi-disciplinary perinatal service in each locality, which provides direct services, consultation and advice to maternity services, and other mental health services and community services In areas of high morbidity, these services may be provided by separate specialist perinatal teams with access to specialist expert advice on the risks and benefits of psychotropic medication during pregnancy and breastfeeding Clear referral and management protocols for services across all levels of the existing stepped-care frameworks for mental health problems, to ensure effective transfer of information and continuity of care

Table 11.2 Primary, secondary and tertiary prevention

Definition in Boyce et al. (2010)	Examples of application to midwifery practice in the context of mental health promotion
Primary prevention This comprises activities designed to reduce the instances of an illness in a population and thus to reduce (as far as possible) the risk of new cases appearing, and to reduce their duration	• Consideration of the stress–vulnerability model • Promoting a woman's autonomy, self-esteem, coping mechanisms, adaptability to change, transitions of identity and ensuring support is available • Sensitive and thorough history taking exploring mental illness, self-harm, drug and alcohol use and any experience of partner violence at the time of booking
Secondary prevention This comprises activities aimed at detecting and treating pre-symptomatic disease	• Screening during pregnancy using the depression and anxiety screening questions (During the past month, have you often been bothered by feeling down, depressed or hopeless? During the past month, have you often been bothered by having little interest or pleasure in doing things?) • Postnatal screening using the above questions and a structured tool such as the Edinburgh Postnatal Depression Scale (EPDS). For further details, see NICE (2014)
Tertiary prevention These are activities aimed at reducing the incidence of chronic incapacity or recurrences in a population, and thus to reduce the functional consequences of an illness, including therapy, rehabilitation techniques or interventions designed to help the patient to return to educational, family, professional, social and cultural life	• All of the recommendations in the NICE guidelines (NICE 2014) • Information and advice giving • Planned pregnancy • Specialist liaison midwife role linking with pharmacists, obstetricians, psychiatrists, community drug and alcohol teams, primary care and service-user groups • Lobbying for specialist post-registration training and specialist service development

MENTAL HEALTH PROMOTION FOR ALL

There remains a risk that mental health promotion is seen as something we only need to do for women who either have a mental illness or are at obvious risk of developing one during or after pregnancy. However, if we use the model of 10 elements of mental health proposed by MacDonald and O'Hara (1998), we could consider that for every interaction at a micro-, meso- and macro-level (Tones & Tilford 2001), there are opportunities, thereby a choice to either promote or demote the mental health of the woman in our care. The micro-level is primarily concerned with the relationship, interactions and interventions between the individual midwife and the woman, her supporters and family and the immediate team. Meso-level interventions are those around the organisation of service delivery, inter-professional liaison and availability of services, for example, and at the macro-level we are concerned with maternal health care funding, priority within the NHS, social trends and issues such as stigma that effect whole populations' views around mental health and mental illness.

The 10 elements of the mental health model attempt to integrate the personal experience of mental health and illness, the impact on family and friends as well as the causal factors of illness in an integrated bio-psycho-social approach. It builds on the work cited above by Albee and Ryan-Finn (1993) and expands the six components of their equation to include environmental, social and self-management/emotional intelligence and maps these across the micro-, meso- and macro-levels.

At the micro, or personal interaction, level, the way in which we care for women can promote their health if we demonstrate woman-centred care and empathy (Figure 11.4). These are not just abstract concepts but the skills we use to make the promoting (rather than demoting) choices. In order to promote a woman's self-esteem, emotional processing and social participation, for example, we need to demonstrate Warmth, Acceptance, Genuineness and Empathy (WAGE) (Rungapadiachy 2008): warmth towards the women, her partner or other family and friends; acceptance of her choices and values; genuineness in your care of her; and empathic responses showing that you have understood, or are attempting to understand, both the content and meaning of what she says and does.

In order to demonstrate empathy, we need not have had the same experience as the woman in our care but be able to imagine what primary emotion she is feeling (fear, happiness, sadness or anger) and be open to knowing what that feels like. We then need to demonstrate that we have understood that emotion. Wiseman (1996) summarises this process as:

- Perspective taking – trying to see things from the woman's point of view
- Staying out of judgement – even when her values seem very different from yours
- Recognising emotion in others and communicating it
- Feeling *with* – making a connection with the woman that acknowledges what she is experiencing

ACTIVITY

Read through the following case study and answer the questions below which should guide you through the principles of applying the 10 elements of mental health in a practical way.

Agnita is a 21-year-old woman who moved to England from Poland with her partner, Gregor, 3 years ago. They both work full-time in a bar owned by Gregor's cousin.

Agnita is expecting her first baby, which was not planned, but they are happy to be pregnant and Gregor has attended both the GP appointments and her first appointment with you as her midwife at about 12 weeks into her pregnancy.

During the appointment, you notice some old scars on Agnita's wrist and when you ask about them briefly, she dismisses them saying 'they are just old childish things', but you think that she seemed uncomfortable talking about them. The rest of the booking is unremarkable and when asked, Agnita states she has no history of physical or mental illness. She has occasionally had too much alcohol in the past but nothing since she thought she might be pregnant. She has never used illicit drugs. Her partner, Gregor, answers a number of the questions for her and corrects her answers on occasion. He is keen to be involved throughout.

Gregor has also asked for your help to give them proof that she is pregnant as they are currently on a waiting list for a housing association flat and need to move out of their flat share where they have one room, but share with four other young people who won't want a baby in the house.

1. First, identify what issues you might want to follow-up with Agnita in order to assess and promote her mental health.

2. Now consider each of the continua within MacDonald and O'Hara's model to plan how you would go about doing this in a way that promotes rather than demotes Agnita's mental health. For example, you may want to ask to see her on her own so that she can answer questions without being interrupted, but how might this impact on her social support or self-esteem. Try to identify an approach for each continuum:

Emotional processing	←——————→	Emotional negligence
Self-esteem	←——————→	Emotional abuse
Environmental quality	←——————→	Environmental deprivation
Social participation	←——————→	Social exclusion
Self-management skills	←——————→	Stress

3. Finally, think about the organisation in which you work or have been on placement. How will you raise these issues on a micro (interpersonal) level with Agnita and with colleagues; what meso or organisational barriers might there be to promoting Agnita's mental health; and at the macro-level, what policies might inform your decision making in practice?

It might be easier to identify the interventions at an individual and organisational level, and in terms of primary promotion of mental health, there are no right or wrong answers to the above exercise. The only thing that is clear from both the NMC (2015) and RCM (2014) is that mental health and psychological well-being must be assessed and promoted. At a macro-level, Khan (2015) makes several recommendations to policy makers and commissioners. Although the report addresses maternal mental health in primary care, they are just as relevant to midwives who are in a position to lobby service managers and commissioners. These include:

- Full implementation of the NICE guidelines on perinatal mental health
- Reducing pressure on workloads in order to allow longer consultations
- Work to reduce stigma around perinatal mental health problems
- Promoting effective liaison between maternity and health visiting services to ensure ongoing assessment of maternal health and attachment
- Fund and provide specialist training around perinatal mental health
- Multi-agency liaison by the various commissioning groups

SUMMARY

This chapter has explored the concepts of mental health and mental illness in order to consider the role of the midwife in promoting mental health and preventing mental illness in women before, during and after pregnancy.

- The NICE guidelines focus on secondary and tertiary prevention of illness and relapse in women who have or are at risk of mental illness, but it is also important for midwives to promote the mental health of all women in their care.
- This can be achieved by reflecting on the impact of pregnancy on the various elements and concepts that challenge all of our vulnerabilities.
- This may often present a balancing act between the needs and pressures of the services in which we work and the individual needs of the women in our care, but the cost of not assessing, screening and promoting perinatal mental health is far too great a risk to both the mother and her child in the long term.
- Both the NMC and RCM are clear that mental health promotion is the responsibility of all midwives.

REFERENCES

Albee, George W. & Kimberly D. Ryan-Finn. 1993. An overview of primary prevention. *Journal of Counselling and Development* 72(2): 115–123.

Boyce, Tammy, Stephen Peckham, Alison Hann & Susan Trenholm. 2010. *A Proactive Approach. Health Promotion and Ill-Health Prevention*. London: The King's Fund.

Honig, Adriaan. 1993. Medication and hearing voices. In Romme, Maurius & Sandra Escher, eds., *Accepting Voices*. London: MIND, pp. 235–243.

Khan, Lorraine. 2015. *Falling through the Gaps: Perinatal Mental Health and General Practice*. London: Centre for Mental Health.

MacDonald, Glenn & Kate O'Hara. 1998. *Ten Elements of Mental Health, Its Promotion and Demotion: Implications for Practice*. London: Society of Health Education & Health Promotion Specialists.

MIND. 2015. *Mental Health Problems*. http://www.mind.org.uk/information-support/types-of-mental-health-problems/mental-health-problems-general/

NICE. 2014. *Antenatal and Postnatal Mental Health: Clinical Management and Service Guidance Clinical Guideline* (Clinical Guideline 192). London: NICE.

NMC (Nursing & Midwifery Council). 2015. *The Code*. London: NMC.

RCM (Royal College of Midwives). 2014. *Maternal Mental Health: Improving Emotional Wellbeing in Postnatal Care*. London: Royal College of Midwives.

Repper, Julie & Rachel Perkins. 2003. *Social Inclusion and Recovery: A Model for Mental Health Practice*. Edinburgh: Balliere Tindall.

Rungapadiachy, Dev M. 2008. *Self-Awareness in Health Care: Engaging in Helping Relationships*. London: Palgrave Macmillan.

Tones, Keith & Silvia Tilford. 2001. *Health Promotion: Effectiveness, Efficiency and Equity*. Third edition. Andover, MA: Cengage.

Tudor, Keith. 1996. *Mental Health Promotion: Paradigms and Practice*. London: Routledge.

Westerhof, Gerban J. & Corrie L. M. Keyes. 2009. Mental illness and mental health: The two continua model across the lifespan. *Journal of Adult Development* 17(2):110–119.

WHO (World Health Organization). 2004. *Promoting Mental Health. Concepts, Emerging Evidence, Practice. Summary Report*. Geneva: WHO.

WHO (World Health Organization). 2014. *Mental Health. A State of Wellbeing*. http://www.who.int/features/factfiles/mental_health/en/

WHO (World Health Organization). 2015. *Mental Disorders*. http://www.who.int/topics/mental_disorders/en/

Wiseman, Theresa. 1996. A concept analysis of empathy. *Journal of Advanced Nursing* 23(6):1162–1167. doi: 10.1007/s10804-009-9082-y

Zubin, Joseph & Bonnie Spring. 1977. Vulnerability: A new view of schizophrenia. *Journal of Abnormal Psychology* 86(2):103–126.

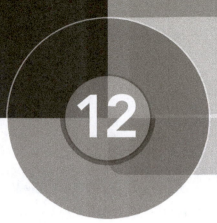

Sexual health promotion in midwifery practice

12

SARAH KIPPS

INTRODUCTION

This chapter will examine the sexual health needs of women during the journey through pregnancy and beyond. Pregnancy and childbirth is a special period in a woman's life and involves significant physical, hormonal, psychological, social and cultural change. As midwives, it is imperative that a holistic approach is taken to the woman's needs, and sexual health is an essential part of comprehensive health care.

Positive sexual health outcomes are seen as important to individuals, and they have also been recognised by the government as a major public health issue. There have been some achievements in sexual health targets, namely decline in teenage pregnancy and more high-risk groups being offered and accepting HIV tests (DoH 2013). But there are still major challenges – there were approximately 440,000 sexually transmitted infection diagnoses made in England in 2014 (Public Health England 2015), up to 50% of pregnancies were unplanned and almost half of adults newly diagnosed with HIV were diagnosed after the point where they should have started treatment (DoH 2013). Midwives are in an ideal position to improve the sexual and reproductive health of women. They have unique access to the private sphere of a woman and her family's life and are able to use targeted measures to address sexual health issues and promote positive sexual health outcomes. However, it has been reported that this area of midwifery practice, namely promoting sexual health, is an area more likely than others to be omitted. This can be for a variety of reasons: midwives feeling unskilled and unprepared to tackle the issue, the fear of uncovering something that the midwife cannot deal with, the perceived idea that new mothers are not interested in contraception and sexual health matters post birth and the idealisation of the new mother as a non-sexual being.

The chapter will discuss the midwife's role during the journey through pregnancy to motherhood and examine how midwives can facilitate positive sexual health promotion throughout this time. This is not without its challenges, but sexual health promotion is an integral part of a midwife's role and delivering this ensures the sexual well-being of the women who are being cared for, as well as their partners and families.

WHAT IS SEXUAL HEALTH?

Sexual health is a multi-faceted, broad concept which is not just narrowly defined by issues such as sexually transmitted infections, pregnancy and contraception but 'is a state of physical, emotional and social well being in relation to sexuality' (WHO 2006). It involves being at ease with one's body, sexual orientation and lifestyle choices. Physical sexual health does not just imply the absence of disease but being enabled to make positive health choices and being able to access services when needed. Sexual health can be altered during pregnancy and after childbirth due to a variety of factors – physical, emotional and psychological. Optimum sexual health outcomes can vary according to the differing needs of individual women and their partners. For some it will be resuming sexual intercourse, for some it will be feeling comfortable in a postnatal body and for others it will be expressing love to their partner in a non-sexual but tender way. The midwives' role in facilitating sexual health is therefore varied and includes anticipating sexual health problems, informing about changes in physical and psychological states that can impact on sexual health, promoting positive sexual health choices and having the ability to recognise and refer on to other agencies if a women needs specialist intervention. The role of the midwife in sexual health, most importantly, is recognising that sexual health is an integral part of holistic care and to omit this part means that women's health needs are not being wholly met.

THE MIDWIFE'S ROLE IN SEXUAL HEALTH PROMOTION

The role of midwives in public health and sexual health promotion is enshrined in professional organisation competencies recognising that midwives, due to their close relationship with women during the maternity episode, are in a unique position to give this information and advice. The Nursing and Midwifery standards (NMC 2009) include a requirement for the qualifying midwife to 'enable women to make informed choices about their health' (23) and to provide care which considers support in the postnatal period while 'facilitating discussion about future reproductive choices' (28). There is also the specific requirement for 'providing advice on contraception' (29). Recent government directives also emphasise the importance of public health stating that midwives will 'embrace a greater public health role' and the public health actions cited include teenage pregnancy and sexual health issues (DoH 2010). Midwives also have a direct role in the antenatal screening programme for HIV and syphilis.

Several studies have indicated that sexual health promotion and advice is not seen as a priority for many midwives and is not given as much attention as other subjects when caring for pregnant and postnatal women (McCance & Cameron 2014; Walker & Davis 2014). Research from nursing and mental health nursing indicates that it was not seen as a priority and highlighted some other reasons why there can be resistance to addressing sexual health needs of patients, and these reasons can be transferred to other health care settings (Lubman et al. 2008; Quinn and Browne 2009).

Reasons given include:

- Embarrassment
- Lack of knowledge
- Fear of offending
- Conservative views
- Not knowing how to broach the subject
- Lack of time

McCance and Cameron (2014) in their study of midwives giving postnatal contraceptive advice also identified with these reasons in their findings. Midwives had the perception that this is a minor part of their role and also stated a perceived lack of training to give adequate advice. Walker and Davis (2014) found a dissonance between what education was given to midwifery students on the subject of sexual health and what they perceived as needed to become competent and confident in the role. This meant that the students engaged in 'safe practice' by avoiding any discussion on sexual health needs or contraception.

There has been extensive work into how to overcome the barriers to initiating a sexual health discussion, and these findings are useful to extrapolate to the work of the midwife when such issues need to be approached, which may be uncomfortable and difficult. One of the first encounters the midwife will have with the woman is at the initial booking interview. This is a time when a comprehensive sexual health assessment can be undertaken.

APPROACHING SEXUAL ISSUES IN PRACTICE

NICE (2006) emphasises that the environment in which antenatal appointments take place should enable women to discuss sensitive issues – this means somewhere private and quiet where there will be no interruptions. There are many issues to discuss at this first appointment and the midwife may well feel that there is so much to cover that sexual health needs are not a priority. It is important to remember that this is the first meeting the pregnant woman has with the midwife, and she may have many unmet needs and questions and she needs to feel listened to in a safe environment where she can explore any concerns or fears. Sensitivity, privacy and confidentiality should be shown at all times. A friendly introduction and eye contact help set the scene and aid comfort and confidence (BASHH 2013). Active listening skills should be employed, avoiding distractions such as looking at the computer screen. It is helpful to start with questions of a less sensitive nature, for example, medical and family history before embarking on other more sensitive questions. 'Signposting' is useful if a more sensitive question is going to be asked, for example: 'I am now going to ask you some questions of a more personal nature. You do not have to answer these questions if you do not wish to but they are useful to assist me in planning your care'. Open-ended questions help the woman to express her thoughts and feelings and have a sense of these thoughts being validated. Closed questions tend to limit the range of responses and make the woman feel not listened to (RCN 2015). It is also imperative to remember as a midwife that many ranges of relationships and sexualities exist and not to assume a heteronormative model. Using expressions such as partner and not assuming heterosexual relationships ensure an inclusive approach is maintained.

It is also important to consider sexually transmitted infection (STI) risk in the pregnant woman and that they carry the same risk from unprotected sexual intercourse as any other woman. The ramifications of undiagnosed STI in a pregnant woman can be very serious, resulting in significant morbidity for the unborn child as well as the woman herself (Rours et al. 2011).

Discussion of blood testing for HIV and syphilis during this appointment is part of the routine, and a query about the need for other tests can be easily and sensitively done. Self-swabs, for chlamydia and gonorrhoea, can be used in private by the woman while producing a urine sample. NICE 2006 do not advocate routine chlamydia screening for pregnant women but do point out that women under the age of 25 should be prioritised because of the high prevalence of this infection in this age group.

It is important to remember that many pregnant woman have fears and worries that they feel are exclusive to them – questions that are universally phrased can help the woman to feel that her worries are shared, for example, many women are worried about being sexually active during pregnancy, do you have any concerns?

It can be useful to use a recognised framework to guide sexual health assessment. The PLISSIT model was developed by Annon in 1976 and was further developed into the Ex-PLISSIT model by Taylor and Davis in 2006. This model has different levels of intervention (Table 12.1).

In the Ex-PLISSIT model, the permission-giving stage is asked for at every stage of the process rather than just at the start; this is what led to the term, Ex-PLISSIT. The model moves

Table 12.1 Ex-PLISSITT model

Permission giving

This is the first step and is aimed at opening up a discussion about sexual health and assessing patients' needs. Here, the midwife may want to ask whether the woman is in a relationship or if they have any concerns about the sexual side of their relationship; they need to make it clear that they are willing to talk about this area. Practitioners need to be explicit about what they are talking about (sex and sexual health) rather than just asking vague questions like 'Do you have any further questions?' This is called explicit permission giving and runs throughout this entire intervention model. Permission is given at all stages.

Limited information

This is where the midwife can give some general information about the effect of pregnancy, illness or medication on sexual function. For example, the increase of progesterone during pregnancy may reduce libido for some women. This gives them an opportunity to correct any inaccurate information women may have such as the myth that sex during pregnancy will harm the baby. Midwives could also back up what they tell patients by offering them written information, for example, booklets or leaflets.

Specific suggestions

Here, the aim is to start solving specific problems a woman may have. It requires taking a detailed history from her and identifying specific problems, for example, pain during intercourse. Midwives may need to refer to another health professional if they feel they do not have enough knowledge or skills to help patients at this level.

Intensive therapy

This is the final stage of the intervention. Intensive therapy requires advanced knowledge and skills on the part of the practitioner. This practitioner will probably have specialist knowledge and skills – it is not an expectation that all midwives should have this as part of their role. However, it is an important part of their role that they know exactly which services are available to refer women to – for example, psychosexual counselling – so that appropriate help can be given.

Source: Adapted from Davis, Sally and Taylor, Bridget. 2006. *Nursing Standard* 21(11): 35–40.

from permission giving to giving limited information to specific suggestion and then to intensive therapy. This therapy is provided by a third party and the midwives' role in this is to have the knowledge to know when a further referral is needed, that is, for psychosexual counselling and to have the resources to be able to do so.

ACTIVITY

Make a list of sexual health issues women may wish to discuss with you in your role as a midwife or a student. Think of how you will approach and respond to these issues and what resources you will use for assistance.

SEXUAL HEALTH ISSUES DURING PREGNANCY AND BEYOND

SEXUAL ACTIVITY IN PREGNANCY

Women during the initial meeting with the midwife may have worries about their sexual health during pregnancy and beyond, and if the initial meeting is perceived as a safe environment to verbalise thoughts and feelings, these worries may be expressed. One issue could be the subject of sex during pregnancy. It is recognised that sexual satisfaction encompasses the environment and stimuli conducive to sexual feelings as well as one's own subjective experience (Basson 2006). Many factors can lead to the changed environment experienced by women during pregnancy. These include physical changes, hormonal changes, psychological changes, fears and myths and cultural beliefs about sexual activity during pregnancy. A body of evidence exists which demonstrates that sexual function declines during pregnancy specifically during the third trimester. This reduction does not resolve immediately post-partum but may persist during the first 3–6 months post-delivery and then steadily recovers (Bartellas et al. 2000; Johnson 2011; Pauleta et al. 2010). Johnson (2011) argues that rather than pathologising these changes, they should be viewed and presented as a normal sequence of events that gradually recovers over time.

Physical and hormonal factors which reduce sexual activity can include fatigue, nausea, back pain and infections, for example, urinary tract infections, candidiasis and vulvar varicose veins. In the third trimester, the sheer weight of the pregnancy and pressure on the bladder and other organs can cause a decrease in sexual frequency and desire and certain sexual practices such as masturbation and oral sex tend to decline during late pregnancy (Table 12.2). If sexual intercourse is desired, adjustments may have to be made to coital positioning (Johnson 2011).

Psychological changes can also affect sexual desire and activity. Pregnancy involves a period of transition; as with all transition, there can be anxiety as well as happiness. Read (2004) points out that not all pregnancy is met with joy and that, even if a baby is planned and wanted, there may be some ambivalence:

"Neither pregnancy nor its absence is inherently desirable. The occurrence of a pregnancy can be met with joy or despair, and its absence can be a cause of relief or anguish. Included in this response will be myths about pregnancy, taboos about sexual activity during pregnancy, fears about the baby and delivery, changes in the relationship with the partner, and beliefs about the roles of motherhood and fatherhood. The woman's changing body shape may cause distress and a sense of unattractiveness."

Read (2004, 561)

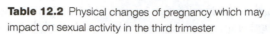

Table 12.2 Physical changes of pregnancy which may impact on sexual activity in the third trimester

Deep engagement of fetal head

Stress urinary incontinence

Haemorrhoids

Weight of partner on uterus

Subluxation of pubic symphysis and sacroiliac joints

Vaginal discomfort/dyspareunia

Pelvic and vaginal vasocongestion

Source: From Johnson, Crista E. 2011. *The Journal of Sexual Medicine* 8: 1267–1284.

Table 12.3 Contraindications to sexual intercourse during pregnancy

Absolute contraindications

Unexplained vaginal bleeding

Placenta previa

Preterm premature dilation of the cervix

Preterm premature rupture of the membranes

Relative contraindications

History of premature delivery

Multiple gestation

Source: From Johnson, Crista E. 2011. *The Journal of Sexual Medicine* 8: 1267–1284.

There also exist fears and myths about sexual intercourse during pregnancy and, of course, there are some conditions, which are contraindications to sexual intercourse (Johnson 2011) (Table 12.3). However, outside of these contraindications, sexual intercourse is safe and acceptable and should be encouraged for women who desire sexual intercourse within their relationship.

A range of post-partum factors can affect sexual well-being. These include mode of delivery and perineal trauma, including episiotomy, perineal tears and lacerations. Severe obstetric morbidity is a predictor of poor general health post-delivery and a delay in the resumption of sexual activity and problems with sexual function (Waterstone et al. 2003). Some evidence suggests a link between operative vaginal birth and impaired sexual health after delivery (Hicks et al. 2004). Dyspareunia was shown in some studies to persist up to 6 months in women who had experienced an operative vaginal birth and an increased delay in resumption of sexual intercourse plus perineal pain, and self-reported perception of sexual health/sexual problems was found in women who underwent operative vaginal birth as opposed to spontaneous vaginal delivery or caesarean section (Hicks et al. 2004). Whilst other studies have indicated that mode of delivery has little impact on resumption of sexual activity or sexual function, there is little evidence in relation to the sexual well-being of partners during the post-partum period (FSRH 2009).

Other factors which can affect sexual function post-delivery include (Woolhouse et al. 2012):

- Fatigue
- Decreased lubrication and vaginal dryness, especially among breastfeeding mothers
- Fear of wakening the baby, especially if the baby sleeps in the mother's bedroom
- Not hearing if the baby cries
- Decreased sense of attractiveness

There is also evidence to suggest that pre-pregnancy sexual health problems are a predictor of altered sexual health after childbirth. Barrett et al. (2000) found that women who experienced dyspareunia before pregnancy had over a fourfold chance of experiencing dyspareunia 6 months after the birth, compared with women who had not experienced dyspareunia before having a baby. This is a small group with specific needs; they could be identified in the antenatal period and offered appropriate help, advice and referral, if required.

PRACTICE POINTS

PHYSIOLOGICAL AND HORMONAL EFFECTS OF BREASTFEEDING ON SEXUAL ACTIVITY

- Low oestrogen levels can result in decreased vaginal lubrication and atrophy of the vaginal epithelium; so during sexual activity, there can be little or no vaginal secretions. This can lead to reduced physical arousal and painful intercourse.
- When a woman is lactating, she may have a milk ejection reflex when she experiences orgasm. She may also find her breast a source of discomfort during lovemaking if they are overly full or leaking milk.
- The nipples of a lactating woman may be sensitive during the act of breastfeeding, yet touching or stimulating of the breasts by her partner may not necessarily evoke the usual sexual desire or a sexual response. Thus, during lactation, the breasts may not be a primary site of sexual response. Some women find the increasing sensitivity of the nipples uncomfortable (Connolly et al. 2005).
- New mothers may struggle with their role as a new mother and their role as a sexual being, and this may cause a clash between her breasts performing a biological function and the sexual connotation of her breasts.
- With a drive to increase breastfeeding rates and prolong duration, it is important that women are informed of the changes that may affect their sexual health and the fact that these changes are normal physiological events.
- Practical advice includes use of vaginal lubricants, oestrogen pessaries and open discussion with partners that can help breastfeeding women feel reassured about their sexual health (FSRH 2009).

Woolhouse et al. (2012) found in their study of women's experiences of sex and intimacy after childbirth that a drop in libido was found to cause feelings of guilt and failure despite it being a very common phenomenon. The authors believe that women have internalised the socially constructed message that mothers can 'be it all', and when faced with the realities of motherhood, feelings of guilt and inadequacy are somewhat inevitable.

Midwives can play an important role in recognising these issues around intimate relationships during pregnancy and beyond and tackling them head on. Johnson (2011) argues for targeted counselling for women on the impact of pregnancy, childbirth and the post-partum period on their sexual health. This should be performed throughout the antenatal period and reinforced by all members of the team. The FSRH (2009) offers the following guidance when counselling women and their partners on sexual function in the postnatal period.

- The time to resume sexual activity will vary between couples.
- There is no set time frame in which sexual activity should have resumed.
- Both partners need to be physically and emotionally ready.
- Some people may experience difficulties with sexual activity following the birth of their child such as dyspareunia caused by perineal trauma and vaginal dryness.
- Sexual desire or sex drive may be low in the first few months.
- Any difficulties or concerns should be discussed with a health professional.

O'Malley and Smith (2013a) feel it is important to consider discussions about sexual health, including changes in sexual health patterns, during the antenatal period and in antenatal classes. This normalises the subject and leads to facilitating open, honest discussion between practitioners, women and their partners. Barrett et al. (2000) concur with this and agree that the antenatal period is an essential time to start discussion about sexual health, and women should be counselled on what to expect in terms of sexual health outcomes. They found that at the 6-week check, it may be taken for granted that women will have resumed sexual intercourse following delivery, so they discuss contraception. However, the quality of women's sexual health is rarely discussed, and if women have not recommenced sexual activity, it may be too early to discover chronic problems with sexual function.

O'Malley and Smith (2013b) believe the postnatal 6-week check is an excellent opportunity to discuss sexual well-being for the majority of women. This can range from advice around specific issues such as recommending lubrication for vaginal dryness and using sexual positions that allow for more shallow penetration or give women more control over penetration, to referring for more in-depth sexual health counselling for those who identify with more ongoing sexual health concerns.

If midwives are able to promote sexual health in every encounter with women from the antenatal period to the post-partum period, there is more of a chance that women will feel that this is an important part of their overall health care and feel empowered to discuss these issues at the 6-week check.

PROMOTING POSITIVE BODY IMAGE

Pregnancy is a time when women face substantial changes to their body shape and weight in a short period of time. Changes in body shape and body image can have a dramatic effect on sexual and intimate relationships. In 2010, the Government Equalities Office report 'Two for the Price of One' acknowledged the pressure that women feel during and after pregnancy to achieve a perfect body. This is not helped by media pictures of celebrities achieving a state of emaciation 6 weeks after delivery. There seems to be a cultural assumption that a mother's job is to present herself as if nothing life changing or body changing has happened (Orbach & Rubin 2014). Some women found that their post-partum bodies left them feeling unattractive and self-conscious. Woolhouse et al. (2012) quote a mother feeling horrified by the thought of having sex with the lights on. However, this is by no means universal and some women are celebrating their sense of empowerment and respect for their bodies following childbirth. Many women have posted pictures of their post-partum bodies at '#takebackpostpartum' celebrating the power of their bodies in giving new life.

Orbach and Rubin (2014), while recognising the heavy workload that midwives face, recommend that they incorporate body image into their consultations and create positive body image models by advertising model diversity in the pictures used around the clinical area ensuring there are pictures of happy, healthy women of all different shapes and sizes and to be mindful of the language used.

PROMOTING ACCESS TO CONTRACEPTIVE COUNSELLING AND TREATMENT

There is no doubt that spacing of children improves the health of mothers and babies (D'Arcangues 2013). Short inter-pregnancy intervals have been linked to increased risk of pre-term birth, low birth weight, small for gestational age and increases in maternal morbidity and mortality (Jackson 2011). During pregnancy, high levels of sex steroid hormones suppress pituitary gonadotrophins. Within 30 days of delivery, placental sex steroid levels decrease and gonadotrophins increase, thus stimulating the activity of the ovaries. The earliest date of ovulation in non-breastfeeding women is thought to be Day 28 and menstruation may return by Week 6. As sperm can live up to 7 days in the genital tract, there is a potential risk of pregnancy from Day 21 after birth, and contraception needs to be started from then on. In women who exclusively breastfeed, suckling disrupts the frequency and amplitude of gonadotrophin pulses and, despite ovarian follicular activity, ovulation is suppressed. Ovulation returns when the frequency and duration of suckling episodes decrease (FSRH 2009).

The FSRH guidelines argue that discussion regarding fertility and contraceptive options should happen both antenatally and postnatally. Prior to childbirth, women and their partners may have greater time to think through their options than immediately after birth when it may not seem like a priority (FSRH 2009).

NICE guidelines advise that methods of contraception should be discussed within the first week of giving birth (NICE 2006). This role usually falls to the midwife when the mother is discharged from the delivery unit. However, research commissioned by the British Pregnancy Advisory Service (BPAS) and Mumsnet of 1000 mothers found that for some women a discussion with a medical professional immediately after giving birth was not appropriate as they felt it was too much information at a time when resuming sex was the last thing on their minds (BPAS 2012).

The survey also revealed that the majority did not discuss postnatal contraception with a health care professional whilst they were pregnant, while more than half did not discuss it until their postnatal check at around 6 weeks or later. Research into midwives' attitudes into giving contraceptive advice postnatally also found the situation to be problematic. The study showed that midwives viewed their role in discussing contraception as a minor one, and due to lack of privacy, time and knowledge would rather signpost women to their general practitioner at the 6-week check (McCance and Cameron 2014).

The issue with waiting to discuss contraception until the 6-week check is the risk that new mothers could become pregnant again before contraception is commenced or women who have not recommenced sexual intercourse feel alienated from the discussion and miss the opportunity to engage with a health care professional at this time. BPAS (2012) also found that the women in the survey commented that there seemed to be a lack of knowledge demonstrated from the health care professional, especially around breastfeeding and contraception, and the information or availability of long-acting reversible contraception (that is, the progestogen-only injection, the progestogen-only sub-dermal implant, the intrauterine copper device and the intrauterine system – 'Mirena').

Sixty-one per cent of women said that there was no discussion with health care professionals whilst they were pregnant regarding plans for contraception after the birth of their baby, and a third (32%) of women who were breastfeeding or planning to breastfeed said that safe contraception when breastfeeding was not discussed or raised at all (BPAS 2012). BPAS (2012) believes as more women are encouraged to breastfeed, it is important that consistent, accurate advice about the effectiveness of this in protecting against pregnancy is offered, and that women can access all the forms of contraception that are safe to use while breastfeeding. Exclusive breastfeeding can work as an effective contraceptive, but only if strict criterion is met about frequency of feeds. The lactational amenorrhoea method (LAM) criteria are that the baby is under 6 months old, the women is amenorrhoeic and is exclusively or almost exclusively breastfeeding. If all these criteria are met, there is only a 2% risk of pregnancy. The risk of pregnancy starts to increase if the frequency of breastfeeding decreases, for example, stopping night feeds, using dummies or supplementary feeding (FSRH 2009).

There are a range of contraceptives that are safe to use while breastfeeding, including progestogen-only methods: pills, implants and intrauterine copper devices and intrauterine system, for example, Mirena, and evidence suggests that progestogen-only methods of contraception do not adversely affect breastfeeding performance when used during lactation (Kapp et al. 2010).

PRACTICE POINTS

Important information to be given to women about postnatal contraception is:

- Contraception is not required before Day 21 post-partum. If starting a hormonal method on or before Day 21, there is no need for additional contraception.
- Non-breastfeeding women should not start a combined method before Day 21 because of the increased risk of thrombosis.
- Use of a combined method, that is, one which contains both oestrogen and progestogen should not be recommended in fully breastfeeding women between 6 weeks and 6 months.
- When starting a hormonal method after Day 21, clinicians should be reasonably sure that the woman is not pregnant or at risk of pregnancy and should advise that she avoids sex or uses additional contraception for the first 7 days of use for a combined method and 2 days for the progestogen-only pill.
- There is no evidence to show that progestogen-only methods affect the volume or quality of breast milk or affect infant growth.
- Post-partum women (breastfeeding and non-breastfeeding) can start the progestogen-only pill at any time post-partum.
- Non-breastfeeding women can start a progestogen-only injectable method at any time post-partum.
- Breastfeeding women should not start a progestogen-only injectable method before Day 21 unless the risk of subsequent pregnancy is high.
- The recommendation for the insertion of the progestogen-only sub-dermal implant is between 21 and 28 days after delivery. However, if more convenient, breastfeeding and non-breastfeeding women can choose to have a progestogen-only implant inserted before Day 21, although this is outside the product licence.
- Intrauterine contraceptive copper devices and intrauterine systems – Mirena – can be fitted from Day 28 post-partum (FSRH 2009).

Contraception choice is also affected by individual preferences, cultural beliefs and attitudes, personal and family health issues and whether the woman is returning to work. Giving the woman an opportunity to explore all the options, her own individual preferences and her suitability for the different methods takes time and knowledge. It may be that the midwife does not have the time to explore all the options fully, but it is imperative that women are given some access to contraceptive advice even if it is signposting to websites, local clinics or providing up to date literature on the subject. A poster presentation in 2015 displayed the results of a survey in Wales which asked women if they wanted to receive contraception in the immediate postnatal period. Eighty-four per cent were interested in receiving contraception prior to discharge with the majority wanting long-acting reversible contraception. The recommendation was to provide a patient-centred postnatal contraception service within the maternity service. This certainly was the case in the past with a contraceptive nurse visiting the postnatal ward on a regular basis (Oliver et al. 2015).

There seems to be very little consensus on the subject of the best time to discuss contraception for the pregnant or new mother. Normalising the subject and including it at every stage along the journey through pregnancy to the postnatal period would cover the differing needs of all women. However, studies into midwives' skills and expertise in the subject do point out that an investment in ongoing skills training in the subject is essential as well as giving midwives the time and space to perform this essential role (McCance & Cameron 2014; Walker & Davis 2014).

SUMMARY

- Sexual health is a broad concept and implies being able to make positive health choices and being able to access services when needed.
- The role of the midwife in sexual health promotion is to recognise that sexual health is an integral part of overall health and its omission would mean that holistic care is not being offered.
- Sexual health can be altered during pregnancy and childbirth in a variety of ways – physical, emotional and psychological.
- The role of midwives in public health and sexual health promotion is enshrined in professional organisation competencies and government directives.
- Sexual health should be discussed in an environment which is private and quiet and midwives should use their communication skills to facilitate a frank and honest discussion which enables the pregnant woman to disclose any fears and worries she may have.
- Pregnant and postnatal women may have concerns surrounding sexual activity in pregnancy and beyond, issues with body image and questions about postnatal contraception.
- Challenges to sexual health promotion can be overcome by training and giving midwives time and space to perform this role.

REFERENCES

Barrett, Geraldine, Elizabeth Pendry, Janet Peacock, Christina Victor, Rance Thakar & Isaac Manyonda. 2000. Women's Sexual Health after Childbirth. *British Journal of Obstetrics and Gynaecology* 107(20): 186–195.

Bartellas, Elias, Joan M. G. Crane, Melita Daley, Kelly A. Bennett, & Donna Hutchens. 2000. Sexuality and Sexual Activity in Pregnancy. *British Journal of Obstetrics and Gynaecology* 107: 964–968.

BASHH (British Association of Sexual Health and HIV). 2013. *UK National Guideline for Consultations Requiring Sexual History Taking*. http://www.bashh.org/BASHH/Guidelines/Guidelines/BASHH/Guidelines/Guidelines.aspx

Basson, Rosemary. 2006. Clinical Practice. Sexual Desire and Arousal Disorders in Women. *New England Journal of Medicine* 354: 1497–1506.

BPAS. 2012. *Mumsnet Bpas Survey Shows Gaps in Contraception*. http://www.bpas.org/about-our-charity/press-office/press-releases/mumsnetbpas-survey-shows-gaps-in-contraception

Connolly, Anne, John Thorp & Laurie Pahel. 2005. Effects of Pregnancy and Childbirth on Postpartum Sexual Function: A Longitudinal Prospective Study. *International Urogynaecology Journal and Pelvic Floor Dysfunction* 16: 263–267.

D'Arcangues, Catherine. 2013. *Family Planning Programmes: Past, Present and Future*. Copenhagen: Entre Nous WHO.

Davis, Sally & Bridget Taylor. 2006. Using the Extended PLISSIT Model to Address Sexual Healthcare Needs. *Nursing Standard* 21(11): 35–40.

DoH (Department of Health). 2010. *Midwifery 2020. Delivering Expectations*. London: DoH.

DoH (Department of Health). 2013. *A Framework for Sexual Health Improvement in England*. London: DoH.

FSRH (Faculty of Sexual and Reproductive Health Care). 2009. *Clinical Guidance. Post Natal Sexual and Reproductive Health*. London: FSRH.

Hicks, Tara L., Susan F. Goodall, Evelyn M. Quattrone & Mona T. Lyndon-Rochelle. 2004. Postpartum Sexual Functioning and Method of Delivery. Summary of the Evidence. *Journal of Midwifery and Women's Health* 49: 430–436.

Jackson, Emily. 2011. Controversies in Postpartum Contraception: When Is It Safe to Start Oral Contraceptives after Childbirth? *Thrombosis Research* 127: 535–539.

Johnson, Crista E. 2011. Sexual Health during Pregnancy and the Postpartum. *The Journal of Sexual Medicine* 8: 1267–1284.

Kapp, Nathalie, Kathryn Curtis & Kavita Nanda. 2010. Progestogen-Only Contraceptive Use among Breastfeeding Women: A Systematic Review. *Contraception* 82: 17–37.

Lubman, Dan I., Susan J. Paxton & Alan P. Brown. 2008. STIs and Blood Borne Viruses: Risk Factors for Individuals with Mental Illness. *Australian Family Physician* 37(7): 531–534.

McCance, Kirsty & Sharon Cameron. 2014. Midwives Experiences and Views of Giving Postpartum Contraception Advice and Providing Long-Acting Reversible Contraception: A Qualitative Study. *Journal of Family Planning and Reproductive Health Care* 40(16): 177–183.

NICE (National Institute for Clinical Excellence). 2006. *Guidelines for Antenatal Care*. London: NICE.

NMC (Nursing and Midwifery Council). 2009. *Standards for Pre Registration Midwifery Education*. http:// www.nmc-org.org/documents/nmc

Oliver, Michelle, Helen Erasmus & Rawaya Al Dabbagh. 2015. Are Women Interested in Receiving Contraception in the Immediate Post Natal Period? *Poster Presentation at the Annual Scientific Meeting*. London: FSRH.

O'Malley, Deirdre & Valerie Smith. 2013a. Altered Sexual Health after Childbirth: Part 1. *The Practising Midwife* 16: 30–32.

O'Malley, Deirdre & Valerie Smith. 2013b. Altered Sexual Health after Childbirth: Part 2. *The Practising Midwife* 16: 27–29.

Orbach, Susie & Holli Rubin. 2014. *Two for the Price of One: The Impact of Body Image during Pregnancy and after Birth*. London: Government Equalities Office Gov. UK.

Pauleta, Joana, Nuno M. Pereira & Luis M. Graca. 2010. Sexuality during Pregnancy. *Journal of Sexual Medicine* 7: 136–142.

Public Health England. 2015. *Health Protection Report.* Vol. 9, pp. 22–26. Public Health England. https://www.gov.uk/government/publications/health-protection-report-volume-9-2015

Quinn, Chris & Graeme Browne. 2009. Sexuality of People Living with Mental Illness: A Collaborative Challenge for Mental Health Nurses. *International Journal of Mental Health Nursing* 18(3): 195–203.

Read, Jane. 2004. ABC of Sexual Health: Sexual Problems Associated with Infertility, Pregnancy and Ageing. *BMJ* 329: 559–561.

Rours, Ingrid J. G., Liesbeth Dujits, Henriette Moll, Lidia Arends, Ronald Groot, Vincent W. Jaddoe, Albert Hofmann et al. 2011. Chlamydia Trachomatis Infection during Pregnancy Associated with Preterm Delivery: A Population-Based Prospective Cohort Study. *European Journal of Epidemiology* 26(6): 493–502.

RCN (Royal College of Nursing). 2015. *Sexual health competencies an integrated career and competence framework for sexual and reproductive health nursing across the UK.* London: RCN.

Walker, Susan & Geraldine Davis. 2014. Knowledge and Reported Confidence of Final Year Midwifery Students Regarding Giving Advice on Contraception and Sexual Health. *Midwifery* 30: 169–176.

Waterstone, Mark, Charles Wolfe, Richard Hooper & Susan. Bewley. 2003. Postnatal Morbidity after Childbirth and Severe Obstetric Morbidity. *British Journal of Obstetric Gynaecology* 110: 128–133.

WHO (World Health Organization). 2006. *Definition of Sexual Health.* http://www.who.int/reproductivehealth/topics/sexual_health/sh_definitions/en/

Woolhouse, Hannah, Ellie McDonald & Stephanie Brown. 2012. Women's Experiences of Sex and Intimacy after Childbirth: Making the Adjustment to Motherhood. *Journal of Psychosomatic Obstetrics and Gynaecology* 33(4): 185–190.

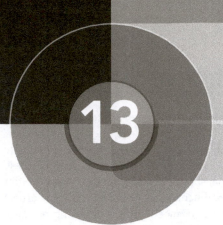

Healthy eating in pregnancy

13

SHEILA O'CONNOR

INTRODUCTION

Nutrition is an essential component of every individual's health. The oft-quoted popular maxim 'you are what you eat' reveals humans' emotional relationship with food. However, the poignancy of this familiar adage is intensified when we consider it in relation to the pregnant woman, as she navigates her way through nutritional advice from diverse sources such as health professionals, family, friends and the Internet. According to the anthropologist Pat Caplan, understanding why people eat what they do entails an understanding of ideas related to the body, health, time, space, social relationships, nature and culture (Caplan 1996). For midwives, the diet of the pregnant woman has always been an important part of their remit. Writing in the seventeenth century, the midwife Jane Sharpe (1671) noted 'two things very useful, good diet moderately taken and convenient labor and exercise of the body' (71). Even though we have long known of the importance of maternal diet, it is telling that research on the subject has increased exponentially only in recent years. Whilst the role of the midwife in public health initiatives such as supporting women experiencing domestic violence and smoking cessation has been highlighted, the midwife's responsibility in supporting women with their diet received much less attention until recently. This burgeoning interest in maternal diet has been undoubtedly shaped by the rise of obesity globally, and for the purpose of this chapter, the concept of an 'obesogenic society' will be employed as a lens of analysis. The rationale for using this framework is shaped by the concept that living in an obesogenic society affects all women, regardless of their body mass index (BMI) and midwives are in a central position to communicate this important public health message to all women.

THE CHANGING ROLE OF THE MIDWIFE AND NUTRITION

The global rise of adult obesity over the past 25 years means that midwives now face a complex task supporting women with their diet. From a public health perspective, the urgency of dealing with maternal obesity has been continually highlighted over the past decade. Systematic literature reviews on antenatal behavioural change interventions for overweight and obese pregnant women have underscored the interest in this subject (Dodd et al. 2010; Oteng-Ntim et al. 2012). However, tackling maternal obesity, a monumental task in itself, is only one aspect of the difficulty facing midwives. The enormity consists of meeting the contrasting needs of underweight and obese women and supporting women within the healthy and overweight categories not to gain excessive gestational weight.

Within both the United Kingdom and internationally, BMI is the key tool employed for monitoring and measuring weight (WHO 1995) (see Table 13.1). Given that being overweight and obese are significant risk factors for cardiovascular disease, diabetes, cancer and premature death, it is hardly surprising that this rise in obesity has been described as a global pandemic. Between 1980 and 2014, the worldwide prevalence of obesity has doubled. In 2014, more than 1.9 billion adults were overweight, and 600 million of these were obese (WHO 2015). Within the United Kingdom, there has also been an increase in both overweight and obesity. From 1993 to 2013, obesity increased from 13.2% to 26% in men and from 16.4% to 23.8% in women. In addition, the proportion of the population that are now either overweight or obese is 67% and 57.2%, respectively, for men and women (HSCIC 2015). This is mirrored by an increased prevalence of childhood obesity since 1995, with 11% of boys and 12% of girls aged between 2 and 15 years now being obese (HSCIC 2015). It has been projected that being overweight or obese will cost the NHS 9.7 billion by 2050, with wider costs reaching 49.9 billion a year (Butland et al. 2007).

From a midwifery perspective, around 50% of women of childbearing age are currently either overweight or obese (NICE 2010). In relation to maternal weight, there has been a notable decrease of women in the ideal BMI range, with first trimester obesity having increased from 7.6% to 15.6% over the past 19 years, and underweight fluctuating at approximately 5% (Heslehurst et al. 2010). In 2007, the Confidential Enquiry into Maternal and Child Health (CEMACH) highlighted the urgency of the situation (Lewis 2007). In this report, more than half of all maternal deaths were among overweight or obese pregnant women,

Table 13.1 Body mass index

Underweight	<18.5
Normal	18.5–24.9
Overweight	≥25.0
Pre-obese	25.0–29.9
Obese	≥30.0
Obese class I	30.0–34.9
Obese class II	35.0–39.9
Obese class III	≥40

Note: Body mass index (BMI) is calculated by taking the individual's weight in kilograms and dividing it by the square of their height [weight (kg)/height (m sq.)] (WHO 1995). Criticisms of employing the BMI classification is that it fails to distinguish fat from bone and muscle, but given the relative ease of calculation, it is understandable that it has become the prominent measure of categorising weight within the health care environment.

with over 15% being morbidly or super morbidly obese. Subsequent reviews have married with these findings (CMACE 2010; Knight et al. 2014).

Excessive gestational weight gain is common during pregnancy (Crozier 2010). Moreover, weight gain in pregnancy is linked to becoming overweight or obese later in life (Rooney and Schauberger 2002; Linné et al. 2004). It is equally important for midwives to consider the small proportion of women who commence pregnancy underweight. Teenagers and women with eating disorders, although a minority, are examples of such groups (Khashan 2010; Micali 2010). Consequently, midwives currently face a complex task supporting the diverse needs of all pregnant women. Moreover, the intricacy of this task has undoubtedly been fashioned by the complicated relationship society has with food and the reasons fuelling the rise of the obesogenic society.

OBESOGENIC ENVIRONMENT

The concept of an obesogenic environment is crucial when examining maternal diet. This is because it aids our understanding of why many women commence their pregnancy within the overweight or obese category and additionally why so many women, across the BMI ranges, put on excessive weight during their pregnancy. Utilising this concept is also a useful method to introduce the topic of diet in pregnancy to all women as it paints a clear picture of how easy it is to eat food that is highly calorific, lacking in nutrition and thereby gain weight quickly. Moreover, by employing this approach, the emphasis is not placed on individual excess and is therefore less stigmatising.

The term obesogenic society was coined by Swinburn et al. in 1999 to express 'the sum of influences, opportunities, or conditions of life have on promoting obesity in individuals or populations' (Swinburn et al. 1999, 564). In comparison to our grandparents and great-grandparents, our everyday life is very different in terms of energy intake and expenditure. Post-industrial Western society has witnessed the rise of a 'toxic food' culture, with the availability of high-calorie and high-fat food making excessive weight gain inevitable (Brownell & Horgen 2004). Changes in food production and processing, the role of the media in advertising, the increasing popularity of fast food restaurants and changes in energy expenditure due to changing work environments and modes of transportation have undoubtedly fuelled this transition (Swinburn et al. 2011; Nestle 2013). A study of obesity in Australia also highlighted how modern and possibly dysfunctional relationship with time also affects our relationship with food. As women become increasingly busier, juggling the demands of work and family life, this speed spills over into family, exercise and leisure times in complicated ways (Banwell et al. 2012). Culturally, excessive weight is often placed at an individual level, and worryingly some obese pregnant women have reported being treated negatively by health care professionals within maternity services (Furber & McGowan 2011). However, the situation is far more intricate than mere individual excess. Acknowledging the pervading obesogenic environment is the first step to supporting all pregnant women with their diet. From a midwifery perspective, alerting pregnant women to the nature of the obesogenic environment can empower them to reflect and make changes to their everyday life.

REFLECTION

REFLECTING ON OUR OBESOGENIC SOCIETY

Compare your everyday life with that of your grandparents and great-grandparents? What was their work? What transport modes did they use? What access did they have to food, etc.? Now think about your everyday life and compare the difference.

WOMEN AND FOOD

Humans have a complex relationship with food which is interwoven with our subjectivity and sense of self (Lupton 1996). A pregnant woman's relationship with food is shaped by many aspects of her everyday life, including embodiment and body image, family and culture, and socio-economic position. From a public health perspective, it is crucial to emphasise this complicated relationship with food, as it then becomes easier to understand why making positive changes to diet is more difficult than other public health initiatives such as smoking cessation. In addition, it also underscores why midwives may have difficulty in broaching the subject of weight with women, particularly if they themselves have a complicated relationship with food.

Research from the social sciences in particular has highlighted women's reflections on embodiment and body image in pregnancy. Ironically, whilst the population has become increasingly heavier in the Western society, expectations on the female body to be an aesthetically pleasing 'thin' have become more pronounced. According to feminist scholars, the post-industrial society has been crucial in the shaping and policing of the female form and a consonant rise of eating disorders (Bordo 1993). Studies that have focused on embodiment in pregnancy have not surprisingly purported diverse findings, with pregnancy offering some women an opportunity to escape social pressures to be thin, whilst fuelling insecurities in others (Bailey 2001; Murray 2014). Moreover, a recent systematic review revealed that obese and overweight pregnant women are more likely to experience elevated antenatal and postnatal depression symptoms, than women in the healthy BMI range (Molyneaux et al. 2014). Clearly, discussing diet and weight with pregnant women is a sensitive subject. Qualitative research has highlighted that heavier women have become upset about the manner on how the subject was raised (Furber & McGowan 2011). In addition, in another qualitative study, some midwives have revealed that they have been reluctant to initiate the subject of weight with heaver women due to the sensitivity of the subject; however, all felt that the risks needed to be discussed (Smith et al. 2012). Frank and sensitive conversations about the importance of a healthy diet in pregnancy and beyond remain essential, whilst also recognising the complexity of feelings around issues of embodiment and body image.

The pregnant woman's partner and family can affect the woman's ability to maintain a healthy diet. Lupton (1996) has highlighted the importance of the family in learning about food as follows:

> It is in the context of the family that the social dimensions of eating and those of emotion are particularly tied together. Food beliefs and behaviours are developed from earliest childhood, and are closely tied to the family unit. (37)

In relation to pregnancy, it is not surprising that the pregnant woman's family wish to ensure that she is nourished. A recent study demonstrates the fundamental role that family play, with some partners giving positive support for lifestyle change and others worrying and insisting that the women needed extra food (Heslehurst et al. 2013). This point highlights that when midwives are discussing nutrition in pregnancy, involving the partner is also crucial and dispelling myths such as eating for two and avoiding physical activity are important public health messages for the entire family. The family/culture diet dynamic is of particular importance in relation to ethnic minorities and migrants. Indeed, there is evidence that obesity rates are higher among Black African and Black Caribbean women in pregnancy with hypertensive disease being more pronounced (Heslehurst et al. 2010). Moreover, migrant groups in particular can be at increased risk of developing obesity, especially as their lifestyle behaviours change as they become more affluent and urbanised (Renzaho et al. 2010). Hence, from a midwifery perspective, it is essential that the dietary support is both relevant and culturally sensitive. Food is an important and enjoyable part of family life, and any change made to diet needs to encompass this central tenant.

It is now well established that social and economic positions affect health (Marmot 2010). Importantly, in relation to maternal diet, low pre-pregnancy BMI, low weight gain during pregnancy and higher maternal obesity have been highlighted within lower socio-economic groups (British Nutrition Foundation and Buttriss 2013). Older research has shown that mothers from low-income families are nutritionally vulnerable and may choose to prioritise their children having food over their own diet (Dobson et al. 1994; Dowler & Calvert 1995). However, low income can affect maternal diet in other ways, with cheap energy-dense food leading to weight gain if over consumed. Research suggests that obese women in England are twice as likely to be living in deprived areas when compared with the non-obese (Heslehurst et al. 2010). Moreover, women with extreme obesity are five times more likely to be living in a deprived area (Heslehurst et al. 2011). In 2006, the government implemented the Healthy Start Scheme (Department of Health 2006), which comprises providing vouchers to low-income families which include a pregnant woman or children under the age of 4 years. However, despite such government initiatives, the vulnerable economic position of many women currently is underscored by a consideration of the current economic downturn. The increased use of food banks over the past 10 years (Lambie-Mumford & Dowler 2014) highlights how women may not necessarily have choice when it comes to what they and their family eat.

ACTIVITY

HEALTHY START VOUCHERS

The vouchers can be exchanged for infant formula, liquid cow's milk and fresh or frozen fruit and vegetables and is accessed via health professionals, for example, midwives or health visitors, who should also ensure that applicants are offered advice and information on healthy eating and breastfeeding.

- With this information in mind, what do you think is the best way for midwives to discuss the use of the vouchers with women?
- Make a map of the area that you are working in. In this map, mark areas such as markets where women can buy fresh and frozen fruit and vegetables.

PRACTICE POINT

Women have a complex relationship with food which is shaped by many aspects of everyday life including body image, family, culture and socio-economic position. Understanding this complicated relationship with food can make it easier to understand why making positive changes to diet may be difficult for some women.

DIET IN PREGNANCY – THE LONG- AND SHORT-TERM HEALTH EFFECTS

The importance of a woman's diet in pregnancy for both her and her developing fetus is very well acknowledged. Epidemiological studies focusing on the Developmental Origin of Health and Disease (DOHaD) have formed a cornerstone in our understanding of the pivotal role of nutrition. Commencing pregnancy either underweight or obese or gaining excessive gestational weight can cause significant health risks for both mother and fetus.

Over the course of the twentieth century, scientific ideas about pregnancy and the developing fetus have changed dramatically. Events of the Second World War in particular such as civilian starvation during sieges and conditions in prisons and camps were crucial to our changing understanding of fetal development (Buklijas 2014). More recently, the theory of fetal programming has been pivotal to our growing understanding of this subject with low birth weight and the pattern of infant growth being linked to Type 2 diabetes and cardiovascular disease in adulthood (Godfrey & Barker 2000). As low birth weight can be related to both maternal undernutrition and overnutrition during pregnancy, the concept of DOHaD clearly has implications for many women (British Nutrition Foundation and McArdle 2013). It is, however, important to stress that research, particularly on maternal obesity and the long-term health consequences for the fetus, continues to grow. The complexity of examining this subject is complicated by a need to discern the 'programmed' propensity in utero from the lived social environment and learned behaviour of later life. In terms of optimising both maternal and fetal health, an overview of existing evidence demonstrates that commencing pregnancy at a healthy weight (BMI 18.5–24.9), gaining an appropriate amount of gestational weight and losing the weight gained in the post-partum period are advantageous for both the short- and long-term health of the mother and her child (NICE 2010). Starting pregnancy underweight or obese has a range of both long- and short-term effects for both the woman and the developing fetus (Abayomi et al. 2007; Heslehurst et al. 2008; Han et al. 2011; Poston 2012) (see Table 13.2). In addition, excessive gestational weight gain is a risk factor for overweight and obesity in subsequent pregnancies (Villamor & Cnattingius 2006).

> **PRACTICE POINT**
>
> There are many adverse outcomes associated with commencing pregnancy, both underweight and obese. NICE recommend that women within the obese category should be educated about the risks associated with this, both for their own health and that of the developing fetus. Of equal importance is for midwives to seek specialised guidance when caring for a woman with an underweight BMI.

CURRENT GUIDELINES AND ADVICE TO PREGNANT WOMEN

In the United Kingdom, the general nutritional advice offered to pregnant women focuses on three main components:

1. Nutritional requirements of pregnancy
2. Food safety
3. Advice pertaining to pregnancy-related conditions (SACN 2011; NHS Choices 2014)

Table 13.2 Consequences of underweight/overweight BMI

Fetal	Woman
Underweight BMI	
Congenital malformations	Anaemia
Placental failure	Fever
Intrauterine infection	Delivery complications
Intrauterine growth restriction	Lack of macro- and micronutrients
Preterm birth	
Breastfeeding difficulties	
Lower birthweight and SGA	
SCBU admission	
Overweight BMI	
Congenital malformations	Hypertension
Macrocosomia	Thromboembolism
Stillbirth	Gestational diabetes
	Pre-eclampsia
	Increased caesarean section
	Increased risk of infection
	Breastfeeding difficulties
Long-term possible consequences for fetus and mother	
Obesity	
Type 2 diabetes	
Cardio vascular disease	

Indeed, these are the aspects of maternal diet with which the midwife has traditionally been most familiar. In addition to this general advice, the past decade has witnessed an expansion on guidance relating to maternal obesity both in the United Kingdom and internationally, reflecting the global concern with obesity.

The dietary recommendations for pregnant women are very similar to the advice presented to the general population – a healthy, varied and balanced diet to ensure adequate intake of energy and nutrients (NICE 2010). This is because metabolic and hormonal changes during pregnancy lead to increased absorption of minerals. However, supplementation of folic acid and vitamin D is recommended in pregnancy.

Women are advised to take a daily supplement of 400 µg of folic acid, before pregnancy and for the first 12 weeks. It is now very well recognised that folic acid supplementation is of crucial importance in protecting against neural tube defects (NTDs). A dose of 5 mg is advised where there is a family history of NTDs (NICE 2008). Vitamin D in adults is maintained by exposure to sunlight rather than by diet and is important for the absorption of calcium. Severe deficiency can result in rickets among children and osteomalacia in adults and children. National surveys have demonstrated that around 20% of adults and up to 25% of children may have low vitamin D stores (NICE 2014). Food safety during pregnancy relates to food preparation and intake. For example, to avoid excessive vitamin A intake, liver and liver products, for example, pâté and fish liver oils, should be avoided. To reduce the intake of mercury, fish such as swordfish, marlin and shark should be avoided and tuna intake should be limited. Actions to avoid the risk of Listeria include avoiding mould-ripened and unpasteurised cheeses and all types of pâté. In addition, midwives also offer dietary guidance in relation to pregnancy-related conditions such as nausea, constipation and anaemia (see further reading NHS choices – common problems in pregnancy).

In addition to the above general advice, the past 10 years has witnessed an expansion in guidance documents such as NICE guidelines on weight management in pregnancy and management of obesity during pregnancy (CMACE-RCOG 2010; NICE 2010). The NICE guidelines focus on beginning pregnancy at a healthy BMI, counselling on healthy lifestyle during pregnancy and a return to a healthy BMI in the postnatal period (NICE 2010). Significantly, these guidelines do not relate to underweight, which may have consequences for this small, but vulnerable group of women. It was also advised that women within the obese category should be educated about the risks associated with obesity, both to their own health and that of the developing fetus. In the United States, specific weight recommendations according to BMI classifications are given (Rasmussen & Yaktine 2009). However, in the United Kingdom, NICE concluded that there was insufficient evidence and that addressing gestational weight gain during pregnancy would result in improvements and they therefore recommended against routine weighing. Maternal anxiety has been cited as a reason against implementing routine weighing. However, a recent cross-sectional survey of maternal weight policies found no empirical evidence to support this (Scott et al. 2012).

Despite this increase in guidance, the task facing midwives remains complex. Heslehurst et al. (2014a) focused on the barriers that health professionals face when implementing pregnancy weight management and obesity guidelines. Guideline dissemination does not mean that the evidence is appropriated and implemented in every day practice. She underlines the lack of knowledge and of uniformity regarding weight management as an issue in care. Weight management was either provided routinely or not at all and was more likely to occur if the woman initiated the conversation. In addition, there was no consistency to the weight gain advice offered. Whilst the emergence of guidelines over the past decade has added to our knowledge of maternal weight management, there seemingly remains a gap between practice and policy.

PRACTICE POINT

Although, within the United Kingdom, there is no specific weight gain guidance during pregnancy, it remains important to give consistent advice and dispel myths such as eating for two and avoiding physical activity.

MOVING FORWARD: THE ROLE OF THE MIDWIFE AND DIET WITHIN AN OBESOGENIC SOCIETY

It is evident from the previous discussions that the subject of tackling maternal diet within an obesogenic society remains in its infancy, with much work still to be done. Recently, attention has focused on antenatal interventions for obese pregnant women, which is understandable considering the risk associated with maternal obesity. However, given the unprecedented rise in obesity, it is apparent that the subject generally needs to be approached in innovative ways. From a public health perspective, pregnancy is an ideal time to broach the subject, as women are regularly engaging with health care practitioners and are motivated for change.

It is not surprising that maternal obesity has been a focus for much research over the past 10 years. Research has ranged from large multi-centred behavioural change antenatal randomised controlled trials to qualitative work centring on experiences of both pregnant women and midwives. In the past year, the result of the UPBEAT trial, a large, behavioural intervention, randomised controlled trial for obese pregnant women, was shown not to reduce gestational diabetes and large-for-gestational-age infants (Poston et al. 2015). However, an improvement in diet and physical activity was noted and the intervention also showed modest reduction in maternal weight gain. From a public health perspective, the results of this study highlight the need for an emphasis to be placed on both the pre-conception and postnatal period when addressing maternal obesity. Nevertheless, it is undoubtedly encouraging that women in the UPBEAT study were able to make positive lifestyle changes during their pregnancy. A key point for consideration is whether this positive change can be translated to all pregnant women and what role could the midwife play. For example, might midwives run antenatal nutritional classes in the second trimester? In order to provide such a service, midwives will need to possess the necessary skills and confidence.

ACTIVITY

DEVELOPING A UNIVERSAL ANTENATAL NUTRITIONAL PROGRAMME

Think about how you might develop an antenatal programme for all women on nutrition.

- What topic areas would you cover? For example, food groups, postnatal weight loss.
- How would you engage the service users when designing the classes?
- How would you enrol the women to the classes?
- Who would run the classes and how would you evaluate them?

Besides including sessions on the importance of diet in the antenatal and postnatal period, the importance of breastfeeding, an important aspect of obesity prevention, could also be emphasised in a universal class. A large UK study examined the relationship between childbearing, breastfeeding and subsequent BMI which concluded that women who breastfed had significantly lower BMIs which remained significant, even after adjusting for confounding variables (Bobrow et al. 2009). Furthermore, meta-analyses have demonstrated that the risk of obesity in babies is reduced in later life by breastfeeding (Arenz et al. 2004; Harder et al. 2005; Owen et al. 2005).

As previously discussed, research has primarily and understandably focused on obese women. Indeed, there is continued evidence that obese women are motivated to change their lifestyles in pregnancy (Heslehurst et al. 2014b). However, as reiterated throughout this chapter, given the obesogenic nature of our environment, midwives should be aiming to support *all* women with their diet in pregnancy. Given the predicted obesity forecasts and consequential long-term health effects, it seems that utilising the public health role and skills of the midwife should be a priority for primary care commissioners.

SUMMARY OF KEY POINTS

- Midwives now face a complex task supporting women with their diet. The enormity consists of the following: meeting the contrasting needs and supporting women within the underweight, healthy, overweight and obesity categories. However, midwives are in a unique position to support women to make positive changes for both themselves and their families.
- The concept of an obesogenic environment is crucial when examining maternal diet. Utilising this concept is a useful method of introducing the topic of diet in pregnancy to all women as it paints a clear picture of how easy it is to consume food that is lacking in nutrition and to gain weight. Moreover, by employing this approach, the emphasis is not placed on individual excess and is therefore less stigmatising.

- The relationship of pregnant women with food is shaped by many aspects of their everyday lives including embodiment and body image, family and culture, and socio-economic position. It is crucial that midwives appreciate this complicated relationship with food, as it then becomes easier to understand as to why making positive changes to diet is difficult.
- Midwives may have difficulty broaching the subject of weight with women, particularly if they themselves have a complicated relationship with food.
- Commencing pregnancy either underweight or obese poses, or gaining excessive gestational weight can cause, significant health risks for both mother and the fetus.
- Guidance relating to maternal obesity, both in the United Kingdom and internationally, reflects the global concern about obesity. However, despite this expansion in maternal dietary recommendations, the task facing midwives in the role of supporting women with their diet remains a challenge.
- Midwives should be aiming to support all pregnant women with their diet, regardless of their BMI, as we all live within an obesogenic society. It is therefore essential that midwives have both the confidence and skills to do this.

REFERENCES

Abayomi, Julie, Helen Watkinson, Joanne Topping & Allan Hackett. 2007. Obesity and underweight among first trimester pregnant women. *British Journal of Midwifery* 15(3):143–147.

Arenz, Stephan, R. Rückerl., Berthod Koletzko & Rudiger von Kries. 2004. Breast-feeding and childhood obesity – A systematic review. *International Journal of Obesity* 28(10) (2):1247–1256.

Bailey, Lucy. 2001. Gender shows: First-time mothers and embodied selves. *Gender & Society* 15:110–129.

Banwell, Cathy, Dorothy Broom, Anna Davies & Jane Dixon. 2012. *Weight of Modernity: An Intergenerational Study of the Rise of Obesity*. Dordrecht: Springer.

Bobrow, Kristy, Maria Quigley, Jane Green, Gillian Reeves & Valarie Beral. 2009. The long-term effects of childbearing and breastfeeding on body mass index in middle aged women results from the Million Women Study. *Journal of Epidemiology and Community Health* 63(Suppl 2):56.

Bordo, Susan. 1993. *Unbearable Weight: Feminism, Western Culture and the Body*. Berkeley: University of California.

British Nutrition Foundation & Judith Buttriss. 2013. *Putting the Science into Practice: Public Health Implications*. West Sussex: Wiley.

British Nutrition Foundation & Harry J. McArdle. 2013. *Normal Growth and Development*. West Sussex: Wiley.

Brownell, Kelly D. & Katherine Battle Horgen. 2004. *Food Fight: The Inside Story of the Food Industry, America's Obesity Crisis, and What We Can Do about It*. Chicago, IL: Contemporary Books.

Buklijas, Tatjana. 2014. Food, growth and time: Elsie Widdowson's and Robert McCance's research into prenatal and early postnatal growth. *Studies in History and Philosophy of Science Part C: Studies in History and Philosophy of Biological and Biomedical Sciences* 47(Part B):267–277.

Butland, Bryony, Susan Jebb, Peter Kopelman, Klim McPherson, Sandy Thomas, Jane Mardell & Vivienne Parry. 2007. *Foresight. Tackling Obesities: Future Choices.* Project report. https://www.gov.uk/government/uploads/system/uploads/attachment_data/file/287937/07-1184x-tackling-obesities-future-choices-report.pdf

Caplan, Pat. 1996. Why do people eat what they do? Approaches to food and diet from a social science perspective. *Clinical Child Psychology and Psychiatry* 1(2):213–227.

CMACE (Centre for Maternal and Child Enquiries). 2010. *Maternal Obesity in the UK: Findings from a National Project.* London: CMACE.

CMACE-RCOG. 2010. *Management of Women with Obesity in Pregnancy.* Centre for Maternal and Child Enquiries and the Royal College of Obstetricians and Gynaecologists. http://www.hqip.org.uk/assets/NCAPOP-Library/CMACE-Reports/15.-March-2010-Management-of-Women-with-Obesity-in-Pregnancy-Guidance.pdf

Crozier, Sarah R., Hazel M. Inskip, Keith M. Godfrey, Cyrus Cooper, Nicolas C. Harvey, Zoë A. Cole & Siân M. Robinson (and the Southampton Women's Survey Study Group). 2010. Weight gain in pregnancy and childhood body composition: Findings from the Southampton Women's Survey. *The American Journal of Clinical Nutrition* 91(6):1745–1751.

Department of Health. 2006. *Healthy Start Vouchers.* http://www.southnorfolkccg.nhs.uk/sites/default/files/pdf/Healthy_Start_-_GP_Presentation_PDF.pdf

Dobson, Barbara, Alan Beardsworth, T. Keil & R. Walker. 1994. *Diet, Choice, and Poverty: Social, Cultural, and Nutritional Aspects of Food Consumption among Low-Income Families.* Loughborough: Family Policy Studies Centre.

Dodd, Jodie M., Rosalie M. Grivell, Caroline A. Crowther & Jeffrey S. Robinson. 2010. Antenatal interventions for overweight or obese pregnant women: A systematic review of randomised trials. *BJOG: An International Journal of Obstetrics & Gynaecology* 117(11):1316–1326.

Dowler, Elizabeth & Claire Calvert. 1995. *Nutrition and Diet in Lone-Parent Families in London.* London: Family Policy Studies Centre.

Furber, Christine M. & Linda McGowan. 2011. A qualitative study of the experiences of women who are obese and pregnant in the UK. *Midwifery* 27(4):437–444.

Godfrey, Keith M. & David J. P. Barker. 2000. Fetal nutrition and adult disease. *The American Journal of Clinical Nutrition* 71(5):1344s–1352s.

Han, Zhen, Sohail Mulla, Joseph Beyene, Grace Liao & Sarah McDonald. 2011. Maternal underweight and the risk of preterm birth and low birth weight: A systematic review and meta-analyses. *International Journal of Epidemiology* 40(1):65–101.

Harder, Thomas, Renate Bergmann, Gerd Kallischnigg & Andreas Plagemann. 2005. Duration of breastfeeding and risk of overweight: A meta-analysis. *American Journal of Epidemiology* 162(5): 397–403.

Heslehurst, Nicola, Sarah Dinsdale, Gillian Sedgewick, Helen Simpson, Seema Sen, Carolyn Dawn Summerbell & Judith Rankin. 2014b. An evaluation of the implementation of maternal obesity pathways of care: A mixed methods study with data integration. *PLoS One* 10(5):e0127122–e0127122.

Heslehurst, Nicola, Helen Moore, Judith Rankin, Louisa Ells, John Wilkinson & Carolyn Summberbell. 2011. How can maternity services be developed to effectively address maternal obesity? A qualitative study. *Midwifery* 27(5):170–177.

Heslehurst, Nicola, James Newham, Gregory Maniatopoulos, Catherine Fleetwood, Shannon Robalino & Judith Rankin. 2014a. Implementation of pregnancy weight management and obesity guidelines: A meta-synthesis of healthcare professionals' barriers and facilitators using the theoretical domains framework. *Obesity Reviews* 15(6):462–486.

Heslehurst, Nicola, Judith Rankin, John Wilkinson & Carolyn Summerbell. 2010. A nationally representative study of maternal obesity in England, UK: Trends in incidence and demographic inequalities in 619 323 births, 1989–2007. *International Journal of Obesity* 34(3):420–428.

Heslehurst, Nicola, Sarah Russell, Sandra McCormack, Gill Sedgewick, Ruth Bell & Judith Rankin. 2013. Midwives perspectives of their training and education requirements in maternal obesity: A qualitative study. *Midwifery* 29(7):736–744.

Heslehurst, Nicola, Helen Simpson, Louisa Ells, Judith Rankin, John Wilkinson, Rebecca Lang, T. J. Brown & Carolyn Summerbell. 2008. The impact of maternal BMI status on pregnancy outcomes with immediate short-term obstetric resource implications: A meta-analysis. *Obesity Reviews* 9(6):635–683.

HSCIC (Health & Social Care Information Centre). 2015. *Statistics on Obesity, Physical Activity & Diet.* England. http://www.hscic.gov.uk/catalogue/PUB16988/obes-phys-acti-diet-eng-2015.pdf

Khashan, Ali S., Philip N. Baker & Louise C. Kenny. 2010. Preterm birth and reduced birthweight in first and second teenage pregnancies: A register-based cohort study. *BMC Pregnancy and Childbirth* 10(1):36.

Knight, Maria, Sara Kenyon, Peter Brocklehurst, Jim Neilson, Judy Shakespeare & Jennifer J. Kurinczuk (eds.) on behalf of MBRRACEUK. 2014. *Saving Lives, Improving Mothers' Care – Lessons Learned to Inform Future Maternity Care from the UK and Ireland Confidential Enquiries into Maternal Deaths and Morbidity 2009–12.* Oxford: National Perinatal Epidemiology Unit, University of Oxford.

Lambie-Mumford, Hannah & Elizabeth Dowler. 2014. Rising use of "food aid" in the United Kingdom. *British Food Journal* 116(9):1418–1425.

Lewis, Gwyneth (Ed). 2007. *Saving Mothers' Lives: Reviewing Maternal Deaths to Make Motherhood Safer – 2003–2005. The Seventh Report on Confidential Enquiries into Maternal Deaths in the United Kingdom.* London: CEMACH.

Linné, Yvonne, Louise Dye, Britta Barkeling & Stephan Rössner. 2004. Long-term weight development in women: A 15-year follow-up of the effects of pregnancy. *Obesity Research* 12(7):1166–1178.

Lupton, Deborah. 1996. *Food, the Body and the Self.* London: Sage.

Marmot, Michael, Jessica Allen, Peter Goldblatt, Tammy Boyce, Di McNeish, Mike Grady & Ilaria Geddes. 2010. *Fair Society, Healthy Lives: Strategic Review of Health Inequalities in England Post-2010.* http://www.instituteofhealthequity.org/projects/fair-society-healthy-lives-the-marmot-review

Micali, Nadia. 2010. Management of eating disorders during pregnancy. *Progress in Neurology and Psychiatry* 14(2):24–26.

Molyneaux, Emma, Lucilla Poston, Sarah Ashurst-Williams & Louise M. Howard. 2014. Obesity and mental disorders during pregnancy and postpartum: A systematic review and meta-analysis. *Obstetrics and Gynecology* 123(4):857.

Murray, Cynthia L. 2014. "It's a wild ride": A phenomenological exploration of high maternal, gestational weight gain. *Health* 6(18):2541–2552.

Nestle, Marion. 2013. *Food Politics: How the Food Industry Influences Nutrition and Health.* Berkeley, CA: University of California Press.

NHS Choices. 2014. *Your Pregnancy and Baby Guide.* www.nhs.uk/conditions/pregnancy-and-baby pages

NICE (National Institute for Health and Clinical Excellence). 2008. *Antenatal Guidelines.* London: Department of Health.

NICE (National Institute for Health and Clinical Excellence). 2010. *Weight Management before, during and after Pregnancy*. London: Department of Health.

NICE (National Institute for Health and Clinical Excellence). 2014. *Vitamin D: Increasing Supplements Use amongst At-Risk Groups*. London: Department of Health.

Oteng-Ntim, Eugene, Rajesh Varma, Helen Croker, Lucilla Poston & Pat Doyle. 2012. Lifestyle interventions for overweight and obese pregnant women to improve pregnancy outcome: Systematic review and meta-analysis. *BMC Medicine* 10(1):47.

Owen, Christopher G., Richard M. Martin, Peter H. Whincup, George Davey-Smith, Matthew W. Gillman & Derek G. Cook. 2005. The effect of breastfeeding on mean body mass index throughout life: A quantitative review of published and unpublished observational evidence. *The American Journal of Clinical Nutrition* 82(6):1298–1307.

Poston, Lucilla. 2012. Maternal obesity, gestational weight gain and diet as determinants of offspring long term health. *Best Practice & Research Clinical Endocrinology & Metabolism* 26(5):627–639.

Poston, Lucilla, Ruth Bell, Helen Croker, Angela C. Flynn, Keith M. Godfrey, Louise Goff, Louise Hayes, et al. 2015. Effect of a behavioural intervention in obese pregnant women (the UPBEAT study): A multicentre, randomised controlled trial. *The Lancet Diabetes & Endocrinology*. http://www.thelancet.com/journals/landia/article/PIIS2213-8587(15)00227-2/fulltext

Rasmussen, Kathleen & Ann L. Yaktine (eds). 2009. *Institute of Medicine and National Research Council Guidelines: Weight Gain during Pregnancy: Reexamining the Guidelines*. Washington DC: The National Academies Press.

Renzaho, Andre, David Mellor, Kelly Boulton & Boyd Swinburn. 2010. Effectiveness of prevention programmes for obesity and chronic diseases among immigrants to developed countries—A systematic review. *Public Health Nutrition* 13(3):438–450.

Rooney, Brenda L. & Charles W. Schauberger. 2002. Excess pregnancy weight gain and long-term obesity: One decade later. *Obstetrics & Gynecology* 100(2):245–252.

SACN (Scientific Advisory Committee on Nutrition). 2011. *Dietary Recommendations for Energy*. London: The Stationary Office.

Scott, Courtney, Christopher Andersen, Natali Valdez, Francisco Mardones, Ellen, Nohr, Lucilla Poston, Katharina Smith, Debbie M, Alison Cooke and Tina Lavender. 2012. Maternal obesity is the new challenge; a qualitative study of health professionals' views towards suitable care for pregnant women with a Body Mass Index (BMI)≥ 30 kg/m². *BMC Pregnancy and Childbirth* 12(1):157.

Sharp, Jane. 1671. *The Midwives Book: Or the Whole Art of Midwifery Discovered:* (1999 Ed.). Oxford: Oxford University Press.

Smith, Debbie M., Alison Cooke, and Tina Lavender. 2012. Maternal obesity is the new challenge; a qualitative study of health professionals' views towards suitable care for pregnant women with a Body Mass Index (BMI)≥ 30 kg/m². *BMC Pregnancy and Childbirth* 12(1):157.

Swinburn, Boyd, Garry Egger & Fezeela Raza. 1999. Dissecting obesogenic environments: The development and application of a framework for identifying and prioritizing environmental interventions for obesity. *Preventive Medicine* 29(6):563–570.

Swinburn, Boyd A., Gary Sacks, Kevin D. Hall, Klim McPherson, Diane T. Finegood, Marjory L. Moodie & Steven L. Gortmaker. 2011. The global obesity pandemic: Shaped by global drivers and local environments. *The Lancet* 378(9793): 804–814.

Villamor, Eduardo & Sven Cnattingius. 2006. Interpregnancy weight change and risk of adverse pregnancy outcomes: A population-based study. *The Lancet* 368:1164–1170.

WHO (World Health Organization). 1995. *Physical Status: The Use of and Interpretation of Anthropometry. Report of a WHO Expert Committee.* http://apps.who.int/iris/bit-stream/10665/37003/1/WHO_TRS_854.pdf

WHO (World Health Organization). 2015. *Obesity and Overweight.* http://www.who.int/mediacentre/factsheets/fs311/en/

FURTHER READINGS

British Nutrition Foundation. http://www.nutrition.org.uk/healthyliving/nutritionfor-pregnancy.html

Weight management before, during and after pregnancy. NICE guidelines [PH27]. Published date: July 2010. https://www.nice.org.uk/guidance/ph27

NHS Choices. Common problems in pregnancy. http://www.nhs.uk/conditions/pregnancy-and-baby/pages/common-pregnancy-problems.aspx#close

NHS Choices. Healthy diet in pregnancy. http://www.nhs.uk/conditions/pregnancy-and-baby/pages/healthy-pregnancy-diet.aspx#close

Managing obesity in pregnant women: An online guide for health professionals. Dr Nicola Heslehurst, NIHR Postdoctoral Research Fellow, Institute of Health & Society, Newcastle University, and Adrian Brown, Specialist Weight Management and Bariatric Dietitian, Heart of England Foundation Trust, Birmingham. http://www.tommys.org/file/Managing-obesity-in-pregnant-women_2013.pdf

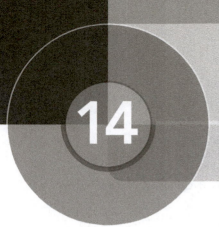

Pelvic floor health during the childbearing years

14

TERESA ARIAS, JANETTE O'TOOLE AND
EMILY NELLIST

INTRODUCTION

The midwife is in a strong position to provide education and support that has the potential to enhance physical, mental and emotional well-being for the woman (DoH 2012). The midwife's public health role is expanding (NMC 2012) and preventative measures, such as maintaining pelvic floor health, should be a component of high quality maternity care according to the joint statement by the Royal College of Midwives (RCM) and the Chartered Society of Physiotherapy (CSP) (Gerrard and ten Hove 2013).

A healthy pelvic floor (PF) is associated with physical and psychological well-being. It has an important role in maintaining urinary and faecal continence, pelvic organ and pelvic lumbar support and aiding the passage of the baby through the vagina during childbirth and enhances sexual function. Pregnancy and childbirth are known to increase the of risk of incontinence with a third of women experiencing urinary incontinence (UI) and approximately a tenth of women experiencing faecal incontinence after childbirth (Boyle et al. 2012).

Pelvic floor muscle exercises (PFMEs) during pregnancy are known to prevent and reduce PF dysfunction (Hay-Smith et al. 2012). Midwives are in an optimal position to provide PF education in the antenatal and postnatal period, and women have reported that they would like to receive this information from their midwives. Midwives, however, have conveyed a lack of confidence in teaching PFMEs and have reported that they would like to have further education on how to improve their effectiveness at instructing women to perform these exercises (Guerrero et al. 2007).

The aims of this chapter are to enhance the midwife's knowledge and understanding of the importance of the role of the PF and improve their confidence in teaching PFMEs. It will cover:

- Incidence of UI
- Functional anatomy of the PF and PF dysfunction
- The impact of pregnancy and childbirth on the PF
- History taking and appropriate referral pathways
- General advice and management strategies for PF dysfunction, current evidence, guidelines and best practice
- How to teach PFMEs
- Common myths relating to PF health
- Case studies

INCIDENCE OF UI

PF dysfunction is common among adults and is more frequently seen in women, its prevalence increasing with age. Accurate incidence rates are difficult to confirm as embarrassment, resulting from incontinence, may lead to underreporting. Studies report a wide range of UI incidence rates between 25% and 45% in women (Milsom et al. 2013). In the United Kingdom, approximately 3.5 million women are affected by UI (Price & Currie 2010). Pregnancy and the post-partum period may be the first time that many experience UI.

FUNCTIONAL ANATOMY OF THE PF COMPLEX

An understanding of the anatomy of the PF is essential for midwives to effectively teach PFMEs. This anatomy should include attention to all the components of the PF, not just the muscle layers, in acknowledgement of the interconnected nature of their function.

The PF spans the outlet of the pelvis and is composed of a complex musculotendinous sling attached to the internal surface of the pelvis. It supports the urogenital organs (bladder, uterus and rectum) and the corresponding openings exiting the pelvis (the urethra, vagina and anus).

It comprises the superficial muscles, the levator ani muscles, fascia, connective tissue, supporting ligaments, nerves and blood vessels which are described in more detail in the following sections (see Figure 14.1).

SUPERFICIAL PELVIC FLOOR MUSCLES

Midwives will be familiar with the superficial pelvic floor muscles (PFMs) as injuries to some of these muscles may be sustained naturally (i.e. perineal tear) or mechanically (as a result of an episiotomy) during vaginal birth. The muscles of the superficial PF are: bulbospongiosus, ischiocavernosus, transverse perinei and external anal sphincter. The main role of the superficial PFMs is to contribute to sexual function. PFMEs have been shown to improve all aspects of sexual function such as sexual desire, arousal, lubrication and orgasm (Zahariou et al. 2008).

LEVATOR ANI MUSCLES

The levator ani is a group of muscles under voluntary control, comprising the ischiococcygeus, iliococcygeus, pubococcygeus and puborectalis muscles. Although the levator ani muscles

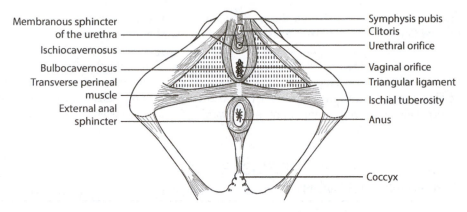

Figure 14.1 Superficial layer of the pelvic floor. (From Bennet, V. Ruth and Linda K. Brown. 1999. The reproductive organs. In V. Ruth Bennet and Linda K. Brown (eds.), *Myles textbook for midwives*. Edinburg: Churchill Livingstone.)

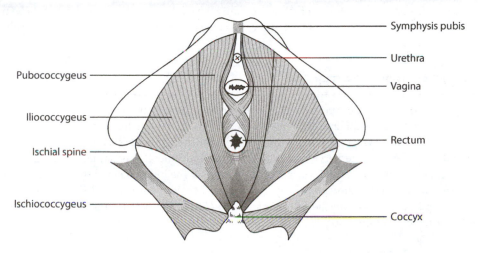

Figure 14.2 Deep layer of the pelvic floor. (From Bennet, V. Ruth and Linda K. Brown. 1999. The reproductive organs. In V. Ruth Bennet and Linda K. Brown (eds.), *Myles textbook for midwives*. Edinburg: Churchill Livingstone.)

are often referred to individually, they are not easily distinguished and perform many of the same functions (Thakar & Fenner 2009). The levator ani, pelvic fascia and the supporting ligaments are known collectively as the pelvic diaphragm (Ashton-Miller & DeLancy 2015) (see Figure 14.2). The levator ani is considered to be the most critical component of the pelvic diaphragm because of its role in protecting the pelvic connective tissue from excessive load (Ashton-Miller & DeLancy 2015). The levator ani has an important role in facilitating vaginal delivery (or birth), defecation, providing support for the spine and the PF in addition to preventing urinary and faecal incontinence and pelvic organ prolapse. Damage to the levator ani could result in an impairing of one or more of these functions.

The levator ani has a resting and active role. At rest, it maintains a constant tone, resulting in closure of the urethra, vagina and rectum by compressing them against the pubic bone. In its active role, contraction of the levator ani initiates a forward and upward movement of the coccyx (Bo et al. 1990), lifts the pelvic organs including the rectum (Raizada and Mittal 2008) and causes further compression of the urethra, vagina and rectum against the pubic bone (Ashton-Miller and DeLancy 2015). This upward and forward movement occurs when the PF contracts, and it is helpful to imagine when instructing women on how to perform PFEs.

During childbirth, the levator ani facilitates the passage of the baby through the pelvis by offering a platform of resistance to the presenting part of the baby which encourages rotation of the baby through the vagina (Coad & Dunstall 2011). The puborectalis muscle (along with the external anal sphincter) is important in maintaining faecal continence (Rao 2004) and has an important role in defecation.

THE FASCIA, CONNECTIVE TISSUE AND SUPPORTING LIGAMENTS

The pelvic fascia encapsulates the levator ani muscles and works with the pelvic ligaments to provide stability to the pelvic organs. The levator ani helps minimise tension on the ligaments and fascia and maintains closure of the openings of the urethra and vagina when working effectively. Damage or weakness of the levator ani may lead to the fascia and ligaments being placed under increasing strain, and over time, this may result in PF dysfunction, such as pelvic organ prolapse.

NERVE SUPPLY OF THE PF

The pudendal nerve is derived from S1-S4. It supplies most of the structures that maintain continence and pelvic support, including the clitoris, urinary sphincter, perineum, vagina and anus. However, the levator ani is supplied by direct branches from the sacral plexus rather than the pudendal nerve. If the nerve supply to the levator ani muscles is damaged, for example, during childbirth, it may result in atrophy (weakening) of the PFMs, leaving the sole support to the fascia alone. As indicated previously, the interconnected nature of the PF function means that the additional strain on the fascia has the potential to impact on the connective tissue contributing to PF dysfunction.

PF DYSFUNCTION

The following definitions for PF dysfunction have been defined by the International Urogynaecological Association (IUGA)/International Continence Society (ICS) Joint Report on the Terminology for Female Pelvic Floor Dysfunction (Haylen et al. 2010). (see Table 14.1)

IMPACT OF PREGNANCY AND CHILDBEARING ON THE PF

Studies have identified that certain factors place women at risk for developing PF dysfunction, including pregnancy and delivery (Viktrup et al. 2006).

Postural changes during pregnancy, increasing abdominal weight and hormonal changes provide additional challenges to the PF (Viktrup et al. 2006; Steen & Roberts 2011). More examples of risk factors are given in Box 14.1.

Specific trauma to the PF can be sustained during vaginal delivery, more commonly assisted delivery. The examples included below demonstrate the different types of injury (Box 14.2).

Table 14.1 Definitions for PF dysfunction as defined by the International Urogynaecological Association (IUGA)/International Continence Society (ICS)

- *Stress (urinary) incontinence:* complaint of involuntary loss of urine on effort or physical exertion, for example, coughing, sneezing, lifting, running
- *Urgency:* complaint of sudden, compelling desire to pass urine which is difficult to defer (with or without urinary leakage)
- *Urgency (urinary) incontinence:* complaint of involuntary loss of urine associated with urgency
- *Mixed (urinary) incontinence:* complaint of involuntary loss of urine associated with urgency and stress incontinence
- *Prolapse symptoms:* may be associated with vaginal bulging (bulge or sensation of something 'coming down'), pelvic pressure (heaviness or dragging), low back ache, splinting/digitation (apply manual pressure to the vagina, perineum or rectum to assist voiding or defecation)
- *Anal incontinence:* complaint of involuntary loss of faeces or flatus
- *Insensible urinary incontinence:* complaint of urinary incontinence where the woman is unaware of how it occurs. This is very important in the immediate postnatal period as it may represent leaking from an over-distended bladder if the bladder is in retention and is unable to empty effectively
- *Sexual dysfunction:* change in normal sensation experienced by the woman during sexual activity such as painful intercourse, vaginal laxity, reduced sexual sensation or reduced sexual pleasure

Source: From Haylen, Bernard T., et al. 2010. *Neurourology and Urodynamics* 29: 4–20.

BOX 14.1: Risk factors for PF damage and PF dysfunction

- Increasing parity (Macarthur et al. 2011)
- Macrosomia (Macarthur et al. 2011)
- Prolonged second stage of labour
- Assisted delivery (Macarthur et al. 2011)
- Very young and older mothers (Thom et al. 2011)
- Previous PF injury
- Women who are overweight or have a high BMI (Danforth et al. 2006; Milsom et al. 2013)
- Chronic constipation (Bassotti and Villanacci 2004)
- High impact exercise, for example, running, star jumps, trampolining (Newman et al. 2013)
- Genetic predisposition such as hypermobility (Buchsbaum et al. 2005)
- Smoking (Danforth et al. 2006)

BOX 14.2: Examples to demonstrate the different types of injury

- Trauma to the connective tissue/fascia/ligaments
- Vascular damage to the pelvic structures as a result of compression by the presenting part of the baby
- Trauma to the pelvic nerves or PFMs
- Injury to the urinary tract (e.g. urethra)

HISTORY TAKING AND REFERRAL PATHWAYS

History taking is an important aspect of the midwife's role in identifying the woman's symptoms and guiding the correct referral pathway (NICE 2013). It is recommended that women are asked about PF health (such as bladder and bowel symptoms) as part of their maternity booking consultation. The early identification of problems will facilitate timely referral to an appropriate health care professional (HCP) such as a woman's health physiotherapist; urogynaecology, colorectal or obstetric teams; community continence service; or a specialist perineal midwife. This may differ between trusts; therefore, it is important for midwives to familiarise themselves with services available to ensure a multi-disciplinary approach to support the woman's physical and emotional needs (NMC 2015).

A full history should include:

- Duration, onset and severity of symptoms
- Impact of symptoms on quality of life
- Checking for haematuria, persistent bladder or urethral pain or recurrent urinary tract infection (UTI) (Price & Currie 2010)

See Box 14.3 for some possible questions you should ask.

Case study 1

Jenny is a 32-year-old woman expecting her first baby. You meet her at the booking appointment at 11 weeks' gestation. Her medical and obstetric history appears normal. She asks whether it is normal to go to the toilet frequently and you explain the hormonal changes in pregnancy and how they result in an increased frequency of micturition in the first trimester.

On further questioning, she tells you that she needs to go to the toilet every hour and often feels that she might not make it in time. This has happened once. She tells you that she has always had a 'weak' bladder, even before pregnancy and dare not run for the bus or she may leak. Try to answer the following questions; refer to answers in Case study 1 – possible answers.

How would you describe Jenny's condition?

What additional information would you like to have?

How might you be able to improve this woman's symptoms?

How might you be able to assess the effectiveness of her attempts at performing PFMEs?

If you decide that her care plan should include a referral to a specialist, who is available to see women with Jenny's symptoms in your unit?

BOX 14.3: Possible questions you can ask about bladder, bowel

Ask women-specific screening questions...

- Do you leak urine when you cough, sneeze, laugh, jump, run?
- Do you leak urine if you are holding too long, and can't make it to the toilet?
- Do you have difficulty holding your wind or bowel movements?
- Do you have a sensation of dragging, bulging, or feeling of something coming down in the vagina?
- Do you suffer from constipation?
- Do you suffer from frequent urinary tract infections?

GENERAL ADVICE AND MANAGEMENT STRATEGIES FOR WOMEN WITH PF DYSFUNCTION

FLUID ADVICE

It is helpful to ask any woman presenting with UI about fluid intake and types of fluid. A high fluid intake may be a risk factor for developing UI (Newman et al. 2013). Monitoring of fluid intake in certain cases may be appropriate.

Although there is some conflicting evidence in relation to the effects of caffeine consumption on UI, the majority of studies do suggest a dose–effect relationship between caffeine and incontinence (Robinson et al. 2014) and recommend that caffeine consumption should be reduced in those women with lower urinary tract symptoms. Caffeine may be found in coffee, tea, green tea, hot chocolate, 'energy' drinks, some cold and flu remedies and over the counter medications. It is important not to have more than 200 mg of caffeine a day. This is equivalent to two mugs of instant coffee or two mugs of tea.

The consumption of carbonated drinks and artificial sweeteners may also be associated with the development or aggravation of urinary urgency or urinary urgency incontinence symptoms (Robinson et al. 2014). Carbonated drinks contain preservatives and anti-oxidants and low concentrations of artificial sweeteners and have also been shown to enhance bladder muscle contraction which is associated with increased urinary urgency, frequency and urinary urgency incontinence (Dasgupta et al. 2006, 2009).

PRACTICE POINT

Recommending fluid modification, a reduction in carbonated drinks and reducing drinks containing artificial sweeteners and caffeine may help improve women's urinary symptoms.

CONSTIPATION

Up to one in four women suffer from constipation during pregnancy (Bradley et al. 2007).

Studies have demonstrated that persistent straining with constipation may result in damage to the pudendal nerve, changes in the PF musculature (Snooks et al. 1985; Amselem et al. 2009), development of uterovaginal prolapse and UI (Spence-Jones et al. 1994). Therefore, it is important to address this problem during pregnancy. Midwives should provide dietary and bowel advice to women to reduce the risk of constipation and to minimise straining on the toilet to protect the PF during pregnancy and in the postnatal period.

DIETARY ADVICE TO AVOID CONSTIPATION

Women should be encouraged to eat a variety of foods including:

- Plenty of fruit and vegetables (fresh, frozen, tinned, dried or a glass of juice) – at least five portions a day.
- Plenty of fibre, found in wholegrain bread, wholegrain cereals, pasta, rice, pulses and fruit and vegetables (NICE 2010).

Constipation is common in pregnancy. Midwives should provide dietary and bowel advice to women to reduce the risk of constipation and minimise straining on the toilet to protect the PF during pregnancy and in the postnatal period.

CORRECT POSITION TO EMPTY BOWELS

Teaching women to sit correctly on the toilet to empty their bowels may help reduce straining on the toilet. This is important to help protect the PF.

- Raise feet (knees higher than hips)
- Lean forward with forearms resting on knees
- Try to 'let go' of *all* muscles
- Gently bulge the tummy muscles and push down gently
- Breathe slowly and gently through the mouth
- Don't strain!!

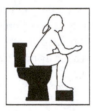

PHYSICAL EXERCISE

Physical exercise is beneficial for women during pregnancy and also in the post-partum period, is not associated with risks to the unborn child and may lead to changes in lifestyle with long-term benefits. In a systematic review, Nascimento et al. (2012) reported that exercise during pregnancy was associated with many health benefits, including prevention of UI.

WEIGHT MANAGEMENT

The incidence of obesity during pregnancy is rapidly increasing in the United Kingdom (Heslehurst et al. 2007). Hernández et al. (2013) demonstrated that high BMI and weight retention at 6 months post-partum increased the risk of UI, whereas post-partum weight loss decreases the risk of incontinence.

Midwives can make a major contribution towards the prevention and rehabilitation of UI in women. Individualised advice about eating and exercise habits may be helpful (NICE 2010) (see Chapter 13).

Case study 2

You meet Michelle at her home 3 weeks after her first baby was born by forceps delivery. You have extended your visits beyond 10 days as Michelle has found breastfeeding her baby particularly challenging and the baby has been putting on weight very slowly. Her episiotomy wound is causing her pain and she reveals that her bowels are 'playing up'. When questioned further, she tells you that she sometimes has to put the baby down quickly as she experiences some faecal urgency. She has always made it to the toilet on time but is worried about going out to meet friends especially since she is unable to control her wind. She started experiencing faecal urgency 3 days after her delivery, and these symptoms have not improved. Try to answer the following questions; refer to answers in Case study 2 – possible answers.

What additional information would you like to have?

How could you support Michelle with her faecal urgency?

If you decide that her care plan should include a referral to a specialist, who is available to see women with Michelle's symptoms in your unit?

ANTENATAL: PF EXERCISES IN PREGNANCY

It is important for midwives to focus on prevention of UI. For many women, the onset of UI is during pregnancy and is strongly predictive of post-partum UI (RCOG 2006). Women should be given information on PF exercises at the booking appointment for maternity care, preferably by 10 weeks' gestation (NICE 2008). Viktrup et al. (2006) found that the prevalence of stress UI in women 12 years after the first pregnancy was significantly higher in women who reported an initial onset of symptoms during the first pregnancy or shortly after delivery, compared with women without initial symptoms. This implies that women who experience urinary symptoms during pregnancy or in the immediate postnatal period are more at risk of experience ongoing UI later in life. Women who engage in PFMEs during pregnancy report fewer symptoms of urinary stress incontinence after giving birth (Sahakian & Woodward 2012). PFMEs both during pregnancy and after delivery can prevent and treat UI (Boyle et al. 2012; Mørkved, Siv & Bø Kari 2014).

PRACTICE POINT

PFMEs should be taught to all women in their first and subsequent pregnancies as a preventative strategy for UI (NICE 2013).

HOW TO TEACH PFMEs

The ability to perform PFMEs correctly is vital to preventing and treating PF dysfunction. It is therefore important that midwives are able to teach women how to perform these exercises correctly and instil confidence in how to perform PFMEs as this may improve compliance with the exercises.

The key to teaching PFMEs successfully is to ensure a correct PFM contraction is being performed from the beginning. Up to 30% of pregnant and postnatal women lack confidence that they are performing PFMEs correctly (Chiarelli et al. 2003). Bump et al. (1991) found that 40% of women were unable to perform an effective PFM contraction with verbal instruction alone.

ACTIVITY

How would you discuss PFMEs with a woman? Write down how you would introduce the subject and include a step-by-step description of how to perform PFMEs in your own language. How does your instruction compare with the one included below?

> **BOX 14.4: Examples of visualisation to use when teaching PFMEs**
>
> - Imagine you are shutting the doors (urethra, vagina and anus) to a lift and going up to the top floor
> - Imagine you are sucking up spaghetti through the urethral, vaginal and anal openings
> - Drawing up the vagina as if it is a lift
> - Imagine a string hanging from the vagina and you are trying to draw it up inside
> - Imagine holding something inside the vagina that is slipping down
> - Imagine the vagina as a cone, wide at the bottom and small at the top, and you are drawing up inside

PROVIDE DIAGRAM/MODEL

In order to perform a correct contraction, the woman needs to first know where the PFMs are. A diagram of the PF or a model of the pelvis is an important aid to illustrate where these muscles are situated.

VERBAL INSTRUCTION

1. **Explain the role of the PFMs and how they work**
   It is important that women understand the impact of weak PFMs and how exercising can prevent and treat problems. Explain the role of the PF in bladder and bowel control, support for the pelvic organs and sexual function (as discussed earlier in this chapter). It is important to check understanding and take steps to meet people's communication needs (NMC 2015).
2. **Explain how to find the muscles and perform a correct contraction**
   Instruct the woman to: 'Imagine you are trying to stop yourself from passing urine and wind from your back passage. Squeeze around the openings and lift inwards'.

Ask her to practice a few contractions on a chair. Encourage her to pull up the PFM, away from the seat of the chair, as strongly as she can, then immediately let go so that these muscles move towards the seat of the chair. It is important to emphasise relaxed breathing throughout.

VISUAL IMAGERY

Visual imagery can be used to help the woman locate and correctly contract their PFMs. Each HCP may use different imagery; these can be varied depending on what suits the HCP and what is acceptable and understood by the woman. A variety of examples have been provided for this reason (Box 14.4).

PF EXERCISES IN THE POSTNATAL PERIOD

At any point of contact, it is important for midwives to screen for symptoms of PF dysfunction, discuss PFMEs and emphasise their importance. The prevalence of UI is high in the first 3 months post-partum with 33% women experiencing symptoms (Thom & Rortveit 2010). Early detection of PF dysfunction, timely referral and prompt initiation (in the first 3 months post-partum) of effective performance of PFMEs is known to increase the likelihood of resolution of UI at 12 months post-partum (Boyle et al. 2012). Those women who report symptoms of UI 3 months post-partum are likely to have ongoing problems without intervention. Early referral to a specialist women's health or PF physiotherapist is recommended as these symptoms may not resolve without treatment.

PFMEs have been shown to reduce the prevalence of UI up to 1 year after delivery (Hay-Smith et al. 2008). In the long term, the evidence is less well defined, but this may be because women go on to have more children or they do not continue with PFMEs.

It is widely accepted that childbirth is a significant risk factor for UI and is the single strongest risk factor for developing pelvic organ prolapse (POP) in later life and the risk increases with each childbirth (Milsom et al. 2013). It is estimated that 50% of parous women develop some degree of POP (Olsen et al. 1997). However, there is often a delay between delivery and onset of POP symptoms. A multi-centred, randomised control trial of 447 women showed that individualised PFMEs were effective at improving prolapse symptoms. PFMEs should therefore be recommended as a first line treatment for women with POP (Hagen et al. 2014).

> **PRACTICE POINT**
>
> Intensive PF muscle training can reduce the incidence and severity of incontinence symptoms in the postnatal period and therefore should be routinely advised by the midwife and postnatal follow up.

PHYSICAL FEEDBACK

Some women will find locating their PFMs difficult as they have never learned to contract these muscles before. Women may benefit from using proprioceptive feedback (physical contact) to help them find the correct muscles.

In sitting, ask the woman to bring their attention to the pressure felt on their perineum against the chair. Ask her to lift the perineum away from chair.

This can also be done in a reclined or lying position by the woman applying pressure on the perineum with her own hand and trying to lift her perineum away from her hand.

VISUAL FEEDBACK

This can be useful for some women to facilitate correct PFM contraction who do not mind looking at their own perineum. By using a mirror they may see the perineum drawing inwards to confirm correct contraction. This may give reassurance to the woman that they are performing the PFMEs correctly, thereby increasing their confidence and compliance.

CARRY OUT A VAGINAL OBSERVATION

A visual observation of a PFM contraction could be done to ensure the correct technique. When a contraction is performed correctly you will observe the perineum drawing inwards and the vagina and anus closing. Give positive feedback at this time to the woman if she is performing the contraction correctly. Some women, including those from some ethnic, religious or cultural groups, may prefer to be examined by a female HCP. Provision for this should be made, if possible (NICE 2013). It is imperative that consent has been gained for any examinations or procedures and consideration should be given to uphold the woman's dignity at all times (NMC 2015).

COMMON ERRORS TO OBSERVE FOR WHEN TRYING TO PERFORM A PFM CONTRACTION

STRAINING AND BEARING DOWN

Ensure the woman does not strain or bear down while attempting a PFM contraction. The seminal research by Bump et al. (1991) and further work by Thompson and O'Sullivan (2003) showed that many women will strain or bear down when attempting to lift their PF. This incorrect technique may weaken not strengthen the PF by stretching connective tissue, increasing the risk of prolapse. If you notice descent or bulging of the perineum/vagina or anus, inform the woman this is incorrect and retry with functional verbal instructions and visual imagery. You can also try the visual and physical feedback suggestions in the above section. If the woman is persistently unable to perform a correct PFM contraction refer on to a women's health specialist physiotherapist.

BREATH HOLDING

Breath holding may be obvious if the woman shuts her mouth and holds her breath. However, some may report dizziness, discomfort or headache which may be due to insufficient breathing or an increase in blood pressure. Encourage the woman to relax her breathing whilst performing PFMEs.

CONTRACTING OTHER MUSCLES

In addition to watching for a PFM contraction, watch for other muscles being contracted at the same time such as abdominals, adductors/abductors (muscles on the inner/outer thighs) and gluteals (buttock muscles) (Bo et al. 1990). Encourage the woman to relax these muscles and to try and only contract the PFMs.

A PFME PROGRAMME

Evidence shows women have the best outcome with an intensive supervised PFM training programme (Hay-Smith et al. 2012). However, there is some inconsistency in the research of what an 'intensive' programme entails. The NICE urinary incontinence guidelines (2013) for women advise a minimum period of 3 months of PFMEs.

A basic PFME programme could consist of three sets of PFMEs per day. With one set consisting of:

- About 8–12 short (pull up and release) contractions. This builds strength and power.
- About 8–12 long holds (pull up and hold) for 3–10 s. This builds endurance.

This is a generalised programme. Should a woman be unable to perform this number of repetitions or hold for 10 s, this programme can be modified and can be reduced according to the woman's ability. Likewise, if the woman can perform this programme easily, then the number of repetitions or holds should be increased.

PFMEs can be performed in any position such as lying, sitting, standing or whilst walking. Within these positions, more variety can be added. Most women will find the exercises easier to perform in lying and sitting positions, so these positions can be encouraged initially. However, standing can also be suggested as a progression, when the woman is more confident at performing these exercises.

> **BOX 14.5: Tips to help with motivation**
>
> - It is important for the HCP to develop rapport with the woman.
> - Good communication skills are paramount to a successful outcome. Helping the woman to understand why the PFMEs are important and how they can help her may help motivate the woman to do them.
> - Explain why they should perform the PFMEs; give the factual evidence of the success of performing PFMEs that is relevant to the individual. For example, reduced UI episodes and increased quality of life.
> - Give the woman written instructions of her PFMEs programme.
> - Encourage the woman to complete an exercise diary to aid adherence and to help her carry out the correct regimen.
> - Many women forget to perform their PFMEs (Mason et al. 2001). Therefore, discuss with them when they will fit the PEMEs into their daily routine. The antenatal appointment may offer an opportunity to include this discussion.
> - Discuss strategies the woman can employ to help remind her to perform the PFMEs, such as placing stickers on cupboard doors, downloading PF mobile phone apps where alarms can be set at certain times during the day to remind the woman to perform the exercises.

It may be helpful for the woman to know that if she experiences no symptoms of PF dysfunction at 6 months post-partum, she can reduce the above programme from three times daily to 2–3 times per week to maintain her PFM fitness. This should be continued indefinitely.

INCLUDE TEACHING 'THE KNACK' AS PART OF THE PFME PROGRAMME

'The knack' is performing a PFM contraction before and during any physical activity that causes an increase in intra-abdominal pressure. For example, coughing, sneezing or lifting (Mantle 2001). Using the knack reduces urethra and bladder descent (Peschers et al. 2001).

Miller et al. (2008) demonstrated that women with stress UI performing the knack before and during a cough significantly reduced their UI. The knack is an important component of PFM rehabilitation as it teaches the woman to use her PF in real-life situations to prevent symptoms from occurring.

MOTIVATION TO PERFORM PFMEs

PFMEs are often unsuccessful because of non-compliance. Effectively promoting adherence to a PFM training programme is one of the major challenges an HCP faces (Box 14.5).

DISPELLING MYTHS

You should practice PFMEs whilst passing urine on the toilet – FALSE
The advice to the woman is to 'imagine' that they are trying to stop urine. The advice is not to actually perform the exercises whilst passing urine. During voiding, the bladder is contracting at very high pressures and contracting the PFMs may increase the risk of ureteric reflux (urine travelling from the bladder up the ureters towards the kidneys).

PF exercises obstructs labour – FALSE

Anecdotally, some obstetricians, midwives and women may believe that antenatal PFMEs may be associated with adverse delivery outcomes while mounting evidence is to the contrary. In a randomised control trial, intensive PFM training has been found to reduce the incidence of prolonged second stage of labour, breech presentation and episiotomy rates (Sherburn 2004).

A Cochrane review by Boyle et al. (2012) assessed delivery outcomes such as caesarean section rates, length of second stage, perineal trauma and episiotomy rates. Women who underwent 16–20 weeks of supervised antenatal PFM training had more favourable delivery outcomes compared with those with routine care.

> **PRACTICE POINT**
>
> PF muscle training during pregnancy facilitates, rather than obstructs, labour.

Urinary incontinence will resolve after I have my baby – FALSE

A study by Buurman and Lagro-Janssen (2012) reported many women believed their problems would improve by themselves. Symptoms that continue 3 months post birth are NOT likely to resolve without intervention. In a systematic review, the incidence of post-partum urinary incontinence in the short term (up to 13 weeks post-partum) did not differ when compared with that in the longer term (up to 52 weeks post-partum) (Thom & Rortveit 2010).

Urinary incontinence is an inevitable consequence of vaginal delivery – FALSE

Research has found that women who engage in PFMEs during pregnancy report fewer symptoms of urinary stress incontinence after giving birth (Sahakian & Woodward 2012). Women who performed PFMEs daily or several times per week during pregnancy were significantly less likely to report symptoms of UI (Mason et al. 2001).

There are no real treatment options – FALSE

There is strong level 1 evidence to support PFM training for women with UI (Neumann et al. 2006; Dumoulin et al. 2010).

This is a problem that affects only older women – FALSE

Very young and older mothers alike demonstrated an increased risk of urinary incontinence (Thom et al. 2011).

Caesarean section is protective against urinary and faecal incontinence – FALSE

Approximately 40% of women who deliver exclusively by caesarean section still report incontinence, and this type of birth confers no benefit in terms of subsequent faecal incontinence (Macarthur et al. 2011).

ADVICE FOR LIFE

Women should be advised that PFMEs should be performed throughout their lives and are important not only during the antenatal and postnatal periods but also lifelong.

Case studies – possible answers

CASE STUDY 1

How would you describe Jenny's condition?

Mixed urinary incontinence

What additional information would you like to have?

What is the impact on her quality of life (work, home, daily activities and sex life)?
Does she report any other symptoms such as heaviness or dragging in the vagina?
What is her bowel function? Does she strain to empty her bowels?
What is her fluid intake?
Does she report a history of persistent or recurrent UTI/ kidney infections?
Is she aware of PFMEs? Does she perform PFMEs? How many? How often?

How might you be able to improve this woman's symptoms?

Demonstrate the anatomy and describe the functions of the PF using a diagram or model
Tell her about the evidence for the effectiveness of PFMEs during pregnancy for urinary incontinence
Use physical or visual feedback to guide her with her PFMEs
Give her a PFME programme
Discuss how she will fit the PFMEs into her daily routine
Give fluid advice and bowel advice as appropriate

How might you be able to assess the effectiveness of her attempts at performing PFMEs?

Carry out a vaginal observation with consent

If you decide that her care plan should include a referral to a specialist, who is available to see women with Jenny's symptoms in your unit?

Review referral pathways to a specialist (e.g. women's health physiotherapist)

CASE STUDY 2

What additional information would you like to have?

When is she experiencing pain? For example, with sitting/opening bowels
Is there any blood in her stools?
What is the stool consistency (i.e. hard, formed, soft)?
Does she have to strain to empty?
What is her current diet?
Is she taking medications? For example, laxatives, softeners or iron tablets
What were her bowels like before and during pregnancy?
Does she report any other symptoms such as urinary urgency, urgency incontinence or heaviness or dragging in the vagina?
Is she aware of PFMEs? Is she able to perform PFMEs effectively? Does she perform PFMEs? How many? How often?
From her medical notes, establish details of perineal injury, for example, third degree tear
Assess the episiotomy wound for healing and exclude infection

How could you support Michelle with her faecal urgency?

Give her appropriate fluid and dietary advice including modification of medications
Initiate or reinforce a PFME programme ensuring correct with visual observation
Arrange for further reviews

If symptoms do not improve within 3 weeks with the advice you have given, further referral is required.

If you decide that her care plan should include a referral to a specialist, who is available to see women with Michelle's symptoms in your unit?

SUMMARY OF KEY POINTS

- The joint statement by the RCM and the CSP (Gerrard & ten Hove 2013) recommends that all women in the antenatal period should be provided with information and advice regarding PFMEs.
- Pregnant women are at risk of developing PF dysfunction such as urinary, bowel, sexual or prolapse symptoms. Midwives should screen all pregnant women and provide advice to prevent development of symptoms and ensure a PFME programme is being performed effectively.
- PFMEs should be taught to women at all points of contact, both in the antenatal and postnatal period. Assumptions should not be made that women are aware of, or know how to perform, these exercises correctly.
- It is imperative to provide clear explanation to all women on how to perform PFMEs, ideally with a visual observation to ensure a correct contraction is being performed.
- Referral pathways to specialised physiotherapy should be developed for women identified at risk of developing PF dysfunction.
- The midwife provides advice and support to women in the childbearing years to enhance PF health. This is important to a woman's physical, mental and emotional well-being.
- Always remember to ask.

REFERENCES

Amselem, Carlos, Malagelada Juan, Puigdollers Aniceto, Azpiroz Fernando, Sala Carmen, Videla Sebastia, Fernández-fraga Xose & Whorwell Peter. 2009. Constipation: A potential cause of pelvic floor damage? *Neurogastroenterology & Motility* 22(2): 150–153. e48.

Ashton-Miller, James & John DeLancey. 2015. Functional anatomy of the pelvic floor. In Bø, Kari, Bary Berghman, Siv Mørkved & Marijke Van Kampen (eds.), *Evidenced based physical therapy for the pelvic floor: Bridging science and clinical practice* (2nd ed.). Edinburgh: Churchill Livingstone, pp. 19–35.

Bassotti Gabrio, Vincenzo Villanacci. 2004. Slow transit constipation: A functional disorder becomes an enteric neuropathy. *World Journal of Gastroenterology* 12(29): 4609–4613.

Bennet, V. Ruth & Linda K. Brown. 1999. The reproductive organs. In Bennet, V. Ruth & Linda K. Brown (eds.), *Myles textbook for midwives*. Edinburg: Churchill Livingstone.

Bo, Kari, Rolf Hagen, Bernt Kvarstein, Jan Jorgensen, Stig Larsen & Kathryn Burgio. 1990. Pelvic floor muscles exercise for the treatment of female stress urinary incontinence: 111. Effects of two different degrees of pelvic floor muscles exercises. *Neurourology and Urodynamics* 9: 489–502.

Boyle, Rhianon, E. Jean C. Hay-Smith, June D. Cody & Siv Mørkved. 2012. pelvic floor muscle training for prevention and treatment of urinary and faecal incontinence in antenatal and postnatal women. *Cochrane Database of Systematic Reviews* 2012(10): CD007471.

Bradley, Catherine, Colleen Kennedy, Anne Turcea, Satish Rao & Irene Nygaard. 2007. Constipation in pregnancy: Prevalence, symptoms, and risk factors. *Obstetrics and Gynecology* 110(6): 1351–1357.

Buchsbaum, Gunhilde M, Erin Duecy, Lindsey Kerr, Li-Shan Huang, MaryAnn Perevich, David Guzick. 2005. Pelvic organ prolapse in nulliparous women and their parous sisters. *Obstetrics & Gynecology* 108(6):1388–1393.

Bump, Richard, W. Glen Hurt, Andrew Fantl & Jean Wyman. 1991. Assessment of Kegel exercise performance after brief verbal instruction. *American Journal Obstetrics and Gynaecology* 165: 322–329.

Buurman, Mirella B.R. & Antoinette Lagro-Janssen. 2012. Women's perception of postpartum pelvic floor dysfunction and their help-seeking behaviour: A qualitative interview study. *Scandinavian Journal of Caring Science* 27(2): 406–413.

Chiarelli, Pauline, Barbara Murphy & Jill Cockburn. 2003. Women's knowledge, practises, and intentions regarding correct pelvic floor exercises. *Neurourology and Urodynamics* 22(3): 246–249.

Coad, Jane & Melvyn Dunstall. 2011. *Anatomy and physiology for midwives* (3rd ed.). Edinburgh: Churchill Livingstone Elsevier.

Dasgupta, Jaydip, Elliot Ruth, Doshani Angie & Tincello Douglas. 2006. Enhancement of rat bladder contraction by artificial sweeteners via increased extracellular Ca2+ influx. *Toxicology and Applied Pharmacology* 217: 216–224.

Danforth Kim, N., Mary K. Townsend, Karen Lifford, Fary C. Cunhan, Neil M. Resnick and Francine Grodstein. 2006. Risk factors for urinary incontinence among middle-aged women. *American Journal of Obstetrics and Gynecology* 194(2): 339–345.

Dasgupta, Jaydip, Elliot Ruth & Douglas Tincello. 2009. Modification of rat detrusor muscle con-traction by ascorbic acid and citric acid involving enhanced neurotransmitter release and Ca2+influx. *Neurourology and Urodynamics* 28: 542–548.

DoH (Department of Health). 2012. *Maternal mental health pathway. Best practice guidelines.* https://www.gov.uk/government/uploads/system/uploads/attachment_data/file/212906/Maternal-mental-health-pathway-090812.pdf (accessed 13 July 2015).

Dumoulin, Chantale, Hay-Smith Jean & Gabrielle Mac Habée-Séguin. 2010. Pelvic floor muscle training versus no treatment, or inactive control treatments for urinary incontinence. *The Cochrane Library* 1. http://onlinelibrary.wiley.com/doi/10.1002/14651858.CD005654.pub3/abstract

Gerrard, Jacque & Ruth ten Hove. 2013. *RCM/CSP joint statement on pelvic floor muscle exercise. Improving health outcomes for women following pregnancy and birth RCM/CSP London.* csp_rcm_pelvicfloorstatement_2013.pdf

Guerrero, Karen, Lloyd Owen, Gillian Hirst & Sherry Emery. 2007. Antenatal pelvic floor exercises: A survey of both patients' and health professionals' beliefs and practice. *Journal of Obstetrics and Gynaecology* 27(7): 684–687.

Hagen, Suzanne, Diane Stark, Cathryn Glazener, Sylvia Dickson, Sarah Barry, Andrew Elders, Helena Frawley, et al. 2014. Individualised pelvic floor muscle training in women with pelvic organ prolapse (POPPY): A multicentre randomised controlled trial. *The Lancet.* 383(9919): 796–806.

Haylen, Bernard T., Dirk de Ridder, Robert M. Freeman, Steven E. Swift, Bary Berghmans, Joseph Lee, Ash Monga, et al. 2010. An International Urogynaecological Association (IUGA)/International Continence Society (ICS) joint report on the terminology for female pelvic floor dysfunction. *Neurourology and Urodynamics* 29: 4–20.

Hay-Smith, Jean, Roselien Herderschee, Chantale Dumoulin & G. Peter Herbison. 2012. Comparisons of approaches to pelvic floor muscle training for urinary incontinence in women: An abridged Cochrane systematic review. *European Journal of Physical and Rehabilitation Medicine* 48: 689–705.

Hernández, Regina, Encarnación RubioAranda & Concepción Tomaś Aznar. 2013. Urinary incontinence and weight changes during pregnancy and post-partum: A pending challenge. *Midwifery* 29(12): e123–e129.

Heslehurst, Nicola, Helen Simpson, Alan Batterham, John Wilkinson & Carolyn Summerbell. 2007. Trends in maternal obesity incidence rates, demographic predictors, and health inequalities in 36 821 women over a 15-year period. *BJOG* 114(2): 187–194.

MacArthur, Christine, Cathryn Glazener, Robert Lancashire, G. Peter Herbison, Don Wilson, and on behalf of the ProLong Study Group. 2011. Exclusive caesarean section delivery and subsequent urinary and faecal incontinence: A 12-year longitudinal study. *British Journal of Obstetrics and Gynaecology: An International Journal of Obstetrics & Gynaecology* 118: 1001–1007.

Mantle, Jill. 2001. Physiotherapy for incontinence. In Cardozo, Linda & David Staskin (eds.), *Textbook of female urology and urogynaecology*. London: ISIS Medical Media, pp. 351–358.

Mason, Linda, Glenn S. Sheila, Irene Walton & Carol Hughes. 2001. The relationship between ante-natal pelvic floor muscle exercises and post-partum stress incontinence. *Physiotherapy* 87(2): 651–661.

Miller, Janis, Carolyn Sampselle, James Ashton-Miller, Son Hong Gwi-Ryung, & John DeLancey. 2008. Clarification and confirmation of the Knack manoeuvre: The effect of volitional pelvic floor muscle contraction to pre-empt expected stress incontinence. *International Urogynecology Journal and Pelvic Floor Dysfunction* 19(6): 773–782.

Milsom, Ian, D. Altman, R. Cartwright, M. C. Lapitan, R. Nelson, U. Sillen & K. Tikkinem. 2013. Epidemiology of urinary incontinence (UI) and other lower urinary tract symptoms (LUTS), pelvic organ prolapse (POP) and anal incontinence (AI). In Paul Abrams, Linda Cardozo, Saad Khoury & Alan Wein (eds.), *Incontinence*. Paris: Health Publications.

Mørkved, Siv & Bø Kari. 2014. Effect of pelvic floor muscle training during pregnancy and after childbirth on prevention and treatment of urinary incontinence: A systematic review. *British Journal of Sports Medicine* 48(Suppl): 299–310.

Nascimento, Simony L., Fernanda Surita, José Cecatti. 2012. *Physical exercise during pregnancy: a systematic review Current Opinion in Obstetrics & Gynecology*: 24(6): 387–394.

Neumann, Patricia B., Karen Grimmer & Yamini Deenadayalan. 2006. Pelvic floor muscle training and adjunctive therapies for the treatment of stress urinary incontinence in women: A systematic review. *BMC Women's Health* 2006(6): 11.

Newman, Diane, Linda Cardozo & Karl-Dietrich Sievert. 2013. Preventing urinary incontinence in women. *Current Opinion in Obstetrics and Gynecology* 25(5): 388–394.

NICE (National Institute for Health and Clinical Excellence). 2008. *Antenatal Care. NICE clinical guideline 62*. London: National Institute for Health and Clinical Excellence.

NICE (National Institute for Health and Clinical Excellence). 2010. *Weight management before, during and after pregnancy. Public health guidance 27*. http://www.nice.org.uk/guidance/ph27/resources/guidance-weight-management-before-during-and-after-pregnancy-pdf

NICE (National Institute for Health and Clinical Excellence). 2013. *The management of urinary incontinence in women NICE clinical guideline 171*. London: National Institute for Health and Clinical Excellence.

NMC (Nursing and Midwifery Council). 2015. *The code: Professional standards of practice and behaviour for nurses and midwives*. London: NMC.

Olsen, Ambre L., Virginia Smith, John Bergstrom, Joyce Colling & Amanda Clark. 1997. Epidemiology of surgically managed pelvic organ prolapse and urinary incontinence. *Obstetrics and Gynecology* 89(4): 501–506.

Peschers, Ursula, D. B Vodusek, Gabi Fanger, Gabriel Schaer, John Delancey & Bernhard Schussler. 2001. Pelvic floor muscle activity in nulliparous volunteers. *Neurourology and urodynamics* 20: 269–275.

Price, Natalie & Ian Currie. 2010. Urinary incontinence in women: Diagnosis and management. *Practitioner* 254(1727): 27–32.

Raizada Varuna and Ravinder K. Mittal. 2008. *Pelvic Floor Anatomy and Applied Physiology Gastroenterology Clinics of North America* 37(3): 493–509.

Rao, Satish. 2004. Pathophysiology of adult fecal incontinence. *Gastroenterology* 126: S14–S22.

Robinson, Dudley, Ilias Giarenis & Linda Cardozo. 2014. You are what you eat: The impact of diet on overactive bladder and lower urinary tract symptoms. *Maturitas* 79: 8–13.

Royal College of Obstetricians and Gynaecology. 2006. *Exercise in pregnancy, statement number 4.* https://www.rcog.org.uk/globalassets/documents/guidelines/statements/statement-no-4.pdf

Sahakian, Josine & Sue Woodward. 2012. Stress incontinence and pelvic floor exercises in pregnancy. *British Journal of Nursing* 21(18): S10–S15.

Sherburn, Margaret. 2004. Pelvic floor muscle training during pregnancy facilitates labour. *Australian Journal of Physiotherapy* 50(4): 258–258.

Snooks, Steven J., P.R. Barnes, M. Swash & M. Henry. 1985. Damage to the innervation of the pelvic floor musculature in chronic constipation. *Gastroenterology* 89: 977–981.

Spence-Jones, Clive, Michael Kamm, Michael Henry & C.N. Hudson. 1994. Bowel dysfunction: A pathogenic factor in uterovaginal prolapse and urinary stress incontinence. *BJOG* 101(2): 147–152.

Steen, Mary & Tanya Roberts. 2011. The consequences of pregnancy and birth for the pelvic floor. *British Journal of Midwifery* 9(11): 693–698.

Thakar, Ranee & Dee Fenner. 2009. Anatomy of the perineum and the anal sphincter. In: Sultan, Abdul H., Ranee Thakar & Dee Fenner (eds.), *Perineal and anal sphincter trauma.* London: Springer, pp. 1–13.

Thom, David H., Jeanette Brown, Michale Schembri, Arona Ragins, Jennifer Creasman & Stephen Van den Eeden. 2011. Parturition events and risk of urinary incontinence in later life. *Neurourology and Urodynamics* 30(8): 1456–1461.

Thom, David H. & Guri Rortveit. 2010. Prevalence of postpartum urinary incontinence: A systematic review. *Acta Obstetricia et Gynecologica Scandinavica* 89(12): 1511–1522.

Thompson, Judith & Peter O'Sullivan. 2003. Levator plate movement during voluntary pelvic floor muscle contraction in subjects with incontinence and prolapse: A cross-sectional study and review. *International Urogynaecology Journal and Pelvic Floor Dysfunction* 14(2): 84–88.

Viktrup, Lars, Guri Rortveit, & Gunnar Lose. 2006. Risk of stress urinary incontinence twelve years after the first pregnancy and delivery. *Obstetrics and Gynecology* 108(2): 248–254.

Zahariou, Athanasios G., Maria V. Karamouti & Polyanthi D. Papaioannouet. 2008. Pelvic floor muscle training improves sexual function of women with stress urinary incontinence. International. *Urogynecology Journal* 19: 401–406.

FURTHER READINGS

Royal College of Obstetricians and Gynaecology. 2006. *Exercise in pregnancy.* Statement number 4. https://www.rcog.org.uk/globalassets/documents/guidelines/statements/statement-no-4.pdf

National Institute for Health and Clinical Excellence. 2007. *Faecal incontinence: The management of faecal incontinence in adults.* http://www.nice.org.uk/guidance/cg49/resources/guidance-faecal-incontinence-pdf (accessed 8 July 2015).

Violence against women and girls

ELSA MONTGOMERY AND HANNAH
RAYMENT-JONES

15

INTRODUCTION

Violence against women and girls is the most widespread form of abuse worldwide and crosses cultural and economic boundaries. The World Health Organization (WHO 2013) reported that approximately 30% of the world's female population has experienced physical or sexual violence. This violence takes on many different forms, including physical, psychological and sexual abuse; domestic violence; female genital mutilation; child marriage and forced marriage; sex trafficking; and 'honour-based' violence. It is a gross violation of human rights. It is also a global public health issue because of the effects on women's physical, psychological and sexual health, and the growing social and economic costs. The adverse health outcomes that women and girls experience as a consequence of abuse lead to an increased use of health care resources (Bonomi et al. 2009). Therefore, health care workers, midwives in particular, frequently and often unknowingly encounter women experiencing or affected by violence.

Maternity services can provide women a safe environment where they can confidentially disclose experiences of violence and receive a supportive response. They can also be a place of distress and lack of control for women who have experienced abuse; therefore, it is imperative that health professionals working in maternity services have an understanding of this complex issue in order to care for women appropriately and strengthen support networks for their future. This chapter discusses domestic violence and childhood sexual abuse (CSA) with a focus on women, pregnancy, maternity services and the role of the midwife.

DOMESTIC VIOLENCE: AN OVERVIEW AND EPIDEMIOLOGY

Domestic violence is defined by the UK government as 'any incident or pattern of incidents of controlling, coercive, threatening behaviour, violence or abuse between those aged 16 or over who are, or have been, intimate partners of family members regardless of gender or sexuality. The abuse can encompass, but is not limited to, psychological, physical, sexual, financial and emotional aspects' (www.gov.uk/domestic-violence-and-abuse#domestic-violence-and-abuse-new-definition). This includes issues of concern to black and minority ethnic communities such as the so-called 'honour-based violence', female genital mutilation and forced marriage. Family members are defined as immediate relatives, whether directly related, in-laws or stepfamily. This definition will be used for the purpose of this chapter.

Table 15.1 depicts different forms of domestic violence with examples.

It is acknowledged that the data on reported incidents of domestic violence, the collection of which have been started only recently by the criminal justice system, merely show the tip of the iceberg as victims of domestic violence are less likely than victims of other violence to report their experiences (Gracia 2004). This reluctance to report incidents may be because of the belief that it is not a matter for police involvement, a 'victim blaming attitude' and a significant fear of reprisal from the perpetrator (Felson et al. 2006).

Although, as the above definition states, people irrespective of gender experience domestic violence, women are considerably more likely to experience repeated and severe forms of violence (Womens Aid 2006). Recent figures from the Crime Survey for England and Wales (ONS 2014) reported that 7% of women and 4% of men have been victims of some kind of domestic abuse in the past year. There were an estimated 406,000 victims of sexual assaults in the past year and nearly 1 million victims of stalkers. More than two-thirds of these were women. The survey also revealed that nearly 5 million women or 30% of the adult female population have experienced some form of domestic abuse since the age of 16. Although there has been a recent fall in the number of domestic violence cases referred to the Crown Prosecution Service, this overall number has steadily risen in the past decade and is now at an all-time high (CPS 2014).

Domestic violence is reported within all socio-economic classes but it is most prevalent within the working and lower-middle social classes (Nagassar et al. 2010). In addition, being male, young, having low educational attainment and a history of abuse are all factors that positively correlate with perpetrators of violence (Coker et al. 2000). Figure 15.1 shows the Duluth 'Power and Control' training model (Pence & Paymar 1993), which was developed by the survivors of domestic abuse to illustrate the many different abusive behaviours of men towards women, and can be used to understand who might be at risk and why. It is stressed however that domestic violence remains common in *all* demographic groups. Similarly, Cook and Bewley (2008) acknowledge there is no 'typical' victim and it is unhelpful, and even stigmatising, to focus attention on one single population, just as it is important not to assume that any individual is at 'low risk'.

Table 15.1 Forms of domestic violence

Forms of domestic violence	Examples
Physical	Slapping, hitting, biting, kicking, beating, choking
Sexual	Forced sexual intercourse and others forms of sexual coercion
Emotional (psychological)	Insults, belittling, constant humiliation, intimidation, tricking, threats of harm, threats to take away children
Control	Isolation from family and friends, monitoring movements, restricting access to financial resources, employment, education or medical care

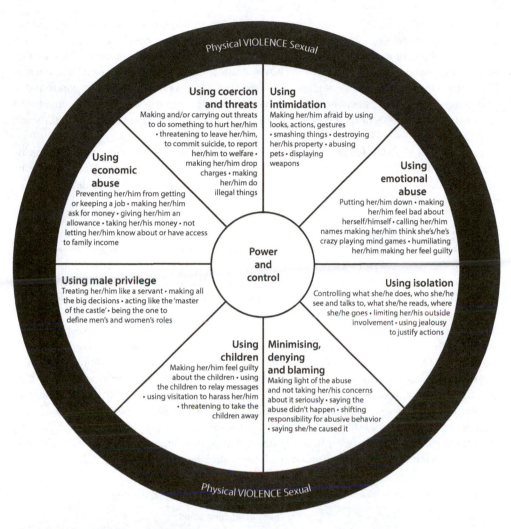

Figure 15.1 Duluth Power and Control Wheel training model.

PREVALENCE OF DOMESTIC VIOLENCE IN PREGNANCY

Estimating the prevalence of domestic violence in pregnancy is difficult and, in addition to genuine diversity, significant variations in estimates across the globe are largely because of different definitions of violence, and when and how women are asked (Gazmararian et al. 1996). Physical domestic violence rates for pregnant women in Canada are reported between 1% and

11% (Daoud et al. 2012) in the United States between 1% and 20% (Gazmararian 1996) and the United Kingdom between 2% and 22% (Bacchus et al. 2004). The prevalence of psychological and sexual abuse of women during pregnancy has also been reported between 13% and 60% (Jahanfar & Malekzadegan 2007). The WHO commissioned a large, multinational study across 15 countries into the prevalence of physical violence reported in pregnancy, which was found to be between 1% and 15%. Between 20% and 50% of these women reported direct trauma to the abdomen, and over 90% of the perpetrators were the biological fathers of the unborn (Ellsberg et al. 2008).

Rodriguez et al. (2001) found that for almost 30% of women who experienced domestic violence, the first incident occurred in pregnancy. The Confidential Enquiry into Maternal Deaths (CMACE 2011) later identified domestic violence as a major factor leading to death in pregnancy and childbirth.

EFFECTS OF DOMESTIC VIOLENCE

Reducing the prevalence of violence against women and girls has been a major public health and human rights initiative across the world for many years (Beydoun et al. 2010). In the United Kingdom alone, the cost of physical health care treatment resulting from domestic violence (including hospital, general practitioner, ambulance and prescriptions) is £1.2 billion (Walby 2009). The associated health consequences are varied and women suffering domestic violence obviously do not all have the same set of symptoms or experiences (Cook & Bewley 2008). It has also been noted that although victims of domestic violence are frequently visiting health care services, they generally do not present with obvious trauma or specific symptoms (Coker et al. 2000). This phenomenon is thought to be because of long-term negative health consequences for victims, even after abuse has ended, manifesting as poor health status, poor quality of life and high use of health services (Bonomi et al. 2009). However, there is a wealth of evidence showing that bruising is one of the most common injuries sustained by women through domestic violence, followed by a multitude of physical and mental health problems listed in Table 15.2.

Table 15.2 Physical and mental health problems associated with domestic violence

Physical health risks	Stress-related/functional disorders	Mental health risks
Bruises and welts	Headaches/migraine	Depression
Lacerations and abrasions, abdominal or thoracic injuries	Irritable bowel syndrome	Anxiety
Fractures/broken bones and teeth	Gastrointestinal symptoms	Phobias
Sight and hearing damage	Fibromyalgia	Suicide
Head injury	Dysmenorrhoea	Alcohol and drug abuse
Attempted strangulation	Dyspareunia	Eating and sleep disorders
Back and neck injury/chronic pain	Various chronic pain syndromes	Physical inactivity
Arthritis	Exacerbation of asthma	Poor self-esteem
Sexually transmitted infections	Angina and chest pain	Post-traumatic stress disorder
Smear abnormalities	Bladder and kidney infections	Smoking
	Stomach ulcers	Self-harm
		Unsafe sexual behaviour
		Cancer worries

The adverse consequences of domestic abuse on children must also be factored into our approach in caring for families experiencing abuse, and looking at interventions to reduce its prevalence. Up to 60% of children directly experience the abuse of their mother including witnessing physical violence and being used in threats or as a spy, and the repercussions, such as removal from the family unit or living in a refuge with their mother (Pinheiro 2006). Children exposed to intimate partner violence have a higher risk of physical, emotional, behavioural and educational problems that persist into adulthood.

The nature of violence can alter during pregnancy, with physical violence aimed directly at the woman's abdomen, and choking, rather than head and musculoskeletal injuries (Bullock et al. 2006). This violence obviously has a direct effect on the mother and the unborn, but it is also known that women who experience violence in pregnancy have an almost 40% higher risk of morbidity, leading to antenatal admission, such as hypertension, premature rupture of membranes and anaemia (Azier 2011). Table 15.3 shows health outcomes found directly and indirectly related to domestic violence in pregnancy (Shah & Shah 2010; Silverman et al. 2006a) and psychological outcomes for women and their children following violence in pregnancy (Almeida et al. 2013; Silverman et al. 2006b).

Of course, this list is not definitive; in fact, more often than not, women demonstrate extraordinary strength and ability to take care of themselves and their infants in spite of often untenable situations (Bancroft et al. 2011).

At its extreme, domestic violence in pregnancy causes death to the mother and the unborn. The review into maternal deaths 2006–2008 (CMACE 2011) reported 34 of the women who died from any cause had features of domestic abuse and had proactively disclosed this abuse to a health care professional either before or during their pregnancy. For some, the abuse was fatal; at least seven women were murdered by a partner or another family member. Overall, 38% of mothers who died and had features of domestic violence presented late for care and did not engage with maternity services. The review continued to recommend that all pregnant women should be asked by a health care professional if they are experiencing, or have ever experienced, domestic violence.

Table 15.3 Health outcomes associated with domestic violence in pregnancy

Physical	Psychological
Hypertension	Depression
Premature rupture of membranes	Anxiety
Preterm labour and birth	Pressured into pregnancy and/or abortion
Fetal distress	Negative attitudes towards pregnancy
Anaemia	Poor relationship with the unborn
Low birth weight	Less likely to breastfeed
Miscarriage	Decreased confidence in ability to parent
Oedema	Childhood behavioural problems
Vomiting and dehydration	
Urinary and renal tract infections	
Weight loss during pregnancy	
Operative delivery	
Placental abruption, antepartum haemorrhage	
Rupture of the uterus, liver or spleen	

IDENTIFYING DOMESTIC VIOLENCE IN PRACTICE

It has long been known that the most effective way to identify domestic violence is by directly asking women; in fact, research has shown that survivors actually want to be asked (Chang et al. 2005). Routine enquiry into domestic violence not only identifies women at risk of a plethora of adverse health outcomes but also raises awareness, reduces stigma and demonstrates an intolerance of violence against women. Almost 20 years ago, it was noted that domestic violence during pregnancy is more common than complications that are routinely screened for in UK maternity services, such as pre-eclampsia and gestational diabetes; yet there was a lack of awareness in maternity services and routine enquiry was uncommon (Mezey & Bewley 1997). Despite a growing responsiveness to recommendations since then, there continues to be reluctance on behalf of some health professionals to embrace enquiry into domestic violence, possibly because they lack the confidence and knowledge to do so (Baird & Salmon 2013).

WHO (2013) stated that all health care providers should be trained to understand the relationship between violence and women's poor health and to be able to respond appropriately. The report identified the importance of maternity services in the identification of violence due to the multiple entry points throughout the antenatal period and the possibility of continuity of care. Women may not disclose on the first occasion they are asked; therefore, it is important to bear in mind the need to make routine enquiries on a number of occasions (Barron 2014). Midwives are in a unique position to offer support and safe referral; however, this is often hampered by the poor coordination of services, inadequate knowledge and by midwives' own experiences, beliefs and attitudes concerning domestic violence and who is at risk (Price et al. 2009). It must be remembered that health professionals, too, are victims of abuse and that domestic abuse occurs across all social classes and within all ethnic groups.

LEARNING ACTIVITY

Thinking about your own practice, how confident do you feel asking women about domestic violence?

How do you ensure a safe environment for the woman when enquiring?

If a woman discloses domestic violence, do you feel confident in follow-up protocol and referral processes?

If a woman you are caring for does not disclose domestic violence but you have concerns about her and her family's safety, what would you do?

The NICE (2010) guidelines for women with complex social factors highlighted five key issues for health care professionals enquiring about and women disclosing violence, and they were the following:

1. Fear of the potential involvement of social services and child custody.
2. Anxiety that her partner will find out she has disclosed the abuse.
3. Insufficient time for health care professionals to deal with the issue appropriately.
4. Insufficient support and training for health care professionals in asking about domestic abuse.
5. Perception of domestic abuse as a taboo subject that should not be discussed.

Recommendations from the WHO (2013) and NICE (2010) continue to focus on the practicalities of routine enquiry, including compulsory education for undergraduate curricula and continued professional development for health care professionals. This education should include a structure to refer women who have disclosed violence for appropriate support and follow-up; this may increase health care professionals' confidence and likelihood to enquire. Figure 15.2 shows a flow chart to ensure safe enquiry.

If appropriate, women should be asked about domestic violence in pregnancy when midwives are taking a social history at booking or at another opportune point during a woman's antenatal period. The CMACE report (2011) recommended women should be seen alone at least once during the antenatal period to facilitate disclosure. This can be difficult for women who are experiencing abuse as controlling partners often accompany them. This scenario can be seen as a warning sign to health professionals, and innovative schemes to identify and direct help towards women in this situation have been set up in trusts across the country. These schemes include women receiving information in toilets, placing a small sticker on their urine pot to alert their midwife or information providing women with a disguised number on a sticker or card for the 24 Hour National Domestic Violence Helpline run by Women's Aid and Refuge. The Helpline is free, staffed 24 h a day by fully trained female helpline workers and all calls are completely confidential.

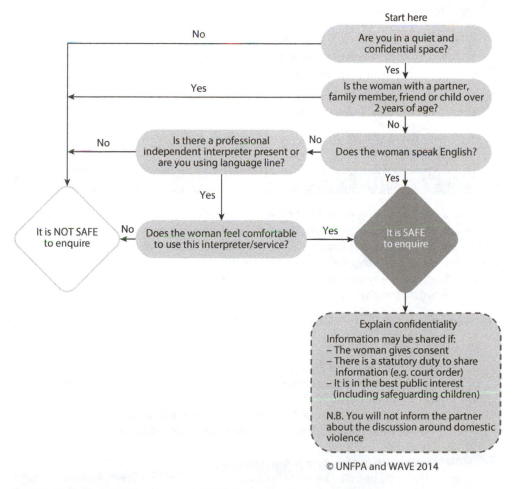

© UNFPA and WAVE 2014

Figure 15.2 Flow chart to ensure safe enquiry.

If, during an appointment, it is deemed safe to proceed, a health professional can broach the subject using direct but open-ended questions. The qualitative study by Chang et al. (2005) identified women want the person asking the question to give a reason for doing so to reduce suspicions and minimise stigma. This reason could be given in the form of discussing routine screening due to the known increased incidence of domestic violence in pregnancy. The women also wanted the health care professional to create a safe and supportive environment, and to be given information around access to support regardless of whether or not they disclose violence. Once it is deemed safe to proceed, a health professional can broach the subject using the following direct but open-ended questions:

- How are things at home?
- Who lives at home with you?
- Are there any problems at home? Tell me about your relationship.
- Does anyone ever try to control what you do?
- Is there somebody that you are frightened of or who hurts you? (NICE 2014)

Hegarty et al. (2008) suggest the following validation statements if a woman chooses to disclose abuse such as:

- Everybody deserves to feel safe at home.
- You don't deserve to be hit or hurt. It is not your fault.
- I am concerned about your safety and well-being.
- You are not alone and help is available.
- You are not to blame. Abuse is common and happens in all kinds of relationships. It tends to continue.

REFERRAL AND SUPPORT – THE MIDWIFE'S ROLE

If a midwife suspects domestic abuse or a woman discloses the same, the midwife must act quickly and appropriately by assessing risk and providing information. This should be carried out in a non-judgemental and sensitive manner, ensuring that the woman is fully informed and involved in the decision-making process (Sohal & Johnson 2014). It is crucial that any action taken does not in any way increase the danger the woman is facing. Barron (2014) suggests the following seven actions that could be taken to ensure safety:

1. For assessing immediate danger, the following questions may be helpful:
   a. Is your partner here with you?
   b. Where are the children?
   c. Is it safe for you to return home today?
   d. Do you have any immediate concerns?
   e. Do you have a place of safety?
   f. If you feel a woman is at immediate risk, do any of the following:
      i. Contact independent domestic violence advisor and safeguarding referral
      ii. Police 999
      iii. Contact a friend/family member not known to the perpetrator
      iv. Contact Refuge (0808 2000 247) for emergency accommodation
2. Give her time to talk about her experience, listen to her and show you believe her.

3. Give her contact numbers and information about how to protect herself and her children.

   The aim of providing information is to give women choices about how to protect themselves and their children and where to go for help. The first option will usually be to signpost the woman to a specialist domestic violence organisation. Contact details for national support services can be found on page 233. It may also be a local service depending on the woman's individual needs. For example, for women who do not speak English, or have safe access to the Internet or a phone. It is important that the midwife giving the information is trained to do so, aware of key sources of information or local services and considers the safety of the woman and her children as part of the process.

4. Do *NOT* give advice on what to do – it is her decision and she will have real reasons behind it

5. Support her in whatever decision she makes

6. Keep detailed records that can only be accessed by relevant professionals. Do NOT document in a woman's hand-held notes

7. Arrange a follow-up appointment and any follow-up referrals that may be helpful- discuss these with the woman.

RECOMMENDATIONS FOR FUTURE SERVICES

The review by Marmot et al. (2008) of social determinants of health encourages the development of partnerships, with those affected by complex social factors working with their health providers. Central to this approach is empowerment through putting in place effective mechanisms that give those affected a real say in decisions that affect their lives, and that recognise their fundamental human rights. These values are echoed in recent UK maternity service policies and guidelines, encouraging women-centred, individualised care, with a focus on choice and continuity of carer (NICE 2010). A recent study of pregnancy outcomes of women with complex social factors, including domestic violence, found women who received a high level of continuity of carer throughout their pregnancy had significantly better outcomes, including less antenatal admissions and more referrals to support services (Rayment-Jones et al. 2015).

The NICE (2010) guidelines recognise that women who are experiencing domestic abuse may have particular difficulties using antenatal care services. For example, the perpetrator of the abuse may try to prevent her from attending appointments, the woman may be afraid that disclosure of the abuse to a health care professional will worsen her situation or anxious about the reaction of the health care professional. To alleviate these concerns, the report called for a reorganisation of maternity services to improve antenatal care for women facing complex social circumstances through the provision of individualised care planning. The recommendations included additional support for women experiencing domestic abuse in their access to antenatal care, provision of flexible services, addressing women's fears about the involvement of social services by providing information tailored to their needs and training health care professionals in the identification and care of women who experience domestic abuse.

CHILDHOOD SEXUAL ABUSE: AN OVERVIEW

Women who access maternity services whilst experiencing domestic violence are more likely than other women to have also experienced CSA. Seng et al. (2008) found that women were three times more likely to be abused as an adult if they had been abused as a child.

Although, unlike those in situations of domestic abuse, survivors of CSA may not be in present danger, but the impact of their childhood experiences can leave them feeling very unsafe during pregnancy and childbirth, and sensitivity will be required from caregivers to prevent retraumatisation (Garratt 2011).

DEFINING CSA

It is complex due to the range of activities that may be encompassed. A useful working definition is that it involves 'forcing or enticing a child or young person to take part in sexual activities, not necessarily involving a high level of violence, whether or not the child is aware of what is happening' (HM Government 2015, 93). Table 15.4 shows the list of activities that may constitute sexual abuse and illustrates that CSA does not necessarily involve contact.

Other issues related to the definition include who the perpetrator is. Some definitions require that the perpetrator is 'significantly older', which usually means a 5-year age gap (Cawson et al. 2000). However, the most recent report on child abuse and neglect from the National Society for the Prevention of Cruelty to Children (NSPCC) identified that nearly 66% of contact sexual abuse was perpetrated by under-18s against other children or young adults (Radford et al. 2011). Of concern is the fact that children had experienced contact abuse by a peer no one else knew in nearly 83% of cases compared with 34% of cases when contact abuse had been perpetrated by an adult. Although the majority of perpetrators are male (Radford et al. 2011), it is increasingly recognised that women also sexually abuse children. Dube et al. (2005) report that of the CSA experienced by women in their study 6% had a female perpetrator.

PREVALENCE

The complexities surrounding the definition of CSA inevitably make determining prevalence complicated too, and there is much variation between studies. For example, in an analysis of 38 articles reporting studies from 21 different countries, Pereda et al. (2009a) found prevalence of up to 53% for women and up to 60% for men. However, this is misleading because all but two studies demonstrated a higher prevalence in women than men. They concluded that CSA is an international problem. This was confirmed by their later work on the prevalence of CSA among student and community samples in which they report a prevalence of approximately 20% in women and 8% in men (Pereda et al. 2009b). These findings

Table 15.4 Defining sexual abuse

Contact	Includes:
	• Assault by penetration (e.g. rape or oral sex)
	• Non-penetrative acts such as masturbation, kissing, rubbing and touching outside of clothing
Non-contact	Includes:
	• Involving children in looking at, or in the production of, sexual images
	• Watching sexual activities
	• Encouraging children to behave in sexually inappropriate ways
	• Grooming a child in preparation for abuse (including via the Internet)

Source: Adapted from HM Government. 2015. *Working Together to Safeguard Children: A Guide to Inter-Agency Working to Safeguard and Promote the Welfare of Children.* London: Crown copyright.

broadly reflect the situation in the United Kingdom. The study for the NSPCC conducted by Cawson et al. (2000) indicated that 21% of girls and 11% of boys had been sexually abused. The update for the NSPCC by Radford et al. (2011) reported that overall, 24% of young people had experienced some form of CSA, and nearly 18% of girls and 5% of boys had experienced contact abuse.

EFFECTS OF CSA ON HEALTH

Similar to women who are victims of domestic violence, those with a history of CSA are likely to have significant health issues and be frequent users of health services (Itzin et al. 2010). The UK government has recognised that these effects are experienced over the whole of an affected person's life (Itzin 2006). They include physical and mental health issues as well as the consequences of increased exposure to domestic violence and abuse. Table 15.5 lists some of the common health issues experienced by women with a history of CSA. It is also common for these women to present with chronic pain conditions which are often unexplained (Seng et al. 2008).

In a small-scale survey of the health needs of survivors of CSA, Montgomery (2015) discovered that 48 of the 49 participants (ranging in age from 18 from 68) had seen their general practitioner at least once in the previous 24 months. Twenty-eight (57%) of them had seen their general practitioner more than six times in the past 24 months. Other health care professionals accessed by these women in the same period are shown in Figure 15.3.

Although 67% had disclosed their history of abuse to the general practitioner, it was much less common for them to have disclosed to other health care professionals. None of this particular group of women had seen a midwife in the previous 24 months but disclosure to midwives is also rare (Burian 1995; Coles & Jones 2009; Montgomery et al. 2015a). The guilt and shame felt by women with histories of CSA are among the reasons for this (Leeners et al. 2006; Montgomery 2012; Seng et al. 2002). The maternity care experiences of women with a history of CSA can be characterised by 'silence' (Montgomery et al. 2015a), and this creates challenges for those providing their care.

CSA AND PREGNANCY

Midwives need not necessarily be aware if the women in their care have a history of CSA, but there are associated risk factors that are worth exploring to help raise awareness and support

Table 15.5 Effects on mental and physical health

Long-term mental health effects	Adverse physical health effects
Depression	Health risk behaviours, e.g., smoking, alcohol and drug misuse
Anxiety	Risky sexual behaviour
Post-traumatic stress disorder	Sexually transmitted infections
Psychosis	Irritable bowel syndrome
Substance abuse	Gynaecological problems
Eating disorders	
Self-harm	
Suicide	

Source: Adapted from Itzin, Catherine. 2006. *Tackling the Health and Mental Health Effects of Domestic and Sexual Violence and Abuse.* London: Crown copyright.

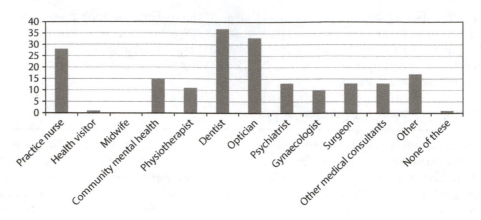

Figure 15.3 Health care professionals accessed by survivors in previous 24 months.

midwives in promoting the health of these women. The physical and mental health effects of CSA have already been mentioned, and women will bring many of these into pregnancy. Figure 15.4 shows the prevalence of various health problems in the 49 women who participated in the survey of survivors' health needs (Montgomery 2015). The latest Confidential Enquiries into Maternal Deaths and Morbidity (Knight et al. 2014) demonstrated that three-quarters of the women who died had pre-existing medical or mental health problems. Seventeen per cent of those who died had mental health problems, and 15% had asthma. Forty-nine per cent were either overweight or obese (Knight et al. 2014). It is not known whether any of these women also had a history of CSA. However, Figure 15.4 shows that a bigger proportion of the women in the survey of health needs had experienced mental health problems, asthma and eating disorders (which incorporated anorexia nervosa, bulimia, obesity and others) than the women who died. Although not all participants were of childbearing age at the time of the survey, it nevertheless suggests that survivors of CSA are a population at increased risk.

Yampolsky et al. (2010) decided that CSA should be considered a risk factor for pregnancy having found that abused women were more likely to be depressed and have symptoms of post-traumatic stress, gynaecological problems and chronic illnesses. They are also more likely to be smokers, unemployed, have an earlier menarche than non-abused women and experience increased levels of discomfort (Grimstad & Schei 1999).

Women with a history of CSA present with more risk factors in pregnancy and an association with premature contractions, cervical insufficiency and premature birth has been suggested (Leeners et al. 2010). Those who have experienced any childhood abuse (emotional, sexual and physical) are more likely to report a variety of common complaints in pregnancy (e.g. heartburn, constipation, nausea and vomiting, backache) (Lukasse et al. 2009). However, despite these risk factors, in general, there is little evidence of worse outcomes for survivors of CSA (Leeners et al. 2006). These findings have been upheld in successive qualitative studies in which most participants appear to have had normal, uncomplicated births (Garratt 2011; Montgomery et al. 2015a; Parratt 1994). So we know that women with a history of CSA have more risk factors in pregnancy than other women although this is not reflected in worse outcomes. They frequently do not disclose their history and may not therefore be distinguishable from other women during their maternity care.

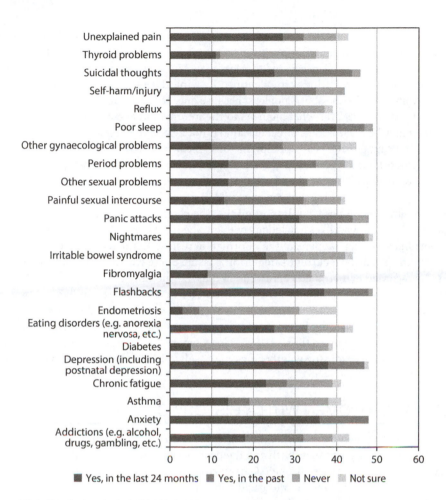

Figure 15.4 Physical and mental health problems.

IDENTIFYING CSA

LEARNING ACTIVITY

Have you ever felt that a woman in your care wanted to tell you something but didn't know how to begin?

How did you respond to her?

How did you feel about the situation?

What did you do to show that you were willing to listen? Could you have done more?

NICE guidelines (2008) state that antenatal care should take place in an environment in which women feel able to discuss sensitive issues such as domestic violence and sexual abuse. Despite recent media attention, CSA is still a taboo subject and although some evidence suggests that screening is acceptable to women (Seng et al. 2008), there is also evidence that women may experience negative reactions if they decide to disclose (Leeners et al. 2006). Women access maternity care at very different stages of understanding and processing their abuse; some may not even remember it (Leeners et al. 2010). Negative responses to a direct question are common, and Seng et al. (2008) discovered that less than 27% of the women with histories of CSA identified in a research setting were identified by clinical screening. It takes a great deal of trust for women to disclose abuse, not least because once they have revealed their history, they potentially lose control over what happens to the information about a very private aspect of their life. It may be that asking a direct question is not helpful in relation to experience of CSA. However, indicating that it is an appropriate topic of conversation should they wish to discuss it is very important. Explaining to women that for some pregnancy can trigger unexpected memories or feelings from childhood and that they are welcome to talk about it if it happens to them may provide an opening if a woman would like to talk.

If a woman does disclose, it is important that the person receiving the disclosure believes the woman's account and acknowledges her courage in sharing it. It is also important that the decision as to what happens to the information rests with the woman – unless she indicates that there may be a current safeguarding issue. Some women will want the information to be recorded in their medical records so that they do not have to repeat the disclosure every time they see someone new. Others will prefer to decide on an individual basis who they trust with the information and will not therefore want it to be documented. Women have spoken about providing little bits of information to test out the response before deciding whether to divulge more (Burian 1995; Montgomery 2012). The way this information is received is key in determining whether a woman feels valued as a person or invalidated and disempowered.

CARING FOR WOMEN WITH A HISTORY OF CSA

Whether or not women choose to disclose their abuse, it is important that they experience sensitive care during pregnancy, birth and the postnatal period. We know that maternity care can be very traumatic for these women (Garratt 2011; Gutteridge 2009). Unlike those suffering from domestic violence, there are no usually outward signs to alert midwives to the issue of CSA. Once domestic violence has been recognised, there is a fairly clear pathway for midwives to follow; however, there is less explicit guidance available for midwives caring for women when a history of CSA is suspected. As midwives may not realise that they are caring for a woman with a history of CSA, 'Universal precautions' (Coles & Jones 2009) are needed. This means that all women are treated in a manner that minimises the risk of trauma for those affected. Essentially, this is the compassionate care to which all midwives aspire (Byrom & Downe 2015). It requires that women are treated with dignity and respect. What is helpful or unhelpful will depend on the woman, how she is at that particular time, her relationship with those providing care, their attitude and the context (Montgomery et al. 2015a).

Feeling safe is equally important for women currently experiencing domestic violence and those who experienced CSA in the past. However, for the latter group of women, 'feeling safe' means not being reminded of their abuse (Montgomery 2013). Unfortunately, even when midwifery care is provided in a sensitive manner, there are many ways in which pregnancy, birth and maternity care can be reminiscent of abuse. Sometimes, this is due to the similarity of bodily sensations experienced or the vulnerability felt during intimate examinations. Sometimes, less immediately obvious situations can trigger memories for women such as hearing footsteps outside the room and wondering who it is and what it means for them (Montgomery et al. 2015b). These situations may not be predicted by the women themselves, which adds an extra layer of complexity in caring for them. Garratt (2011, 189) suggests that 'the most useful guide to providing appropriate care for a woman with a history of abuse is the woman herself' and this is sound advice.

LEARNING ACTIVITY

Think of a high-risk woman for whom you have provided care in labour.
What did you do that helped her to feel in control?
Could you have done anything else?

Although women report feeling violated again by their experience of childbirth (Garratt 2011; Kitzinger 1992), it can also be an affirming, healing process. Control is pivotal in determining how women experience their maternity care (Montgomery 2013). Sensitive care in which women get to know and trust those caring for them, are viewed as partners in their care and during which midwives both listen to them and hear the messages they are trying to convey can help a woman to change her perception of herself and appreciate the good her body can do.

PRACTICE POINTS

- Women may not respond to a direct question about abuse but need to know they can talk about it if they want to.
- Recognise and respond sensitively to a woman's distress even if she does not want to name abuse.
- Control is of paramount importance for these women.

SUMMARY

- Both domestic abuse and CSA are complex issues which severely impact on women's physical and mental health.
- Midwives are in a unique position to identify domestic abuse due to the nature of antenatal care and the known increased incidence of abuse in pregnancy.
- Inquiry should only take place in a safe and private environment when a woman is on her own.
- Women should be given information on how to access support and protect themselves and their children in a safe way.
- Few women disclose CSA.
- Women want to 'feel safe' and for those with a history of CSA this means not being reminded of their abuse.

REFERENCES

Almeida, Clementia, Eduardo Sá, Flavia Cunha, & Ermelinda Pires. 2013. Violence during pregnancy and its effects on mother–baby relationship during pregnancy. *Journal of Reproductive and Infant Psychology* 31(4): 370–380.

Azier, Anna. 2011. Poverty, violence, and health: The impact of domestic violence during pregnancy on newborn health. *Journal of Human Resources* 46(3): 518–538.

Bacchus, Lorraine, Gill Mezey, Susan Bewley, & A. Haworth. 2004. Prevalence of domestic violence when midwives routinely enquire in pregnancy. *British Journal of Obstetrics and Gynaecology* 111(5): 441–445.

Baird, Kathleen & Debra Salmon. 2013. A five year follow-up study of the Bristol pregnancy domestic violence programme to promote routine enquiry. *Midwifery* 29: 1003–1010.

Bancroft, Lundy, Jay Silverman & Daniel Ritchie. 2011. *The Batterer as Parent: Addressing the Impact of Domestic Violence on Family Dynamics* (2nd ed). LA: Sage.

Barron, Jackie. 2014. Sources of referral and support for domestic violence. In Susan Bewley, & Jan Welch (eds.), *ABC of Domestic and Sexual Violence*. Oxford: Wiley Blackwell.

Beydoun, Hind A., Ban Al-Sahab, May A. Beydoun & Tamim Hala. 2010. Intimate partner violence as a risk factor for postpartum depression among Canadian women in the Maternity Experience Survey. *Annals of Epidemiology* 20(8): 575–583.

Bonomi, Amy E., Melissa L. Anderson, Frederick P. Rivara & Robert S. Thompson. 2009. Health care utilization and costs associated with physical and nonphysical-only intimate partner violence. *Health Services Research* 44: 1052–1067.

Bullock, Linda, Tina Bloom, Jan Davis, Erin Kilburn & Mary Ann Currie. 2006. Abuse disclosure in privately and Medicaid-funded pregnant women. *Journal of Midwifery Womens Health* 51: 361–369.

Burian, Jennifer. 1995. Helping survivors of sexual abuse through labor. *Maternal Child Nursing* 20: 252–256.

Byrom, Sheena & Soo Downe. 2015. *The Roar Behind the Silence*. London: Pinter & Martin.

Cawson, Pat., Corrine Wattam, Sue Broker & Graham Kelly. 2000. *Child Maltreatment in the United Kingdom: A Study of the Prevalence of Child Abuse and Neglect*. London: NSPCC.

Chang, Judy., Michelle Decker, Kathryn Moraco, Sanda Martin, Ruth Petersen & Pamela Fraiser. 2005. Asking about intimate partner violence: Advice from female survivors to health care providers. *Patient Education and Counseling* 59(2): 141–147.

CMACE (Centre for Maternal and Child Enquiries). 2011. Saving mothers' lives: Reviewing maternal deaths to make motherhood safer: 2006–08. The Eighth Report on Confidential Enquiries into Maternal Deaths in the United Kingdom. *British Journal of Obstetrics and Gynaecology* 118(1): 1–203.

Coker, Ann L., Paige Hall Smith, Robert E. McKeown & Melissa J. King. 2000. Frequency and correlates of intimate partner violence by type: Physical, sexual and psychological battering. *American Journal of Public Health* 90: 553–559.

Coles, Jan & Kay Jones. 2009. Universal precautions: Perinatal touch and examination after childhood sexual abuse. *Birth* 36(3): 230–236.

Cook, Joanna & Susan Bewley. 2008. Acknowledging a persistent truth; domestic violence in pregnancy. *Journal of the Royal Society of Medicine* 101(7): 358–363.

CPS (Crown Prosecution Service). 2014. *Violence against Women and Girls Crime Report 2013–2014*. http://www.cps.gov.uk/publications/docs/cps_vawg_report_2014.pdf

Daoud, Nihaya, Marcelo L. Urquia, Patricia O'Campo, Maureen Heaman, Patricia A. Janssen, Janet Smylie & K. Thiessen. 2012. Prevalence of abuse and violence before, during, and after pregnancy in a national sample of Canadian women. *American Journal of Public Health* 102(10): 1893–1901.

Dube, Shanta R., Robert F. Anda, Charles L. Whitfield, David W. Brown, Vincnet J. Felitti, Maxia Dong & Wayne H. Giles. 2005. Long-term consequences of childhood sexual abuse by gender of victim. *American Journal of Preventive Medicine* 28(5): 430–438.

Ellsberg, Mary, Henrica A. F. M. Jansen, Lori Heise, Charlotte H. Watts & Claudia Garcia-Moreno, WHO Multi-country Study on Women's Health and Domestic Violence against Women Study Team. 2008. Intimate partner violence and women's physical and mental health in the WHO multi-country study on women's health and domestic violence: An observational study. *Lancet* 371: 1165–1172.

Felson, Richard B., Steven F. Messner, Anthony W. Hoskin & Glenn Deane. 2006. Reasons for reporting and not reporting domestic violence to the police. *Criminology* 40: 617–648.

Garratt, Lis. 2011. *Survivors of Childhood Sexual Abuse and Midwifery Practice.* Oxford: Radcliffe Publishing.

Gazmararian, Julie A., Suzanne Lazorick, Alison M. Spitz, Terri J. Ballard, Linda E. Saltzman & James S. Marks. 1996. Prevalence of violence against pregnant women. *JAMA* 275: 1915–1920.

Gracia, Enrique. 2004. Unreported cases of domestic violence against women: Towards an epidemiology of social silence, tolerance, and inhibition. *Journal of Epidemiology & Community Health* 58: 536–537.

Grimstad, Hilde & Berit Schei. 1999. Pregnancy and delivery for women with a history of child sexual abuse. *Child Abuse and Neglect* 23(1): 81–90.

Gutteridge, Kathryn. 2009. 'From the deep' surviving child sexual abuse into adulthood: Consequences and implications for maternity services. *MIDIRS Midwifery Digest* 19(1): 125–129.

Hegarty, Kelsey, AngelaTaft & Gene Feder. 2008. Violence between intimate partners; working with the whole family. *British Medical Journal* 337:a839.

HM Government. 2015. *Working Together to Safeguard Children: A Guide to Inter-Agency Working to Safeguard and Promote the Welfare of Children.* London: Crown copyright.

Itzin, Catherine. 2006. *Tackling the Health and Mental Health Effects of Domestic and Sexual Violence and Abuse.* London: Crown copyright.

Itzin, Catherine, Ann Taket & Sarah Barter-Godfrey. 2010. *Domestic and Sexual Violence and Abuse: Findings from a Delphi Expert Consultation on Therapeutic and Treatment Interventions with Victims, Survivors and Abusers, Children, Adolescents, and Adults.* Melbourne: Deakin University.

Jahanfar, Shayesteh & Zahra Malekzadegan. 2007. The prevalence of domestic violence among pregnant women who are attended in Iran University of Medical Science Hospitals. *Journal of Family Violence* 22(8): 643–648.

Kitzinger Sheila. 1992. Birth and violence against women generating hypotheses from women's accounts of unhappiness after childbirth In Roberts Helen Womens Health Matters. Routledge: London.

Knight, Marian, Sara Kenyon, Peter Brocklehurst, Jim Neilson, Judy Shakespeare & Jennifer J. Kurinczuk (eds.) on behalf of MBRRACEUK. 2014. *Saving Lives, Improving Mothers' Care – Lessons Learned to Inform Future Maternity Care from the UK and Ireland Confidential Enquiries into Maternal Deaths and Morbidity 2009–12.* Oxford: National Perinatal Epidemiology Unit, University of Oxford.

Leeners, Brigitte, Hertha Richter-Appelt, Bruno Imthurn & Werner Rath. 2006. Influence of childhood sexual abuse on pregnancy, delivery, and the early postpartum period in adult women. *Journal of Psychosomatic Research* 61(2): 139–151.

Leeners, Brigitte, Ruth Stiller, Emina Block, Gisela Gorres & Werner Rath. 2010. Pregnancy complications in women with childhood sexual abuse experiences. *Journal of Psychosomatic Research* 69(5): 503–510.

Lukasse, Mirjam, Berit Schei, Siri Vangen & Pal Øian. 2009. Childhood abuse and common complaints in pregnancy. *Birth* 36(3): 190–199.

Marmot, Michael, Sharon Friel, Ruth Bell, Tanja A. J. Houweling, Sebastian Taylor & Commission on Social Determinants of Health. 2008. Closing the gap in a generation: Health equity through action on the social determinants of health. *The Lancet* 372(9650): 1661–1669.

Mezey, Gill & Susan Bewley. 1997. Domestic violence in pregnancy. *British Journal of Obstetrics and Gynaecology* 104: 528–531.

Montgomery, Elsa. 2012. Voicing the silence: The maternity care experiences of women who were sexually abused in childhood. PhD diss., University of Southampton.

Montgomery, Elsa. 2013. Feeling safe: A metasynthesis of the maternity care needs of women who sexually abused in childhood. *Birth* 40(2): 88–95.

Montgomery, Elsa. 2015. *CIS'ters Survey of Health Needs.* Healthwatch Hampshire. http://www.healthwatchhampshire.co.uk/sites/default/files/community_cash_fund_-_healthwatch_report_-_20-04-15.pdf

Montgomery, Elsa, Catherine Pope & Rogers Jane. 2015a. A feminist narrative study of the maternity care experiences of women who were sexually abused in childhood. *Midwifery* 31(1): 54–60.

Montgomery, Elsa, Catherine Pope & Rogers Jane. 2015b. The re-enactment of childhood sexual abuse in maternity care: A qualitative study. *BMC Pregnancy and Childbirth* 15: 194.

Nagassar, R. P., J. M. Rawlins, N. R. Sampson, J. Zackerali, K. Chankadyal, C. Ramasir & R. Boodram. 2010. The prevalence of domestic violence within different socio-economic classes in Central Trinidad. *West Indian Medical Journal* 59(1): 20–25.

NICE (National Institute of Clinical Excellence). 2008. *Antenatal Care Routine Care for the Healthy Pregnant Woman.* London: RCOG.

NICE (National Institute of Clinical Excellence). 2010. *Pregnancy and Complex Social Factors: A Model for Service Provision for Pregnant Women with Complex Social Factors.* London: NICE.

NICE (Nation Institute of Clinical Excellence). 2014. Domestic violence and abuse: multiagency working Public health guideline. https://www.nice.org.uk/guidance/ph50/resources/domestic-violence-and-abuse-multiagency-working-1996411687621

ONS (Office for National Statistics). 2014. *Crime Survey for England and Wales.* Statistical bulletin: Crime in England and Wales, Year Ending June 2014. http://www.ons.gov.uk/ons/rel/crime-stats/crime-statistics/period-ending-june-2014/stb-crime-stats--year-ending-june-2014.html

Parratt, Jenny. 1994. The experience of childbirth for survivors of incest. *Midwifery* 10: 26–39.

Pence, Ellen & Michael Paymar. 1993. *Education Groups for Men Who Batter. The Duluth Model.* New York: Springer.

Pereda, Noemí, Georgina Guilera, Maria Forns & Juana Gomez-Benito. 2009a. The international epidemiology of child sexual abuse: A continuation of Finkelhor (1994). *Child Abuse and Neglect* 33: 331–342.

Pereda, Noemí, Georgina Guilera, Maria Forns & Juana Gomez-Benito. 2009b. The prevalence of child sexual abuse in community and student samples: A meta-analysis. *Clinical Psychology Review* 29: 328–338.

Pinheiro, Paulo Sérgio. 2006. *World Report on Violence against Children.* Geneva: United Nations.

Price, Sally, Kathleen Baird & Debra Salmon. 2009. Asking the question: Antenatal domestic violence. *Midwifery: Best Practice* 5: 125.

Radford, Lorraine, Susana Corral, Christine Bradley, Helen Fisher, Claire Bassett, Nick Howat & Stephen Collishaw. 2011. *Child Abuse and Neglect in the UK Today.* London: NSPCC.

Rayment-Jones, Hannah, Trevor Murrells & Jane Sandall. 2015. An investigation of the relationship between the caseload model of midwifery for socially disadvantaged women and childbirth outcomes using routine data – A retrospective, observational study. *Midwifery* 31(4): 409–417.

Rodriguez, Eunice, Katryn E. Lasch, Pinky Chandra & Jennifer Lee. 2001. Family violence, employment status, welfare benefits, and alcohol drinking in the United States: What is the relation? *Journal of Epidemiology and Community Health* 55(3): 172–178.

Seng, Julia S., Kathleen J. H. Sparbel, Lisa K. Low & Cheryl Killion. 2002. Abuse-related posttraumatic stress and desired maternity care practices: Women's perspectives. *Journal of Midwifery & Womens Health* 47(5): 360–370.

Seng, Julia S., Mickey Sperlich & Lisa K. Low. 2008. Mental health, demographic, and risk behavior profiles of pregnant survivors of childhood and adult abuse. *Journal of Midwifery and Women's Health* 53(6): 511–521.

Shah, Prakesh S. & Jyotsna Shah. 2010. Maternal exposure to domestic violence and pregnancy and birth outcomes: A systematic review and meta-analyses. *Journal of Women's Health* 19(11): 2017–2031.

Silverman, Jay G., Michele R. Decker, Elizabeth Reed & Anita Raj. 2006a. Intimate partner violence victimization prior to and during pregnancy among women residing in 26 US states: Associations with maternal and neonatal health. *American Journal of Obstetrics and Gynecology* 195(1): 140–148.

Silverman, Jay G., Michele R. Decker, Elizabeth Reed & Anita Raj. 2006b. Intimate partner violence around the time of pregnancy: Association with breastfeeding behavior. *Journal of Women's Health* 15(8): 934–940.

Sohal, Alex & Medina Johnson. 2014. Identifying domestic violence and abuse. In Bewley, Susan & Jan Welch (eds.), *ABC of Domestic and Sexual Violence*. Chichester: Wiley Blackwell.

Walby, Sylvia. 2009. The Cost of Domestic Violence Up-date 2009 Lancaster University. www.lancs.ac.uk/fass/doc_library/ sociology/Cost_of_domestic_ violence_update.doc

WHO (World Health Organization). 2013. *Violence Against Women: A 'Global Health Problem of Epidemic Proportions'. New Clinical and Policy Guidelines Launched to Guide Health Sector Response*. http://www.who.int/mediacentre/news/releases/2013/violence_against_women_20130620/en/

Womens Aid. 2006. *Who Are the Victims of Domestic Violence?* http://www.womensaid.org.uk/domestic-violence articles.asp?section=00010001002200410001&itemid=1273

Yampolsky, Lee, Rachel Lev-Wiesel & Itzahk Z. Ben-Zion. 2010. Child sexual abuse: Is it a risk factor for pregnancy? *Journal of Advanced Nursing* 66(9): 2025–2037.

FURTHER READING AND INFORMATION

CIS'ters, http://cisters.org.uk

CIS'ters is a charity that provides emotional support for females aged 18+ who (as children/teens) were raped/sexually abused/exploited by a member of their immediate and/or extended family. They offer female survivors the opportunity to explore painful issues and their associated anxieties in a confidential environment.

The Lancet Series on Violence Against Women and Girls covers the evidence base for interventions, discuss the vital role of the health sector in care and prevention, show the need for men and women to be involved in effective programmes, provide practical lessons from experience in countries and present a call for action with key recommendations and indicators to track progress (Ellsberg et al. 2014).

24-hour National Domestic Violence Freephone Helpline 0808 2000 247

(Run in partnership between Women's Aid and Refuge)

NAPAC, http://napac.org.uk

National Association of People Abused in Childhood

Women's Aid, http://www.womensaid.org.uk

Women's Aid is the national charity for women and children working to end domestic abuse. The charity informs policy and empowers survivors by listening and responding to their needs. They are a federation of over 220 organisations who provide more than 300 local services to women and children across the country. The website includes the 'Women's Aid Survivors Handbook' available in pdf format in 11 languages

Refuge, http://www.refuge.org.uk

Respect Phoneline, http://www.respectphoneline.org.uk 0808 802 4040

For perpetrators of domestic abuse. A confidential and anonymous helpline for anyone concerned about his or her violence and/or abuse towards a partner or ex-partner.

The Survivors' Trust, http://www.thesurvivorstrust.org/about-tst

The Survivors Trust (TST) is a national umbrella agency for over 135 specialist rape, sexual violence and childhood sexual abuse support organisations throughout the UK and Ireland.

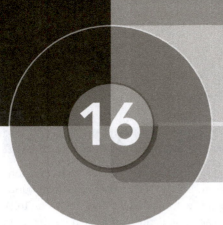

16

Smoking, pregnancy and the midwife

FABIANA LORENCATTO AND JAMES M HARRIS

INTRODUCTION

As discussed throughout this book, midwives play a key role in public health and health promotion. One area where there is clear potential for midwives to realise their public health and health promotion potential is 'smoking cessation', that is, advising and encouraging clients, and their families, on stopping the use of tobacco products. Midwives are in a key position to motivate and encourage healthier lifestyles. Intervention during this key period of a woman's life could have a long-lasting impact on her health and well-being, and that of her wider family, well beyond the pregnancy and post partum period.

While the health messages related to smoking are well known, many people within the United Kingdom continue to smoke, and many women who smoked prior to pregnancy will continue to smoke after the baby is born. This can create a variety of conflicts for some midwives – 'How do we foster a relationship of trust while questioning habitual behaviours?', 'Should midwives contribute to the increasingly anti-social treatment of smokers, during a time when women's stress levels and personal identities are in flux?' This chapter aims to consider these questions, alongside providing knowledge about the effects of smoking and why women smoke, and offering evidence-based aids in providing smoking cessation advice.

This chapter outlines the facts related to smoking in pregnancy and the evidence around what strategies might work best to help pregnant women to stop smoking. The current policy guidelines on this topic will be explored as will be some of the barriers to midwives in providing this health promotion advice. The last part of the chapter will look at the steps a midwife might take to ask, advise and assist a pregnant woman to stop smoking.

BACKGROUND: SMOKING IN PREGNANCY

Smoking remains a leading preventable cause of mortality and morbidity. Cigarettes contain approximately 600 chemicals and produce an additional 4,000 chemical compounds once lit, many of which are carcinogenic or poisonous (e.g. formaldehyde, arsenic) (Box 16.1). Approximately, 40% of all deaths among the middle-age population are caused by smoking, and smoking is estimated to reduce a smoker's life expectancy on average by 10 years (Doll et al. 2005). Smoking is also closely linked with psychological disorders, with a smoking prevalence of approximately 60%–80% in those suffering from psychosis (Banham & Gilbody 2010). In addition, smoking negatively affects the health of non-smokers through secondary smoke that is passively inhaled (Öberg et al. 2011). In England, cigarette smoking is estimated to cost the National Health Service (NHS) £2.7 billion annually (Callum et al. 2011).

In addition to these general risks, there are several serious consequences for both the mother and the baby specifically associated with maternal smoking during pregnancy. Women who smoke during their pregnancy expose their fetus to all the toxins and poisons mentioned above. Some of the numerous negative consequences associated with maternal smoking during pregnancy include complications during labour, risk of miscarriage, premature and stillbirths, low birth weight and sudden infant death syndrome (SIDs) (Agrawal et al. 2010). The negative consequences associated with maternal smoking during pregnancy also extend beyond birth through childhood. Children exposed to tobacco in the womb are at an increased risk of experiencing respiratory infections; asthma; problems of ear, nose and throat; psychological and behavioural difficulties (i.e. attention and hyperactivity problems and disruptive, negative behaviours); heightened risk of obesity, early onset of adult diabetes and high blood pressure; and detrimental effects on educational performance (Montgomery & Ekbom 2002; Lawlor et al. 2004; Oken et al. 2008; Lumley et al. 2009; Ekblad et al. 2010). Compared with women who do not smoke during pregnancy, the costs of complications and poor infant health outcomes attributable to smoking are substantial; it is estimated that savings to the NHS from reducing smoking in pregnancy are £4 for every £1 spent (NICE 2010).

Despite the well-established risks associated with smoking, approximately one in five of the current English population are smokers (Smoking in England 2015). There are two principal sources of data that provide information on the prevalence of smoking in pregnancy in England: Smoking at Time of Delivery (NCSCT 2013) and the Infant Feeding Survey

BOX 16.1: Contents of cigarettes

- Ammonia (cleaning fluid)
- Formaldehyde (preserves dead bodies)
- Shellac (varnish)
- Hydrogen cyanide (industrial pollutant)
- Arsenic (deadly poison)
- Cadmium (used in batteries)
- Benzene (petrol fumes)
- Acetone (nail polish remover)

(McAndrew et al. 2012). Both sources indicate that the prevalence of smoking in pregnancy has decreased over recent years. Nonetheless, many women who smoke struggle to quit when they become pregnant, and approximately 26% of pregnant women in the United Kingdom continue to smoke immediately before or during pregnancy, of which 13% continue to smoke through to the point of delivery (McAndrew et al. 2012). These prevalence statistics are similar to those from other high-income countries (Tong et al. 2009). It is of note that due to social pressure and stigma, it is likely that many women may under-report their smoking behaviour during pregnancy; consequently, prevalence statistics are likely to be an underestimate of the true smoking rates in this population group (Shipton et al. 2009; Brose et al. 2013a).

There is a range of factors that influence the likelihood of maternal smoking during pregnancy. For example, younger mothers (i.e. <20 years) are five times more likely to smoke than older mothers aged 35+ (45% vs. 9%, respectively) (Penn & Owen 2002). Similarly, mothers who are less educated and work in routine and manual occupations are four times more likely to smoke than those who are educated and work in managerial/professional occupations (29% vs. 7%, respectively). There are also marked geographical variations in smoking prevalence throughout the United Kingdom, with the lowest prevalence being in central London (1.9%) and the highest in Blackpool (27.5%) (Orchard 2014). Moreover, partners also have a strong influence over the likelihood of women smoking and/or quitting during pregnancy. It is estimated that 38% of mothers in England live in a household where at least one person smokes, typically their partner, and the likelihood of maternal smoking in pregnancy significantly increases for women who have a partner who smokes. It has also been demonstrated that women whose partners smoke encounter greater difficulties when trying to quit, and higher rates of subsequent relapse (Fang et al. 2004).

Alongside the influence that partner smoking has on the likelihood of the woman smoking, it is important to also note the risk for a fetus or newborn being in a household where someone smokes. Research has shown that, when compared with non-smoking households, babies have more chance of dying of SIDs if the father smokes than if the mother smokes, perhaps because smoking fathers tend to smoke more than the mother, thereby exposing the child to more harmful chemicals (Blackburn et al. 2005). It is therefore important for health professionals to consider the smoking behaviour of the whole household, not just that of the pregnant woman herself.

PRACTICE POINTS

- Cigarettes contain over 4,000 chemicals once lit, many of which are poisonous.
- Smoking has been shown to contribute to miscarriages, preterm births, stillbirths, low birth weights and deaths in infancy.
- Less than 2% of pregnant women in Westminster smoke. Over 27% of pregnant women in Blackpool smoke.
- Partner smoking is of equal, or greater, risk to a newborn than maternal smoking.

Given the damage smoking can have on both mother and the baby, it is vital that pregnant smokers are adequately supported to quit for good. When asked, a large proportion of adult smokers (around 70%) report that they are actually interested in quitting and would like support to do so (Orleans 2007). There is a range of interventions currently available to support smokers who are trying to quit. These broadly fall into two categories: (1) pharmacological interventions and (2) behavioural support interventions.

PHARMACOLOGICAL INTERVENTIONS

Pharmacological interventions to aid smoking cessation include medications such as varenicline (i.e. Champix), bupropion (i.e. Zyban) and the numerous forms of nicotine replacement therapy (NRT) products (i.e. the patch, inhaler, lozenge, gum, microtab and nasal spray). NRT products can be used individually or combined with other modalities (i.e. slow-acting NRT products such as the transdermal patch, combined with faster-acting products such as the gum, inhaler or nasal spray). Pharmacological interventions work by targeting the underlying biological dependence to nicotine and by providing relief from nicotine cravings and withdrawal symptoms. There is substantial evidence illustrating the effectiveness of these different types of pharmacological interventions in the general population (Brose et al. 2013a; Stead et al. 2013).

However, there is limited, good evidence for the safety and efficacy of pharmacological interventions in pregnant smokers (Brose 2014). Medications such as varenicline and bupropion have not been evaluated in pregnant smokers (Tobacco Use and Dependence Guideline Panel 2008). While some studies indicate marginal benefits of NRT use in pregnancy (Myung et al. 2012), a systematic review of randomised controlled trials highlights that the evidence for NRT's efficacy and safety in this population group is inconclusive (Coleman et al. 2012). Women and their care providers need to consider the risks of continued smoking compared with the risks of taking medicines to help quit smoking.

More recent evidence from clinical practice supports the finding that a combination of a slow-acting form of NRT with a faster-acting NRT product (i.e. nicotine patch + gum) can significantly increase the likelihood of pregnant smokers successfully quitting smoking (Brose et al. 2013b). It is hypothesised that this occurs due to the more rapid metabolism of nicotine during pregnancy, meaning that a stronger dose of nicotine delivered via a combination of both NRT products is required to achieve significant relief from cravings and withdrawal symptoms (Brose et al. 2013b). Although combination NRT exposes the fetus to higher levels of nicotine, NRT arguably remains a much safer alternative to actual smoking, as NRT products deliver nicotine without the additional exposure to carbon monoxide(CO) and the thousands of harmful chemical compounds present in cigarettes and cigarette smoke (West et al. 2003). There is thus a critical need for more high-quality research to establish what the safest and most effective medications are to help pregnant women to successfully quit smoking (Brose 2014).

ACTIVITY

- Find out what the protocol for prescribing NRT and other 'stop smoking medications' are in your trust.
- Is there an option for medication if an individual is an inpatient?

BEHAVIOURAL SUPPORT INTERVENTIONS

Unlike pharmacological interventions, there is good evidence that behavioural support interventions can help pregnant smokers to successfully quit smoking (Lumley et al. 2009). Quitting smoking is challenging, and providing psychosocial support is imperative in the early stages of any attempt to quit smoking (Brose 2014). Psychosocial behavioural support interventions for smoking cessation can be brief or intensive. Brief advice – often called 'Very Brief Advice' or VBA – is given by first-line health care professionals, such as midwives and general practitioners. Detailed description of the process involved is discussed later but also see behaviour change theory in Chapter 6). Intensive behavioural support is typically delivered by a trained, dedicated stop smoking advisor, and consists of advice, discussion and targeted activities that aim to minimise a smoker's motivation to smoke, facilitate relapse prevention and coping, and optimise the use of smoking cessation medications and social support (West & Stapleton 2008). Behavioural support for smoking cessation can be delivered through various modalities, including face-to-face individual and group support sessions, telephone, Internet and smartphone applications, and is consistently shown to be a highly cost-effective, life-preserving intervention in the general population (Shahab & McEwen 2009).

Given their effectiveness, behavioural support interventions have been widely implemented in clinical practice. For instance, in England, a network of 152 NHS Stop Smoking Services represent a unique, national initiative to offer support to smokers who are motivated to quit. These services offer medications, alongside free, weekly one-to-one or group meetings with a trained specialist practitioner, which follows a structured, withdrawal-oriented behavioural therapy approach (Bauld et al. 2010). In general, smokers engaging with these services are four times more likely to successfully quit than those attempting to quit unaided (Judge et al. 2005). Many NHS Stop Smoking Services also offer specialist behavioural support tailored to the unique needs of specific population groups, including pregnant women. Of the 21,839 pregnant women setting a quit date with a NHS Stop Smoking Service in 2011/2012, 27% successfully quit at 4 weeks' follow-up (Health and social care information centre 2012).

Behavioural support interventions are complex, comprising multiple component behaviour change techniques (Michie et al. 2009). In order to more precisely answer the question 'what works to help pregnant smokers quit', recent research has aimed to identify which specific components of behavioural support interventions for pregnant smokers are linked to better outcomes (i.e. 'the active ingredients'). While the assessment of the effectiveness of the various different components of behavioural change techniques is complex, researchers have devised an evidence-based approach that has been shown to help pregnant women to stop smoking. These findings are detailed in the remainder of this chapter.

Furthermore, 'cutting down' as opposed to stopping 'cold turkey' (i.e. abruptly and completely) can initially appear an attractive, more achievable option to many smokers. Indeed, 69% of pregnant women presented with both options would prefer to try and gradually reduce their smoking. However, there is evidence that pregnant smokers who have been advised to gradually cut down, as opposed to stopping smoking completely, were much less likely to successfully quit long term (8% vs. 36%, respectively) (NICE 2010). Therefore, an additionally important component of behavioural support interventions for pregnant smokers involves emphasising the importance of stopping smoking completely, rather than gradually cutting down.

CURRENT GUIDELINES, POLICY AND RECOMMENDATIONS

There is a national target to reduce the rate of women smoking at the time of delivery to 11% (Department of Health 2011). In 2010, NICE published guidelines on 'quitting smoking in pregnancy and following childbirth'. This guidance emphasises that any pre-conceptual care meetings and routine antenatal appointments are potential opportunities to intervene with women considering pregnancy and pregnant smokers. The guidance also outlines recommendations for midwives and stop smoking services on how to identify and where to refer pregnant smokers; the different options and type of support that could be offered to assist them in quitting; and the necessary training and competencies required of the professionals delivering such support. The Royal College of Midwives (RCM 2015) recognises the importance of targets for the reduction of pregnant smokers, noting that a rate of 1 in 10 babies being born to a smoking mother is unacceptable. However, they also note the importance of resources, such as training and adequate staffing levels, to aid these targets.

Given the state of the current evidence for smoking cessation medications in pregnancy, clinical guidelines surrounding pharmacological interventions in pregnant smokers are cautious in nature (Brose 2014). Many smoking cessation medications are contraindicated in pregnancy, thereby limiting the pregnant smoker's choice of medications to support their attempt to quit. For example, varenicline and bupropion are not licensed for use in this population group (NICE 2010). Current NICE guidance recommends that NRT should only be used with pregnant smokers if it is deemed necessary, and the advantages of its use are judged to outweigh any potential disadvantages. It also recommends that NRT should only be considered for use with pregnant smokers in instances where a pregnant woman has initially tried to quit without pharmacological support but failed to do so (NICE 2010). In other countries, any use of NRT in pregnancy is not recommended (i.e. USA; Department of Health and Human Services). It is important to note that this is not because there is evidence of any harm caused by NRT when compared with smoking cigarettes, but rather a lack of evidence showing no harm. As with many pharmacological treatments, testing via randomised control trials with pregnant women pose ethical problems.

In terms of behavioural interventions, NICE guidance emphasises the important role midwives have in supporting pregnant women to quit. See Box 16.2.

Although this NICE guidance was published 5 years ago, there is evidence that its uptake and implementation in clinical practice has been limited (NCSCT 2013).

PRACTICE POINTS

- A combination of pharmacological and behavioural approaches increases the likelihood of a successful quit attempt by 40%.
- Behavioural interventions are complex and multi-layered, but there is strong evidence of appropriate techniques to be used to help pregnant women to stop smoking.
- Some smoking cessation medications have not been proven to be safe for use in pregnancy; this is because of the ethics of medicine testing in pregnancy rather than a suggested harm. It is assumed that taking these medications would be less harmful than continuing to smoke.

BOX 16.2: NICE (2010) recommendations for midwives supporting smoking cessation

- Identifying pregnant smokers by assessing, documenting and discussing exposure to tobacco smoke by conducting a CO-monitoring test.
- Providing brief, opportunistic smoking cessation advice, including information about the risks to the unborn child of smoking whilst pregnant, and the hazards of secondhand smoke exposure (i.e. via partners who smoke) to both mother and baby.
- Offering and arranging a referral to a NHS Stop Smoking Service.
- At the subsequent appointment(s), checking whether the woman took up her referral, and her progress with smoking cessation (NICE 2010).

BARRIERS FOR THE MIDWIFE WHEN PROVIDING SMOKING CESSATION ADVICE

Considering the wide-ranging ramifications of smoking in pregnancy and around newborns, and the strong evidence base on how to support women to quit smoking, it is important to consider what barriers are stopping midwives from following the recommendations of NICE. The provision of smoking cessation advice from midwives has been shown to be inconsistent, with some studies showing over two-thirds of midwives never advising women to stop smoking (Condliffe et al. 2005). This section will use the research literature to identify these barriers and address them to help uptake of smoking cessation advice.

SMOKING CESSATION AND THE IMPACT ON THE MOTHER–MIDWIFE RELATIONSHIP

Some midwives are worried that giving smoking cessation advice could impact on the relationship they have with their clients, and they feel it is not a midwife's job to make women feel guiltier than they may already do about smoking in pregnancy:

> Yeah, and I think you've got to be really careful not making them feel incredibly guilty by asking about smoking. But I mean they do feel bad enough already without you saying 'well it's going to make your baby small, and won't be as good at school'… And you don't want to alienate the women. You actually want her to continue to receive your care so it's kind of a fine line between telling her what the research says about smoking but also maintaining that relationship with her.
>
> **McLeod et al. (2003, 290)**

This position of finding a balance between maintaining the client–midwife relationship and yet providing health promotion advice has been repeated in other studies on the topic (Beenstock et al. 2012; Herberts & Sykes 2012). It is understandable why midwives may be wary of risking this relationship. However, part of the role of the midwife is public health education, which includes advising on avoiding discussions on the harms of smoking is contradicting this role.

Nonetheless, some women have felt guilty after talking to their midwives about their smoking behaviours, and that this could impact on the midwife–client relationship (McLeod et al. 2003; Herberts et al. 2012; Beenstock et al. 2012). It is therefore important to note that the NICE guidelines do not involve pressurising women to quit. Smoking cessation advice may be viewed in the same way as providing dietary, alcohol and place of birth advice – a midwife's role is to provide information to facilitate an informed decision from women, but not to coerce or make decisions for them. Without being provided with evidence-based information, women may unwittingly cause harm to themselves and their baby.

It is clear that communication needs to be woman-centred and non-judgemental (NICE 2010); however, more positive results may be seen if practitioners take an opt-out approach rather than an opt-in one (Brose 2014). Women can always decline the help of the smoking cessation service when they are contacted, but they cannot accept their help if they are never referred to in the first place.

Studies have shown that pregnant smokers do however want advice on smoking cessation and often suggest that midwives provide insufficient advice (Ussher et al. 2004). Midwives are well placed to provide initial support and facilitate access to more dedicated support if needed or desired by the pregnant woman but lack confidence or training to do this which is discussed below.

INADEQUATE TRAINING AND A LACK OF SELF-EFFICACY

Another key barrier to midwives providing stop smoking advice – a lack of knowledge and training, alongside a lack of belief in their ability to deliver the advice (self-efficacy):

"Lack of self-confidence and knowledge is visible, so my message about smoking cessation is not strong enough, the client doesn't listen and then I feel like I can do nothing to influence her decision."

De Wilde et al. (2015, 70)

This lack of knowledge and self-efficacy has been evident in many other studies which have shown that a lack of confidence in providing information can influence whether or not a health professional actually provides the information (Aquilino et al. 2003; Condliffe et al. 2005). It may be the case that the current focus on the medical issues surrounding pregnancy means that limited time is given to midwifery curricula to teaching communication skills and increasing knowledge on issues such as smoking cessation. Indeed, significant gaps have been identified in the current curricula of UK nursing, medical and optometry schools regarding the teaching of issues related to smoking and smoking cessation (Raupach et al. 2009; Richards et al. 2014). The curricula often focuses on teaching students the harmful health effects of smoking but provide little to no practical skills training for delivering evidence-based smoking cessation interventions in clinical practice.

This barrier is easier to address – easy to access online training packages are available for all health professionals, see further resources at the end of the chapter for more information. A study by Brose et al. (2012) has shown that health professionals' self-efficacy and knowledge increase significantly after completing the modules.

INSTITUTIONAL BARRIERS

The NICE guidelines (2010) for antenatal care stipulate 29 different activities required from the midwife during the 'booking visit' – a pregnant woman's initial appointment with a midwife.

This ranges from educating on how the baby develops and providing dietary advice, to discussing genetic screening tests and ascertaining risk factors for the pregnancy. These appointments vary in length, depending on trust and practitioner. There is little surprise that time pressures and competing priorities often come up as key barriers for not providing smoking cessation advice.

"You've got all these other factors you're supposed to be giving information on...as well as making referrals and sometimes...there's something else that they [the clients] really want to talk about."

Aquilino et al. (2003, 329)

While the time pressures of the booking appointment are well documented, we suggest that the health benefits of smoking cessation are so great that they should be given time within the booking appointment. When following the VBA process outlined below, this can be conducted in less than 4 min. It is for individual practitioners to decide if these 4 min equate to a valuable use of their time.

THE ROLE OF THE MIDWIFE IN PLANNING SMOKING CESSATION CARE

This section aims to explain specifically what a midwife should do in relation to smoking cessation. Ascertaining smoking status at the booking appointment is an important first step, but smoking cessation advice should not be restricted to this appointment only. Once it is established the woman is a smoker, this (as is every contact with the woman) is an opportunity to provide VBA (McEwen 2015).

Figure 16.1 provides an outline of the VBA steps – Ask, Advise, Act – that should be taken. These are then discussed in greater detail below. These guidelines are adapted from 'Smoking Cessation: A Briefing for Midwifery Staff' (McEwen 2015). The VBA process is a theoretically designed approach to promoting smoking cessation (Michie et al. 2011). A meta-analysis of various different brief opportunistic approaches has shown that this approach is more successful in promoting attempts to stop smoking than just advising people to stop smoking, or only offering smoking cessation advice when requested (Aveyard et al. 2012).

ASK

When taking the full medical history at the booking appointment, past and present smoking status should be explored (McEwen 2015). Past and present smoking status relates to tobacco smoking only and not to electronic cigarettes (e-cigarettes). If a woman reports that she is using an e-cigarette, confirm that she is no longer using tobacco as well. If she is not using tobacco, her current smoking status should be recorded as a non-smoker. As e-cigarettes are relatively new, longitudinal harm data are limited, but it is assumed that the harm caused will be less than tobacco smoking and comparable to taking NRT medications (Goniewicz et al. 2014).

It is important to ask women about their smoking status at least once each trimester and to record any advice given (NICE 2014; McEwen 2015). This ensures that stopping smoking is deemed important throughout the pregnancy and not just at the initial visit. Pregnant women

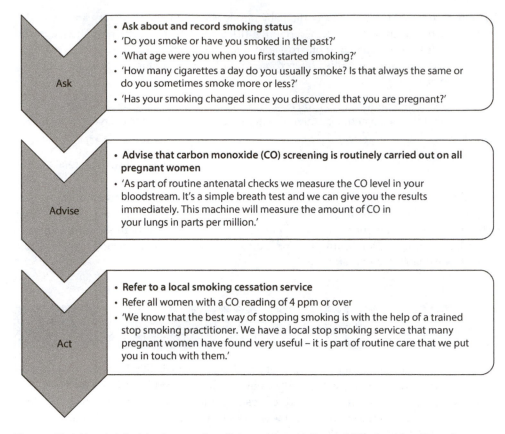

Figure 16.1 Very brief advice intervention. (Adapted from McEwen, 2015, Smoking Cessation, a Briefing for Midwifery Staff. NCSCT. http://www.ncsct.co.uk/usr/pub/NCSCT_midwifery_briefing.pdf)

who stop smoking prior to conception, or in the initial stages of pregnancy, may well relapse and so it is important that the topic is raised repeatedly, even with those who are recorded as ex-smokers or non-smokers.

ADVISE

CO is a poisonous gas contained within cigarettes. It impacts on oxygen transport, which reduces the oxygen available for the developing fetus. It increases the miscarriage risk and slows fetal growth and development. NICE guidelines have recommended the use of CO monitors in antenatal appointments since 2010 on all women. It is also present in exhaust fumes and faulty gas appliances (i.e. boilers). There have been documented cases of a faulty boiler being identified due to routine antenatal CO monitoring.

CO monitoring is a quick, non-invasive test. The woman holds her breath for 15 s to allow the CO in the blood to pass into the air in her lungs. She then blows into the machine until it indicates enough breath has been expelled. The recommended cut off for detecting smoking in pregnant women is four parts per million (4 ppm). While CO screening is a good indication of recent smoking, it does not usually detect smoking from more than 48 h prior.

This is because CO is expelled from the body rapidly and can be seen as a positive motivator for pregnant smokers wanting to quit – very soon after they stop smoking, the fetus will be exposed to less CO. If the woman confirms that she is a non-smoker, and the CO reading is less than 4 ppm, you can reassure the woman that this is a normal reading and move on with the appointment.

If the CO reading is above 4 ppm, then the midwife should explore if the woman is a smoker. This should be done sensitively, especially if she has already stated that she is a non-smoker. Point out that exposure to tobacco smoke is the most common reason that CO is found during a breath test, and ask if she or anyone else in the household smokes. Note that electronic cigarettes alone will not cause an increase in CO, and a high reading may indicate that the woman is combining e-cigarette use with tobacco smoking. If she reveals that she is a smoker, explain that a normal reading is between 1 and 4 ppm, and she is over that limit, and explain that this level is harmful to her baby.

If the woman has a high reading, but states she is not currently smoking, then there are other possible reasons for the high reading – this could be due to exposure to a faulty gas boiler, car exhausts or to a paint stripper. These are all serious exposures in pregnancy, and you should give the woman the Gas Safety Advice Line number (0800 300 363). Alternatively, someone who is lactose intolerant but has recently consumed dairy may emit some CO in their breath which could explain the reading.

ACT

Once a smoking status is identified, the next step is to identify the woman's motivations to quit smoking. Pregnant women tend to be highly motivated to make positive behaviour changes, and simply informing a woman that there is a local service that others have found useful can motivate them to want to quit. If a woman informs you that she has reduced her smoking, it is worth exploring this further. If she has done this because she feels it will reduce the harms to the baby, it is important to point out that cutting down does not offer any significant health advantages, and stopping is the only way she can eliminate the risk to her baby. If the woman feels she is able to stop smoking, or is reluctant to receive help, then the midwife can advise that this is her choice, but that the stop smoking service will be able to talk this through with her. While no one can force her to stop, it is important that she has all the facts and help at hand. A referral does not mean a commitment to quitting, and she would be free to withdraw at any time.

This is also a good time to explore if there are other smokers in the household. The support of family and friends is crucial, especially anyone who lives with her. A joint referral can be made, thereby increasing the woman's likelihood of quitting and reducing the risk of SIDS.

Ensure that any referrals agreed upon are actioned to ensure help is received. Remember, the role of the midwife is to refer on, not to provide the smoking cessation advice. As with all health care interventions, documentation of the findings and subsequent discussions should be made in the notes. This will enable positive reinforcement in subsequent visits of quit attempts, or enable midwives to revisit the topic if a referral is declined. Following this, you can move on with the appointment.

REFERENCES

Agrawal, Arpana, Jeffrey F. Scherrer, Julia D. Grant, Carolyn E. Sartor, Michele L. Pergadia, Alexis E. Duncan, Pamela A. Madden, Jon Randolph, Theodore Jacob Kathleen Bucholz & Hong Xian. 2010. The effects of maternal smoking during pregnancy on offspring outcomes. *Preventive Medicine* 50(1): 13–18.

Aquilino, Mary Lober, Cynthia M. Goody & John B. Lowe. 2003. WIC providers' perspectives on offering smoking cessation interventions. *MCN: The American Journal of Maternal/Child Nursing* 28(5): 326–332.

Aveyard, Paul, Rachna Begh, Amanda Parsons & Robert West. 2012. Brief opportunistic smoking cessation interventions: A systematic review and meta-analysis to compare advice to quit and offer of assistance. *Addiction* 107(6): 1066–1073.

Banham, Lindsay & Simon Gilbody. 2010. Smoking cessation in severe mental illness: What works? *Addiction* 105(7): 1176–1189.

Bauld, Linda, Kirsten Bell, Lucy McCullough, Lindsay Richardson & Lorraine Greaves. 2010. The effectiveness of NHS smoking cessation services: A systematic review. *Journal of Public Health* 32(1): 71–82.

Beenstock, Jane, Falko F. Sniehotta, Martin White, Ruth Bell, Eugene M.G. Milne & Vera Araujo-Soares. 2012. What helps and hinders midwives in engaging with pregnant women about stopping smoking? A cross-sectional survey of perceived implementation difficulties among midwives in the northeast of England. *Implementation Science* 7(1): 36.

Blackburn, Clare, Sheila Bonas, Nicholas Spencer, Chris Coe, Alan Dolan & R. Moy. 2005. Parental smoking and passive smoking in infants: Fathers matter too. *Health Education Research* 20(2): 185–194.

Brose, Leonie S. 2014. Helping pregnant smokers to quit. *BMJ* 348: g1808.

Brose, Leonie S., Andy McEwen & Robert West. 2013a. Association between nicotine replacement therapy use in pregnancy and smoking cessation. *Drug and Alcohol Dependence* 132(3): 660–664.

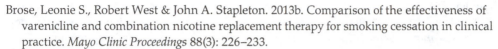

Brose, Leonie S., Robert West & John A. Stapleton. 2013b. Comparison of the effectiveness of varenicline and combination nicotine replacement therapy for smoking cessation in clinical practice. *Mayo Clinic Proceedings* 88(3): 226–233.

Brose, Leonie S., Robert West, Susan Michie, Jennifer Kenyon & Andy McEwen. 2012. Effectiveness of an online knowledge training and assessment program for stop smoking practitioners. *Nicotine & Tobacco Research* 14(7): 794–800.

Callum, Christine, Seán Boyle & Amanda Sandford. 2011. Estimating the cost of smoking to the NHS in England and the impact of declining prevalence. *Health Economics, Policy and Law* 6(4): 489–508.

Coleman, Tim, Catherine Chamberlain, Mary-Anne Davey, Sue Cooper & Jo Leonardi-Bee. 2012. Pharmacological interventions for promoting smoking cessation during pregnancy. *The Cochrane Library*. http://onlinelibrary.wiley.com/doi/10.1002/14651858.CD010078/abstract

Condliffe, Leona, Andy McEwen & Robert West. 2005. The attitude of maternity staff to, and smoking cessation interventions with, childbearing women in London. *Midwifery* 21(3): 233–240.

Department of Health. 2011. *Healthy lives, healthy people: A tobacco control plan for England.* London: The Stationery Office.

De Wilde, Katrien, Inge Tency, Sarah Steckel, Marleen Temmerman, Hedwig Boudrez & Lea Maes. 2015. Which role do midwives and gynecologists have in smoking cessation in pregnant women? – A study in Flanders, Belgium. *Sexual & Reproductive Healthcare* 6(2): 66–73.

Doll, Richard, Richard Peto, Jillian Boreham & Isabelle Sutherland. 2005. Mortality from cancer in relation to smoking: 50 years observations on British doctors. *British Journal of Cancer* 92(3): 426–429.

Ekblad, Mikael, Mika Gissler, Liisa Lehtonen & Jyrki Korkeila. 2010. Prenatal smoking exposure and the risk of psychiatric morbidity into young adulthood. *Archives of General Psychiatry* 67(8): 841–849.

Fang, Wei Li, Adam Goldstein, Anne Butzen, S. Allison Hartsock, Katherine Hartmann, Margaret Helton & Jacob Lohr. 2004. Smoking cessation in pregnancy: A review of post-partum relapse prevention strategies. *The Journal of the American Board of Family Practice* 17(4): 264–275.

Goniewicz, Maciej, Jakub Knysak, Michal Gawron, Leon Kosmider, Andrzej Sobczak, Jolanta Kurek, Adam Prokopowicz, Magdalena Jablonska-Czapla, Czeslawa Rosik-Dulewska, Christopher Havel, Peyton III Jacob & Neal Benowitz. 2014. Levels of selected carcinogens and toxicants in vapour from electronic cigarettes. *Tobacco Control* 23: 133–139.

Health and social care information centre. 2012. Statistics on NHS stop smoking services-England, April 2011 to March 2012. http://www.hscic.gov.uk/catalogue/PUB07011

Herberts, Carolina & Catherine Sykes. 2012. Midwives' perceptions of providing stop-smoking advice and pregnant smokers' perceptions of stop-smoking services within the same deprived area of London. *Journal of Midwifery & Women's Health* 57(1): 67–73.

Judge, Ken, Linda Bauld, John Chesterman & Janet Ferguson. 2005. The English smoking treatment services: Short-term outcomes. *Addiction* 100(Suppl 2): 46–58.

Lawlor, Debbie A., Jake M. Najman, Jonathan Sterne, Gail M. Williams, Shah Ebrahim & George Davey Smith. 2004. Associations of parental, birth, and early life characteristics with systolic blood pressure at 5 years of age findings from the Mater-University study of pregnancy and its outcomes. *Circulation* 110(16): 2417–2423.

Lumley, Judith, Catherine Chamberlain, Therese Dowswell, Sandy Oliver, Laura Oakley & Lyndsey Watson. 2009. Interventions for promoting smoking cessation during pregnancy. *The Cochrane Library*. http://www.ncsct.co.uk/usr/pub/interventions-for-promoting-smoking-cessation-during-pregnancy.pdf

McAndrew, Fiona, Jane Thompson, Lydia Fellows, Alice Large, Mark Speed & Mary J. Renfrew. 2012. Infant feeding survey 2010. *Leeds: Health and Social Care Information Centre*. http://www.hscic.gov.uk/catalogue/PUB08694/Infant-Feeding-Survey-2010-Consolidated-Report.pdf

McEwen, Andy. 2015. *Smoking cessation: A briefing for midwifery staff.* NCSCT. http://www.ncsct.co.uk/usr/pub/NCSCT_midwifery_briefing.pdf

McLeod, Deborah, Cheryl Benn, Susan Pullon, Anne Viccars, Sonya White, Timothy Cookson & Antony Dowell. 2003. The midwife's role in facilitating smoking behaviour change during pregnancy. *Midwifery* 19(4): 285–297.

Michie, Susan, Charles Abraham, Craig Whittington, John McAteer & Sunjai Gupta. 2009. Effective techniques in healthy eating and physical activity interventions: A meta-regression. *Health Psychology* 28(6): 690.

Michie, Susan, Natasha Hyder, Asha Walia & Robert West. 2011. Development of a taxonomy of behaviour change techniques used in individual behavioural support for smoking cessation. *Addictive Behaviors* 36(4): 315–319.

Montgomery, Scott M. & Anders Ekbom. 2002. Smoking during pregnancy and diabetes mellitus in a British longitudinal birth cohort. *BMJ* 324(7328): 26–27.

Myung, Seung-Kwon, Woong Ju, H.-S. Jung, C.-H. Park, Seung-Won Oh, Hg Seo & H. S. Kim. 2012. Efficacy and safety of pharmacotherapy for smoking cessation among pregnant smokers: A meta-analysis. *BJOG: An International Journal of Obstetrics & Gynaecology* 119(9): 1029–1039.

NCSCT (National Centre for Smoking Cessation and Training). 2013. *Smoking in pregnancy survey report*. http://www.networks.nhs.uk/nhs-networks/smoking-cessation-in-pregnancy/documents/ncssct-cic-sip-survey-2.pdf (accessed 9 April 2013).

NICE (National Institute for Health and Clinical Excellence). 2010. *How to stop smoking in pregnancy and following childbirth.* http://www.nice.org.uk/nicemedia/live/13023/49345/49345.pdf

NICE (National Institute for Health and Clinical Excellence). 2014. *Antenatal care.* https://www.nice.org.uk/guidance/cg62

Öberg, Mattias, Maritta Jaakkola, Alistair Woodward, Armando Peruga & Annette Prüss-Ustün. 2011. Worldwide burden of disease from exposure to second-hand smoke: A retrospective analysis of data from 192 countries. *The Lancet* 377(9760): 139–146.

Oken, Emily, Emily Levitan & Matthew Gillman. 2008. Maternal smoking during pregnancy and child overweight: Systematic review and meta-analysis. *International Journal of Obesity* 32(2): 201–210.

Orchard, Craig. 2014. *Adult smoking habits in great Britain, 2013.* http://www.ons.gov.uk/ons/rel/ghs/opinions-and-lifestyle-survey/adult-smoking-habits-in-great-britain—2013/stb-opn-smoking-2013.html

Orleans, C. Tracy. 2007. Increasing the demand for and use of effective smoking-cessation treatments: Reaping the full health benefits of tobacco-control science and policy gains – In our lifetime. *American Journal of Preventive Medicine* 33(6): S340–S348.

Penn, G. & L. Owen. 2002. Factors associated with continued smoking during pregnancy: Analysis of socio-demographic, pregnancy and smoking-related factors. *Drug and Alcohol Review* 21(1): 17–25.

Raupach, Tobias, Lion Shahab, Sandra Baetzing, Barbara Hoffmann, Gerd Hasenfuss, Robert West & Stefan Andreas. 2009. Medical students lack basic knowledge about smoking: Findings from two European medical schools. *Nicotine & Tobacco Research* 11(1): 92–98.

RCM. 2015. *'We must strive to reduce smoking at time of delivery even further' say midwives.* https://www.rcm.org.uk/news-views-and-analysis/news/ 'we-must-strive-to-reduce-smoking-at-time-of-delivery-even-further'-s-0

Richards, Becky, Ann McNeill, Emma Croghan, Jennifer Percival, Deborah Ritchie & Andy McEwen. 2014. Smoking cessation education and training in UK nursing schools: A national survey. *Journal of Nursing Education and Practice* 4(8): 188.

Shahab, Lion & Andy McEwen. 2009. Online support for smoking cessation: A systematic review of the literature. *Addiction* 104(11): 1792–1804.

Shipton, Debra, David Tappin, Thenmalar Vadiveloo, Jennifer Crossley, David Aitken & Jim Chalmers. 2009. Reliability of self-reported smoking status by pregnant women for estimating smoking prevalence: A retrospective, cross sectional study. *BMJ* 339: b4347.

Smoking in England. 2015. *Latest information on smoking and smoking cessation in England.* http://www.smokinginengland.info/

Stead, Lindsay F., Diana Buitrago, Nataly Preciado, Guillermo Sanchez, Jamie Hartmann-Boyce & Tim Lancaster. 2013. Physician advice for smoking cessation. *Cochrane Database of Systematic Reviews* 2013(5): CD000165.

Tobacco Use and Dependence Guideline Panel. 2008. *Treating tobacco use and dependence: 2008 update.* Rockville, MD: US Department of Health and Human Services.

Tong, Van, Jaime Jones, Patricia Dietz, Denise D'Angelo & Jennifer Bombard. 2009. Trends in smoking before, during, and after pregnancy: Pregnancy risk assessment monitoring system (PRAMS), United States, 31 sites, 2000–2005. *MMWR* 58(SS04): 1–29.

Ussher, Michael, Robert West & Nicola Hibbs. 2004. A survey of pregnant smokers' interest in different types of smoking cessation support. *Patient Education and Counseling* 54(1): 67–72.

West, Robert., Ann McNeill & Martin Raw. 2003. *Meeting Department of Health smoking cessation targets. Recommendations for primary care trusts.* London: Health Development Agency.

West, Robert & J. Stapleton. 2008. Clinical and public health significance of treatments to aid smoking cessation. *European Respiratory Review* 17(110): 199–204.

FURTHER READINGS

Further information on the VBA's, including example scripts and difficult conversations, can be found in the NCSCT's briefing document on the topic: http://www.ncsct.co.uk/usr/pub/ NCSCT_midwifery_briefing.pdf

E learning modules for health professionals on giving smoking cessation advice can be found here: http://elearning.ncsct.co.uk/england.

Index

Note: Page numbers in *italics* indicate figures and tables.